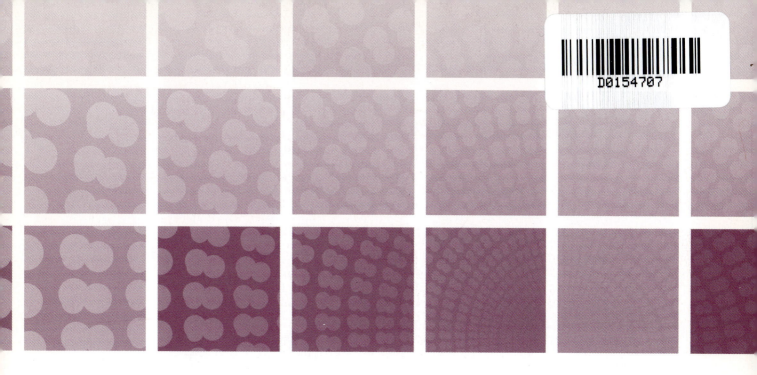

Coding Exam Success

Coder's Guide to Passing the CPC and CCS-P Exams

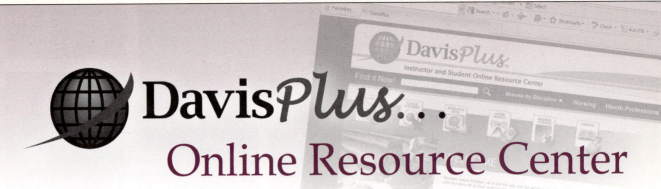
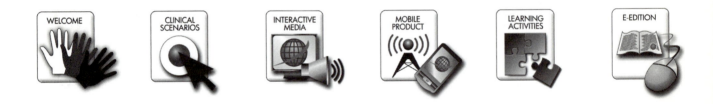
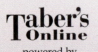
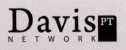
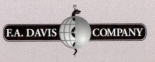

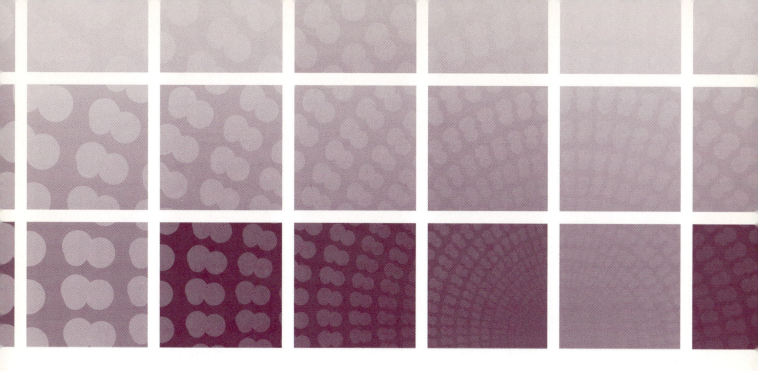

Coding Exam Success

Coder's Guide to Passing the CPC and CCS-P Exams

Jacqueline Thelian, CPC, CPC-I

President
Medco Consultants, Inc.
Fresh Meadows, New York

F.A. Davis Company • Philadelphia

F. A. Davis Company
1915 Arch Street
Philadelphia, PA 19103
www.fadavis.com

Printed in the United States of America

Last digit indicates print number: 10 9 8 7 6 5 4 3 2 1

Senior Acquisitions Editor: Andy McPhee
Manager of Content Development: George W. Lang
Development Editor: Vicki Hoenigke
Manager of Art and Design: Carolyn O'Brien

As new scientific information becomes available through basic and clinical research, recommended treatments and drug therapies undergo changes. The author(s) and publisher have done everything possible to make this book accurate, up to date, and in accord with accepted standards at the time of publication. The author(s), editors, and publisher are not responsible for errors or omissions or for consequences from application of the book, and make no warranty, expressed or implied, in regard to the contents of the book. Any practice described in this book should be applied by the reader in accordance with professional standards of care used in regard to the unique circumstances that may apply in each situation. The reader is advised always to check product information (package inserts) for changes and new information regarding dose and contraindications before administering any drug. Caution is especially urged when using new or infrequently ordered drugs.

REVIEWERS

Karen R Baker, CPC, CPC-H, CPC-I, MCS-P, CCAT, CCT, PCS, FCS
Clinical Documentation Educator
Cooper University Hospital
Revenue Cycle Education
Cherry Hill, New Jersey

Joanne Becker, RHIT, CCS, CCSP, CPC, CPCI
Associate Director
University of Iowa Healthcare
Joint Office for Compliance
Iowa City, Iowa

Linda I. Bingham, BBA
Instructor
Carrington College
Medical Billing and Coding Program
Phoenix, Arizona

Darlene Boschert, BS, CPC-I, CPC-H, NCMA, CMT
Director
Career Institute of Florida
Allied Health Department
St. Petersburg, Florida

Tina L. Cressman, MALS, CPC-I, CPC-H-I, CPC-P, CCS-P, MCS-P, MCS-I, CMC
Director, Managed Care Education
Cooper University Hospital
Cooper University Physician Administration
Cherry Hill, New Jersey

Linda H. Donahue, RHIT, CCS, CCS-P, CPC
Instructor, Coding
Delgado Community College
Health Information Technology Program
Allied Health Department
New Orleans, Louisiana

Sandra M Erlewine, CPC, CMA (AAMA)
Instructor
Yakima Valley Community College
Allied Health Technology
Yakima, Washington

Tammy T. Gant, CPC, CMA (AAMA), RHIT, CAHI
Medical Assisting Program Director
Surry Community College
Business Technologies Division
Dobson, North Carolina

Heather D. Gatton, CPC, CPC-H, CPC-P, CFPC, CPMA, MCS-P
Senior Compliance Auditor
Cooper University Hospital
Camden, New Jersey

Carolyn M. Hutt, CPC, CPC-I, CCS-P
Practice Administrator
Fort Worth, Texas

Jaci Johnson, CPC, CPMA, CEMC, CPC-H, CPC-I
President
Practice Integrity, LLC
Henrico, Virginia

Cynthia R. Lundquist, BS
Director, Medical Office Programs
Maric College—Stockton Campus
Department of Education
Stockton, California

Eva Ruth Oltman, MS, CPC, CMA (AAMA)
Division Chair of Allied Health; Professor
Allied Health Department
Jefferson Community and Technical College
Louisville, Kentucky

ACKNOWLEDGMENTS

This book was made possible by the help and support of many people.

My thanks to the people at F.A. Davis who made up "Team Thelian" for their dedication and contribution to the book. Special thanks to Andy McPhee, Senior Acquisitions Editor, for taking the chance on making my dream a reality; to my talented Development Editor Vicki Hoenigke, for her insight, patience, and ability to take my words and transform them into eloquent sentences; and, of course, to the personable and just plain enjoyable Virgil Lloyd, Promotions Manager.

I also thank my family, Victor, Gregory, Melanie, Colette, and John, for their unwavering support and constant encouragement. Special thanks to two people who cheered me on and had the vision to see in me what I could not see in myself: Linda Fisher, my dear friend and mentor: thank you for taking me under your wing; and my husband, Victor (a.k.a. the Bear): it is your love that makes all things possible...you are my True North.

CONTENTS IN BRIEF

CONTENTS IN DETAIL

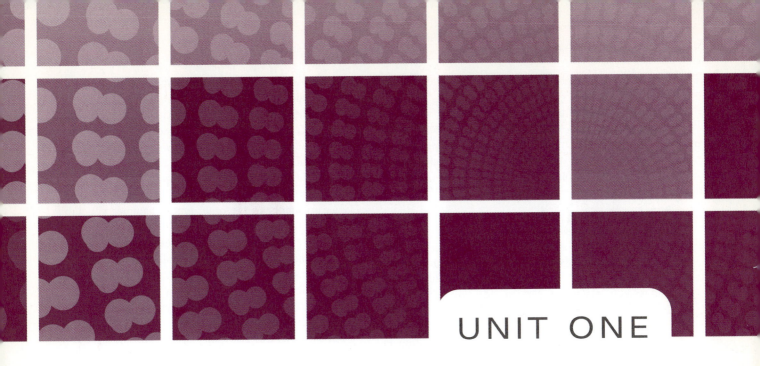

UNIT ONE

Introduction to the Exam

CHAPTER 1

Coding Basics

Medical Coding is an art. The medical coder (artist) paints a picture of the physician-patient encounter by translating the written word into numeric codes. The numeric codes are then sent to the insurance company on a CMS1500 claim form (the canvas) and if properly coded returns back to the physician in the form of a reimbursement check.

As with any artist, certain tools are necessary to paint the picture properly. The same is true for medical coding. The coder's paint palette consists of CPT (*Current Procedural Terminology*), ICD-9-CM (*International Classification of Diseases "9th Revision" Clinical Modification*) and HCPCS (*Healthcare Common Procedure Coding System*) codes. The finishing touches are applied by use of CPT and HCPCS modifiers.

Just as the artist uses light as a resource, the medical coder utilizes Web sites and publications from various government, state, and specialty societies.

Let's take a look at the medical coder's basic "tools of the trade" and "resources."

Tools of the Trade

Every profession has certain tools they use to help with their job. In the coding profession, our tools are the books and resource materials we use to code. You will find there are many books written for our industry, but if you look closely you will notice that there are just a few that need to be purchased. Much of the additional information and resources required can be found for free on line at source Web sites such as the Centers for Medicare and Medicaid Services (CMS), the Office of Inspector General (OIG), and so on.

As you read through this study guide and move forward with your coding career, I hope that you will take the time to "customize" your coding books (tools). Customizing your books by highlighting key information or writing in notes in your own words that help to clarify certain coding guidelines not only give you the edge when taking the certification test but, each year as you copy your notes from one set of books to the next, you will be giving yourself a review of the coding rules and regulations. You will also find that, after a period of time, you will no longer need to copy some of the notes because they will become ingrained in your memory.

The Coder's Top Three Tools

The certification examination is an open book test. You are allowed to use three coding books for the examination:

■ *Current Procedural Terminology (CPT)*
■ *International Classification of Diseases, 9th Revision Clinical Modification (ICD-9-CM)*
■ *Healthcare Common Procedure Coding System (HCPCS)*

These books are considered your "tools of the trade". (Information on the publications is given at the end of this chapter in the "Learn More About It" section.)

Not coincidentally, after you have passed the examination and earned your certification, these three books are also the main books required for your career as a professional coder. These books are updated yearly with new codes, revised codes, and deleted codes. The CPT book is

usually available for purchase in October for the upcoming year, and the updated codes become effective in January. The ICD-9-CM book is updated every year and, unlike CPT, the new ICD-9-CM codes, which are published usually in August, go into effect in October of the current year. The HCPCS book is also updated every year, and the new codes go into effect in January.

There are many different versions of these books. Just like a carpenter has a "favorite" type of hammer, you will find the favorite version (type) of book you prefer. Different versions have different looks, feel, and information in them. The prices of the books will also vary, so in some cases cost is a consideration. It is important to remember that all books contain all the codes and guidelines; the difference is in the type of book and the features included in the book.

For example, CPT has a standard version and a professional edition. Let's look at some of the differences:

CPT Standard	CPT Professional Edition
Not spiral-bound	Spiral-bound
Not index-tabbed	Index-tabbed
No anatomical illustrations	Includes anatomical illustrations
No medical prefixes, suffixes, and roots	Includes medical prefixes, suffixes, and roots
Printed in black and white	Printed in color

As you can see, there are differences in the type of book produced (spiral-bound) and the various features included in the book (anatomical illustrations). The same is true for the ICD-9-CM and HCPCS books.

Look at your books as an investment in your coding career, so a trip to the bookstore is well worth the effort. I recommend you go to a bookstore before purchasing your books to actually get the feel of the book and look at the different versions of the books. Find the version that is best for **you**. Once you have determined the version you want to purchase, you can then price-shop on line. I have found the *Professional CPT, Expert ICD-9-CM,* and *Standard HCPCS* are excellent versions that include helpful additional features. I also prefer a spiral-bound book as it allows you to open the book to one side and lay it flat, which is also helpful when coding.

You should always keep the old versions of your CPT, ICD-9-CM, and HCPCS books as the *older versions are extremely valuable*. Often, CMS and insurance carriers can go back several years when auditing a physician or physician practice group. In these cases, it is imperative to have the correct year of coding manual to match with the correct year of notes in question.

Other Helpful Resources

While the CPT, ICD-9-CM, and HCPCS books are mandatory for coding, two other books are strongly recommended:

■ **A medical dictionary.** There are a number of medical dictionaries on the market at all different levels. Some include color illustrations or a CD; some are large and hardcover, some smaller and softbound. A good medical dictionary at your level of understanding is the best investment you can make, so take your time and look at many different types before making this purchase. My preference is *Taber's Cyclopedic Medical Dictionary;* it is hardbound, tabbed, written at an appropriate level, and includes color illustrations and a CD that brings the words in the dictionary to life with pictures, videos, and pronunciation of the medical words.

■ **A medical abbreviation book.** This is a valuable tool as many providers document their notes with medical abbreviations. A good medical abbreviation book can be found for as little as $30 online and is also available in a small compact version (*Medical Abbreviations* by Neil M Davis).

As you move forward with your coding career, you may also consider the following books/publications, *CPT Changes: An Insiders View* and *the CPT Assistant.* Both publications are referenced throughout the CPT book and provide additional information about the CPT codes. These two publications will be discussed in detail in Chapter 6, "Current Procedural Terminology."

■ **The 1995 and 1997 Documentation Guidelines.** These guidelines can be downloaded for free from the CMS Web site (http://www.cms.hhs.gov/MLNEdwebGuide/25_EMDOC.asp). It is recommended you print these out, bind them, and keep them with your coding books as they will be referenced often throughout your coding career. (These guidelines will be reviewed in Chapter 8, Evaluation and Management Codes.)

Many of the other reference materials or resources relating to compliance can be found on line for free and will be referenced as we review compliance in the next section.

Compliance

Compliance, simply stated, is defined as establishing a business environment that adheres to the principles of business practice as identified by *state and federal regulations and recommendations.*

When we think of compliance, the **Centers for Medicare and Medicaid Services (CMS)** immediately comes to mind; however, there are also state rules and regulations that must be followed. For example, Medicaid, No Fault, and Workers Compensation have rules and regulations at the state level.

There are also **Medicare Administrative Contractors (MACs).** These are entities contracted by CMS that are responsible for the receipt, processing of claims, and payment for Medicare fee-for-service claims at the *local level.* They are also the primary contact for physicians, and they perform services such as appeals, provider outreach and education, provider enrollment, financial management, reimbursement, payment safeguards, and information systems security. Most important, they publish **Local Coverage Determinations (LCDs).**

An LCD is a MAC-developed coverage policy pertaining to services or items at the local level. The LCDs contain coding and utilization guidelines such as required documentation, what type of professional can perform the service, how often the service can be performed, and what provides medical necessity for the service (covered ICD-9-CM codes).

LCDs are developed for various reasons, some of which are: to define the appropriate use of new technology, to address high-volume or high-dollar services, and to address services with an abuse or potential abuse history. All of your LCDs can be found free of charge by going to the CMS Web site and searching the term Local Coverage Determination. Remember to be sure to search for the LCD for your local jurisdiction.

If you are unable to find an LCD for a particular CPT code on the CMS Web site, you can search for a **National Coverage Determination (NCD).** NCDs provide the same type of information in an LCD but are written at the *national level.*

If you are unable to find coding guidance in either an LCD or NCD, you can then search the **Medicare Carrier Manual (MCM)** or the **Medicare Internet Only Manual (IOM).** All of this coding guidance is available online from the source (Medicare, MAC, and so on) at no cost.

Many of these policies are frequently updated by CMS, MAC, or the insurance carrier, so it is important to stay updated. Medicare has a Medicare Learning Network called MedLearn. The MedLearn network includes information on the Internet, national educational articles, brochures, fact sheets, Web-based training, and videos to provide education, all for free. You can access the MedLearn Network by going to http://www.cms.hhs.gov/mlngeninfo/

Although several of the insurance carriers will follow Medicare rules, it is important to always check with the insurance carrier to be sure you are following their specific rules and regulations. Many of the various insurance carriers have their provider manuals on line and will often send bulletins with updated information to the providers either by mail or e-mail.

Another source of compliance information is the **Office of Inspector General (OIG)** Web site (http://oig .hhs.gov/). The OIG conducts and supervises audits and investigations relating to the CMS programs and operations and also looks to prevent and detect fraud and abuse.

Each year, usually by November, the OIG Web site will publish their "Work Plan" for the upcoming year. This work plan includes a listing of services and items they will review in the upcoming year. It is a valuable tool as it provides a "heads up" for providers as to what the OIG will be reviewing/auditing and allows physicians to take an internal look at these services/items to be sure they are compliant in their documentation and coding practices for these services/items.

The OIG Web site also has a compliance program. With the recent passage of the Patient Protection and Affordable Care Act of 2010, which was signed into law on March 23, 2010, compliance programs became mandatory for certain types of health-care providers that bill Medicare, Medicaid, and other federally funded programs. A compliance program is also considered "preventive medicine" for the practice. The compliance program for individuals and small physician practices contains seven components that provide a basis by which physicians can create a compliance program.

Both the OIG's Work Plan and Compliance Program can be downloaded from the OIG's Web site.

Learn More About It

As you begin to utilize your coding skills in the workplace, you will find that the Internet and various Web sites are instrumental in keeping you updated about the rules and regulations for coding and compliance. These Web sites provide accurate information directly from reputable sources and, best of all, the information is *free.* So let's start to get familiar with some of the sites.

Visit the following Web sites, and learn how to navigate the sites. Remember to bookmark any areas of interest as you browse the site for future reference. Anytime you visit a new Web site, ask yourself:

1. Was the site easy to navigate?
2. Were you able to search the site and find what you were looking for?
3. How would you rate the information on each of the sites?
4. How will you use these sites in the future?
5. Did you remember to bookmark the sites as one of your coding favorites?

Recommended Web Sites

The 1995 and 1997 Documentation Guidelines

http://www.cms.hhs.gov/MLNEdwebGuide/25_ EMDOC.asp

MedLearn Network

http://www.cms.hhs.gov/mlngeninfo/

Office of Inspector General

http://oig.hhs.gov/

Centers for Medicare and Medicaid Services

http://www.cms.gov/

Recommended Books

CPT Professional Edition (Current Procedural Terminology (CPT) Professional)

Author: American Medical Association

Publisher: American Medical Association

ISBN: 978-1-60359-119-5

ICD-9-CM Expert for Physicians, Vols. 1 and 2

Author: Ingenix

Publisher: Ingenix

ISBN: 978-1-60151-261-1

HCPCS Level II (Standard Edition)

Author: Ingenix

Publisher: Ingenix

ISBN: 978-1-60151-155-3

Taber's Cyclopedic Medical Dictionary, Indexed, 21st Ed.

Author: Donald Venes

Publisher: F A Davis Co; 21st edition (February 2, 2009)

ISBN-10: 0803620535

ISBN-13: 978-0803620537

CPT Changes : An Insider's View

Author: American Medical Association

Publisher: American Medical Association

ISBN: 978-1-60359-120-1

CPT Assistant

Newsletter, 8½ × 11

Author: American Medical Association

To order, go to AMABookstore.com

Acronyms and Abbreviations

CMS– **C**enters for **M**edicare and Medicaid **S**ervices

LCD– **L**ocal **C**overage **D**etermination

MAC– **M**edicare **A**dministrative **C**ontractor

MCM– **M**edicare **C**arrier **M**anual

NCD– **N**ational **C**overage **D**etermination
OIG– **O**ffice of **I**nspector **G**eneral

TAKE THE CODING CHALLENGE

1. CPT stands for:
   a. Common procedural terminology
   b. Certified physician terminology
   c. Current procedural terminology
   d. Current procedure translation

2. A Local Coverage Determination can be found:
   a. On the Centers for Medicare and Medicaid Web site
   b. On a Medicare Administrative Contractor's Web site
   c. In the *Medicare Carrier Manual*
   d. All of the above

3. New ICD-9-CM codes go into effect:
   a. In October
   b. As soon as the insurance carriers update their systems
   c. In January
   d. The codes are published in October but go into effect in January

4. HCPCS stands for:
   a. Healthcare Current Physician Coding System
   b. Healthcare Common Professional Coding System
   c. Healthcare Common Procedure Coding System
   d. Healthcare Current Professional Coding System

5. OIG stands for:
   a. Office of Insurance Guidelines
   b. Office of Inspector General
   c. Official Insurance Guidelines
   d. Official Inspector General

6. A sample compliance program can be found on the following Web site:
   a. OIG
   b. CMS
   c. MAC
   d. All of the above

7. The OIG Work Plan includes:
   a. Compliance components for physician practice
   b. National Coverage Determinations
   c. A list of services/items that are targeted for review/audit in the upcoming year
   d. All of the above

8. All CPT, ICD-9-CM, and HCPCS book should be updated:
   a. Varyingly, depending on the book
   b. Only when the code changes effect your physician's specialty
   c. Every 2 years, as the codes do not change that often
   d. Yearly; each year codes are added, deleted, and revised

9. At the end of each year, you should:
   a. Update your coding books
   b. Keep all your coding books
   c. Discard *and* update your coding books
   d. Keep *and* update your coding books

10. MAC stands for:
    a. Medicare Administrative Contractor
    b. Medical Administrative Contractor
    c. Medicare Administrator Carrier
    d. Medicare Advantage Carrier

Answers and Rationales

1. The correct answer is **c.**, Current Procedural Terminology. This information can be found on the front cover of the CPT book.

2. The correct answer is **a.**, an LCD is written at the local level; however, it is located on the Centers for Medicare and Medicaid Services Web site; **b.** is incorrect; one would think an LCD would be found on the local carrier's Web site; however, all LCDs are centrally located on the CMS Web site; **c.** is incorrect as the *Medicare Carrier Manual* does not include local rules and regulations.

3. The correct answer is **a.**, new ICD-9-CM codes are effective and need to be reported in October for all carriers.

4. The correct answer is **c.**, Healthcare Common Procedure Coding System. Although this is not easily located within the HCPCS book, it is recommended you write this on the front page of your HCPCS book for future reference.

5. The correct answer is **b.**, Office of Inspector General.

6. The correct answer is **a.**, the OIG Web site includes a sample compliance program.

7. The correct answer is **c.**, the OIG Work Plan includes a list of services/items that are targeted for review/audit in the upcoming year; **a.** is incorrect: the OIG *Web site* includes a sample compliance program, which is separate and distinct from the Work Plan and has a different purpose; **b.** is incorrect as National Coverage Determinations are located on the CMS Web site.

8. The correct answer is **d.**, the CPT, ICD-9-CM, and HCPCS books should all be updated yearly as every year there are codes that are added, deleted, or revised. Whereas it may be true that a particular specialty (e.g., Cardiovascular) may not have any changes in its particular section of CPT, there are other sections of CPT that are utilized by all specialties, such as the Evaluation and Management section, the Medicine section, modifiers, and so on. Therefore, it is important that all three books be updated yearly.

9. The correct answer is **b.**, CMS and other insurance carriers can go back several years when auditing a provider; therefore it is imperative to keep all outdated coding books.

10. The correct answer is **a.**, Medicare Administrative Contractor.

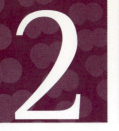

Anatomy and Medical Terminology

Anatomy is the science that studies the structural organization of living things. The human body is made up of *cells* (the basic unit of all living things), *tissues* (groups of cells that perform a specific task), *organs* (groups of two or more tissues working together to perform specific body functions), and *organ systems* (groups of organs working together to perform body functions).

The human body has five cavities, each of which contains an orderly arrangement of internal organs. The cavities are: cranial, spinal, thoracic or chest, abdominal, and pelvic. The cavities are lined with membranes (a thin layer of tissue). There are four types of membranes: mucous, serous, synovial, and meningeal. Membranes also cover an organ or a structure.

The human body is a fascinating structure with the ability to run on automatic pilot and with organ systems working together in perfect harmony.

Let's take a look at the various organ systems and how they work.

Integumentary System

The largest organ system in the human body, the integumentary system, includes the skin, glands, hair, and fingernails. The skin covers the body and provides protection, regulation of body temperature, and water balance. The skin is divided into three separate layers: the epidermis, the dermis, and the subcutaneous tissue (Fig. 2.1). The skin includes two types of glands: the sweat glands (sudoriferous) and the oil glands (sebaceous). There are two types of sweat glands: eccrine, which produce sweat, and apocrine, which produce body odor. The hair has two separate structures: the follicle and the shaft. The nails provide protection for the nerve endings in the fingertips and toes. The nail is divided into six separate parts: root, nailbed; nail plate, eponychium (cuticle), perionychium (soft tissue surrounding the border of the nail), and hyponychium (the area between the nail plate and the fingertip).

Anatomical Terms Related to the Integumentary System

Collagen: A protein that connects and supports other bodily tissues.

Epithelium: Membranous tissue that lines the internal organs, cavities, and surfaces of structures throughout the body.

Melanin: A pigment that gives the skin and hair their natural color.

Stratum corneum: A layer of dead cells in the epidermis that forms a barrier to retain moisture.

Subcutaneous tissue: The deepest layer of the skin, which contains fat cells (adipose cells or lymphocytes), connective tissue, blood vessels (venule, arteriole), and nerves.

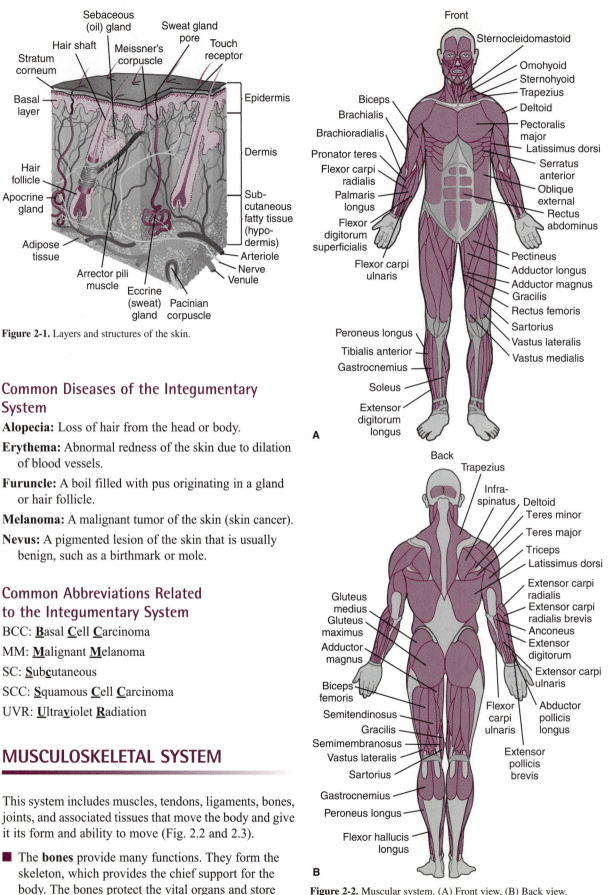

Figure 2-1. Layers and structures of the skin.

Common Diseases of the Integumentary System

Alopecia: Loss of hair from the head or body.

Erythema: Abnormal redness of the skin due to dilation of blood vessels.

Furuncle: A boil filled with pus originating in a gland or hair follicle.

Melanoma: A malignant tumor of the skin (skin cancer).

Nevus: A pigmented lesion of the skin that is usually benign, such as a birthmark or mole.

Common Abbreviations Related to the Integumentary System

BCC: **B**asal **C**ell **C**arcinoma

MM: **M**alignant **M**elanoma

SC: **S**ub**c**utaneous

SCC: **S**quamous **C**ell **C**arcinoma

UVR: **U**ltra**v**iolet **R**adiation

MUSCULOSKELETAL SYSTEM

This system includes muscles, tendons, ligaments, bones, joints, and associated tissues that move the body and give it its form and ability to move (Fig. 2.2 and 2.3).

■ The **bones** provide many functions. They form the skeleton, which provides the chief support for the body. The bones protect the vital organs and store

Figure 2-2. Muscular system. (A) Front view, (B) Back view.

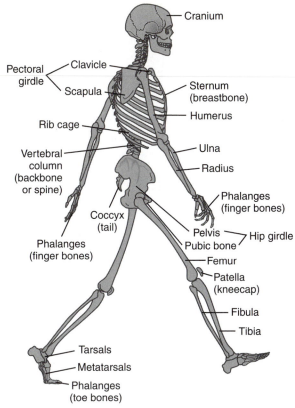

Figure 2-3. Skeletal system.

calcium, phosphorus, magnesium salts, and marrow (which produces blood cells).

■ **Ligaments** are strong bands of connective tissue that bind bones together at the joints.

■ **Tendons** are bands of fibrous connective tissue connecting a muscle to a bone. They act like an elastic band, allowing body movement.

■ **Muscles** are the contractile tissue of the body whose primary function is to provide power. Muscles also provide form and produce heat for the body. There are three types of muscles: skeletal (muscle that moves extremities and external areas of the body), cardiac (muscle that is in the walls of the arteries), and smooth (e.g., muscle found in the bowel).

■ The **joints** are the locations where two or more bones make contact; they provide a flexible connection between the bones.

Anatomical Terms Related to the Musculoskeletal System

Clavicle: Also called the collar bone; it is the flat bone located between the shoulder and the neck.

Deltoid: The muscle covering the shoulder joint that provides for flexibility, extension, and rotation of the arm.

Maxilla: The bones on either side of the upper jaw that provide support to the canines and cheek teeth.

Soleus: A powerful broad flat muscle located in the back of the calf (lower leg) that controls postural stability.

Sternum: Also called the breast bone; it is the long flat bone located in the center of the thorax (chest).

Common Diseases of the Musculoskeletal System

Bursitis: Inflammation of the bursa (small fluid-filled sacs that ease friction between tendons and bones) resulting in swelling and pain.

Crepitation: A grating, clicking, rattling, or crackling sound produced by the rubbing of bone fragments.

Effusion: An abnormal collection of fluid in various spaces of the body (e.g., the knee)

Kyphosis: Also called "hunch-back"; this is the abnormal backward cure of the vertebral column.

Torticollis: Also called a "stiff neck"; spasms in the neck muscles causing the head to tilt to one side, causing difficulty in rotating the head.

Common Abbreviations Related to the Musculoskeletal System

DJD: **D**egenerative **J**oint **D**isease

Extremity: **Ext** (UE = **U**pper **E**xtremity, LE = **L**ower **E**xtremity)

FROM: **F**ull **R**ange **O**f **M**otion

MS: **M**usculoskeletal

OA: **O**steoarthritis

Respiratory System

This system comprises the nose, mouth, nasal passages, nasal pharynx, pharynx, larynx, trachea, bronchi, bronchioles, air sacs (alveoli) of the lungs, and muscles of respiration (Fig. 2.4). The primary function of the respiratory system is to supply the blood with oxygen in order for the blood to deliver oxygen to all parts of the body.

Anatomical Terms Related to the Respiratory System

Bronchi: Large hollow air passages that carry air into the lungs.

Diaphragm: A sheet of muscle that extends across the bottom of the rib cage and separates the thoracic cavity from the abdominal cavity. Its function is to pull the lungs open and push them closed for inhalation and exhalation.

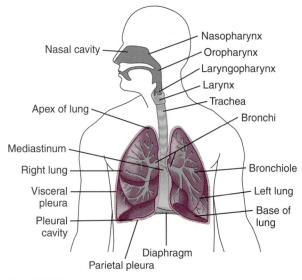

Figure 2-4. Respiratory system.

Glottis: The true vocal cords and the opening between them. This is where the voice tone is generated.

Nasopharynx: The area of the upper throat that lies behind the nose.

Oropharynx: The area of the throat that is at the back of the mouth.

Common Diseases of the Respiratory System

Asbestosis: A chronic inflammatory lung disease caused by the inhaling of asbestos particles.

Emphysema: A chronic, irreversible disease of the lungs whereby the small air sacs (alveoli) of the lungs become damaged, resulting in decreased respiratory function. Smoking is a common cause of emphysema.

Nasopharyngitis: Also known as the "common cold"; it is a viral infectious disease of the upper respiratory system.

Pleurisy: Inflammation of the membranes around the lungs, resulting in fever, coughing, and difficulty breathing.

Pneumothorax: Air outside the lung and within the chest cavity, resulting in collapse of the lung.

Common Abbreviations Related to the Respiratory System

CLD: <u>C</u>hronic <u>L</u>ung <u>D</u>isease

COPD: <u>C</u>hronic <u>O</u>bstructive <u>P</u>ulmonary <u>D</u>isease

CPAP: <u>C</u>ontinuous <u>P</u>ositive <u>A</u>irway <u>P</u>ressure

OLB: <u>O</u>pen <u>L</u>ung <u>B</u>iopsy

RAD: <u>R</u>eactive <u>A</u>irway <u>D</u>isease

Cardiovascular System

The cardiovascular system comprises the heart, blood vessels (arteries, veins, and capillaries) or also called the "vasculature," and the cells and plasma that make up the blood (Fig. 2.5). The primary function of the cardiovascular system is to circulate blood throughout the body via a network of vessels to provide oxygen and nutrients to individual cells and to help dispose of metabolic wastes (Fig. 2.6).

Anatomical Terms Related to the Cardiovascular System

Aorta: A large artery that carries oxygen-enriched blood from the left ventricle of the heart to branch arteries.

Atrium: The upper chamber of each half of the heart.

Mitral valve: Also known as "bicuspid valve"; the mitral valve separates the two chambers on the left side of the heart; it prevents blood from backing up into the atrium and the lungs.

Tricuspid valve: A valve with three cusps located between the right atrium and right ventricle; it prevents the backflow of blood into the right atrium.

Ventricle: The lower pumping chambers of the heart.

Common Diseases of the Cardiovascular System

Angina: Pain in the heart from insufficient flow of blood to the heart muscle.

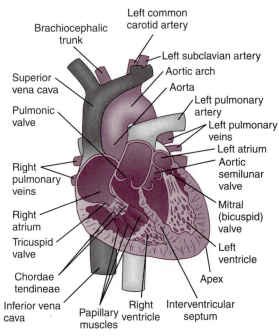
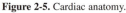

Figure 2-5. Cardiac anatomy.

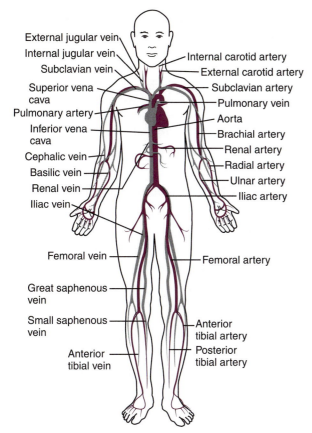

Figure 2-6. Circulatory system.

Cerebrovascular accident: Also known as a "stroke"; a blood vessel or clot (thrombus) in the brain that deprives the brain tissue of oxygen.

Endocarditis: An infection of one of the four heart valves.

Myocardial infarction: The death of heart tissues due to lack of oxygen for an extended period.

Transichemic attack: Also called "mini-strokes"; caused when a small blood clot blocks an artery to the brain for a short period.

Common Abbreviations Related to the Cardiovascular System

BMI: **B**ody **M**ass **I**ndex

CAD: **C**oronary **A**rtery **D**isease

CVA: **C**erebro**v**ascular **A**ccident

RRR: **R**egular **R**ate and **R**hythm (heart)

TIA: **T**ransient **I**schemic **A**ttack

Lymphatic System

The lymphatic system consists of lymph organs (e.g., bone marrow, spleen, and thymus), lymph vessels, and lymph nodes that are located throughout the body (Fig. 2.7). The lymphatic system is responsible for draining fluid back into the bloodstream from the tissues, filtering lymph and the blood, and fighting infection.

Anatomical Terms Related to the Lymphatic System

Axillary lymph nodes: Lymph nodes located in the armpit that drain the lymph channels from the breast.

Bone marrow: The soft and spongy tissue that fills the cavities of the bones.

Cisterna chyli: The origin of the thoracic duct.

Lymph: A transparent, watery bodily fluid containing white blood cells.

Thoracic duct: This is a major duct of the lymphatic system that drains lymph from the entire body (with the exception of the right upper quadrant) and returns it to the left subclavian vein.

Common Diseases of the Lymphatic System

Autoimmune lymphoproliferative syndrome: A disease by which an unusually high number of white blood

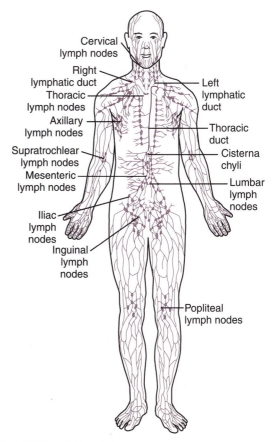

Figure 2-7. Lymphatic system.

cells accumulate in the lymph nodes, liver, and spleen, leading to enlargement of these organs.

Castleman's disease: Benign tumors that develop in the lymph node tissue at a single site or throughout the body.

Lymphadenitis: Inflammation of the lymph nodes.

Lymphatic falariasis: A parasitic disease caused by microscopic worms in the lymph system.

Mesenteric lymphadenitis: Inflammation of the lymph nodes in the membrane that attaches the intestine to the abdominal wall.

Common Abbreviations Related to the Lymphatic System

ALPS: **A**utoimmune **L**ympho**p**roliferative **S**yndrome

CD: **C**astleman's **D**isease

LAG: **L**ymph**a**ngio**g**ram

LN: **L**ymph **N**ode

PLND: **P**elvic **L**ymph **N**ode **D**issection

Digestive System

As shown in Figure 2.8, the digestive system comprises the mouth, esophagus, stomach, small intestine, large intestine (the colon), rectum, anus, and ancillary organs (pancreas, liver, and gallbladder). The primary function of the digestive system is to break down the food into smaller parts that the body will use to build and nourish cells and provide energy.

■ The **small intestine** is divided into three sections: duodenum (first third), jejunum (second third), and ileum (distal third).

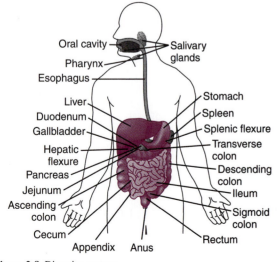

Figure 2-8. Digestive system.

■ The **large intestine** begins at the iliac region of the pelvis and consists of four portions: ascending, transverse, descending, and sigmoid or pelvic colon.

■ The **ancillary organs** include the pancreas, which produces digestive enzymes that are secreted into the intestines; the liver, which produces bile (a digestive juice), and the gallbladder, which stores and secretes bile to help the body digest fats.

Anatomical Terms Related to the Digestive System

Cecum: A blind sac that opens into the colon.

Duodenum: The first part of the small intestine, extending from the stomach to the jejunum, which breaks down food.

Esophagus: The tubular portion of the digestive tract that connects the mouth to the stomach.

Ileum: The longest portion of the small intestine responsible for digestion and the absorption of nutrients.

Jejunum: The part of the small intestine that connects the duodenum and ileum.

Common Diseases of the Digestive System

Crohn's disease: An inflammation of the gastrointestinal tract (from the mouth to the anus) most commonly affecting the lower part of the small intestine.

Dyspepsia: Also known as "indigestion"; the feeling of fullness during a meal and/or uncomfortable fullness after a meal accompanied by burning or pain in the upper abdomen.

Gastroparesis: A disorder of the stomach that causes the stomach to take too long to empty, resulting in bacterial overgrowth from the fermentation of the food and in some cases the hardening of the food, which may cause an obstruction.

Helicobacter pylori: A spiral-shaped bacterium in the stomach that damages the stomach, causing inflammation and peptic ulcers.

Stomach ulcer: An open sore or erosion in the lining of the stomach.

Common Abbreviations Related to the Digestive System

HSM: **H**epato**s**pleno**m**egaly

LFT: **L**iver **F**unction **T**est

GERD: **G**astro**e**sophageal **R**eflux **D**isease

GIST: **G**astro**i**ntestinal **S**tromal **T**umor

IBS: **I**rritable **B**owel **S**yndrome

Urinary System and Reproductive System

Urinary System

The urinary system comprises the kidneys, ureters, bladder, and urethra. The primary function of the urinary system is to produce, store, and eliminate urine (Figs. 2.9 and 2.10).

■ The **kidneys** have multiple functions. Primarily, they filter waste products from the blood; they also regulate blood pressure by maintaining a steady level of electrolytes.

■ A **ureter** is a tube leading away from the kidney to the urinary bladder, whose function is the movement of urine.

■ The function of the **bladder** is to store and release urine.

■ The **urethra** is the tube through which urine passes when emptying the bladder.

Reproductive System

The **female reproductive system** is divided into two parts: external and internal. The external part of the reproductive system consists of the vulva, the mons pubis, labia, and clitoris (Fig. 2.11). The internal organs are the vagina, uterus, fallopian tubes, and ovaries (Fig. 2.12).

The **male reproductive system** is likewise divided into external and internal parts (Fig. 2.13). The external male reproductive organs include the penis and scrotum. The internal organs include the vas deferens, testes, and seminal vesicles. The primary function of the reproductive system, whether male or female, is to produce offspring.

Anatomical Terms Related to the Male and Female Reproductive Systems

Cervix: The narrow entryway between the vagina and the uterus.

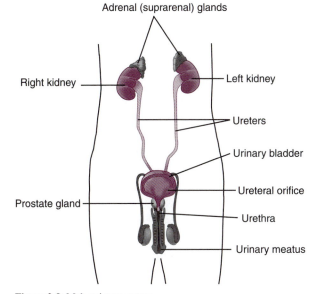

Figure 2-9. Male urinary system.

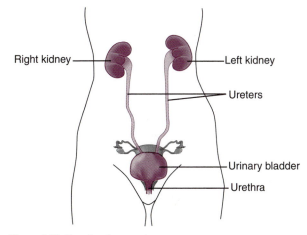

Figure 2-10. Female urinary system.

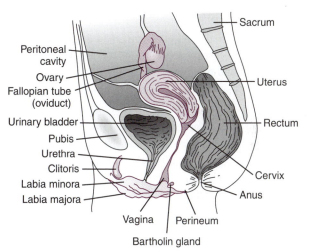

Figure 2-11. Sagittal section of the female reproductive system.

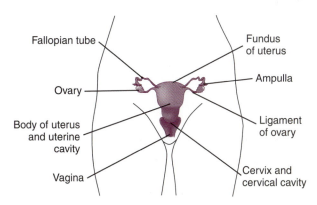

Figure 2-12. Anterior view of female reproductive system.

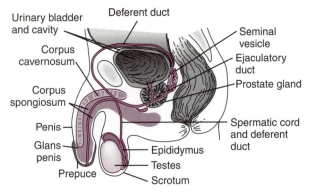

Urinary bladder and cavity
Corpus cavernosum
Corpus spongiosum
Penis
Glans penis
Prepuce
Deferent duct
Seminal vesicle
Ejaculatory duct
Prostate gland
Spermatic cord and deferent duct
Epididymus
Testes
Scrotum

Figure 2-13. Male reproductive system.

Epididymis: Tightly coiled tubes attached to the top of the testis, where sperm is stored during maturation.

Fallopian tube: A tube through which the eggs from the ovary pass to the uterus.

Labia majora: The outer folds of skin (lips) that cover and protect the female genitalia.

Labia minora: The smaller inside folds of skin (lips) located between the labia majora and the external genitalia.

Ovary: The female reproductive organ that contains the eggs necessary for reproduction and produces estrogen and progesterone.

Prepuce: The foreskin or sheath of skin that covers the penis.

Prostate gland: The male sex gland that produces a fluid that forms part of the semen.

Testes: The male reproductive glands located in the scrotum that produce testosterone and sperm.

Vas deferens: The ducts by which sperm passes from the testis to the urethra.

Common Diseases of the Urinary and Male and Female Reproductive Systems

Amenorrhea: The absence of menstruation in a woman of reproductive age; not related to menopause.

Benign prostatic hypertrophy: Swelling or enlargement of the prostate gland.

Cryptorchidism: Also known as "hidden testicle"; the failure of one or more of the testes to descend into the scrotum.

Cystitis: Inflammation of the bladder and ureters.

Dysmenorrhea: Painful menstrual periods.

Dysuria: Painful or difficult urination.

Endometriosis: The tissue that normally lines the inside of the uterus (endometrium) becomes implanted outside the uterus; this is one of the most common gynecological diseases.

Hematuria: The presence of blood in the urine.

Hydrocele: A fluid-filled sac surrounding the testis, resulting in swelling on the side of the scrotum.

Kidney stones: Also known as calculus of the kidney; hard, solid pellets that form in the urinary tract.

Menorrhagia: Heavy menstrual period with excessive bleeding.

Polycystic kidney disease: A genetic disorder of the kidneys by which numerous fluid-filled cysts form in the kidneys.

Testicular torsion: The spermatic cord gets twisted around the testicle, cutting off the supply of blood to the testicle.

Varicocele: Dilated and twisted veins of the testis.

Vulvovaginitis: An inflammation of the vulva and vagina; commonly caused by irritating substances (bubble bath) or poor hygiene.

Common Abbreviations Related to the Urinary and Male and Female Reproductive Systems

CKD: Chronic Kidney Disease

CX: Cervix

DRE: Digital Rectal Examination

DUB: Dysfunctional Uterine Bleeding

ED: Erectile Dysfunction

ESRD: End-Stage Renal Disease

GU: Genitourinary

HPV: Human Papillomavirus

HRT: Hormone Replacement Therapy

IVP: Intravenous Pyelogram

KUB: Kidneys, Ureters, Bladder

PID: Pelvic Inflammatory Disease

PSA: Prostate-Specific Antigen

STD: Sexually Transmitted Disease

UTI: Urinary Tract Infection

Endocrine System

The endocrine system comprises glands located throughout the body (Fig. 2.14). The glands produce and secrete hormones that have an impact on the function of the body. The endocrine system is responsible for growth and development, tissue function, reproduction, metabolism, and even plays a part in regulating mood.

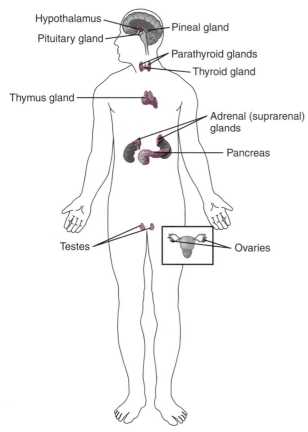

Figure 2-14. Endocrine system.

Anatomical Terms Related to the Endocrine System

Hypothalamus: Part of the brain located above the pituitary gland that connects the endocrine system to the nervous system and is responsible for regulating the release of hormones, body temperature, food intake, and sleep.

Parathyroid gland: Small glands located within the lobe of the thyroid that control the supply of calcium to the body.

Pineal gland: A small endocrine gland in the brain that secretes the hormone melatonin, which assists with the regulation of wake/sleep cycles.

Thymus gland: The thymus gland is located behind the breast bone and plays an important role in the development of the immune system of the body. As people age, the thymus gland decreases in size.

Thyroid gland: One of the largest endocrine glands in the body, it helps to regulate growth and metabolism

Common Diseases of the Endocrine System

Diabetes: The inability of the body to produce or metabolize the human hormone insulin, resulting in high glucose levels, frequent urination, and excessive thirst.

Gestational diabetes: The elevation of blood glucose during pregnancy.

Goiter: An abnormally enlarged thyroid gland.

Hyperglycemia: Excess glucose in the blood.

Hypothyroidism: An underactive thyroid (insufficient production of thyroid hormones) causing a reduced metabolic rate, tiredness, and lethargy.

Common Abbreviations Related to the Endocrine System

DM: **D**iabetes **M**ellitus

GH: **G**rowth **H**ormone

GTT: **G**lucose **T**olerance **T**est

HGH: **H**uman **G**rowth **H**ormone

TSH: **T**hyroid-**S**timulating **H**ormone

Nervous System

This system includes a large network of nerve fibers that traverse the body (Fig. 2.15). The nervous system includes the brain (Fig. 2.16) and spinal cord, called the central nervous system (CNS), and the peripheral nervous system (PNS). The primary function of the nervous system is to act as a central intelligence station for the body by receiving signals (sensory input), processing signals (integration), and performing actions (output). The nervous system regulates subconscious body functions and provides an internal method of communication by sending signals from one part of the body to another.

Anatomical Terms Related to the Nervous System

Brachial plexus: A network of nerves originating from the neck and running down to the shoulder, arm, hand, and fingers.

Cerebellum: A portion of the brain located in the back of the head responsible for the coordination of movement and balance.

Obturator nerve: Arises from the ventral divisions of the second, third, and fourth lumbar nerves; responsible for the innervations of the skin of the medial aspect of the thigh.

Peripheral nervous system: Extends outside the central nervous system (the brain and spinal cord) and connects the central nervous system to the limbs and organs.

Spinal cord: A long thin tube-like structure of nervous tissue that runs from the base of the skull down the back; its function is to carry messages from the brain to the rest of the body (e.g., touch, pain, and signals telling the muscles to move).

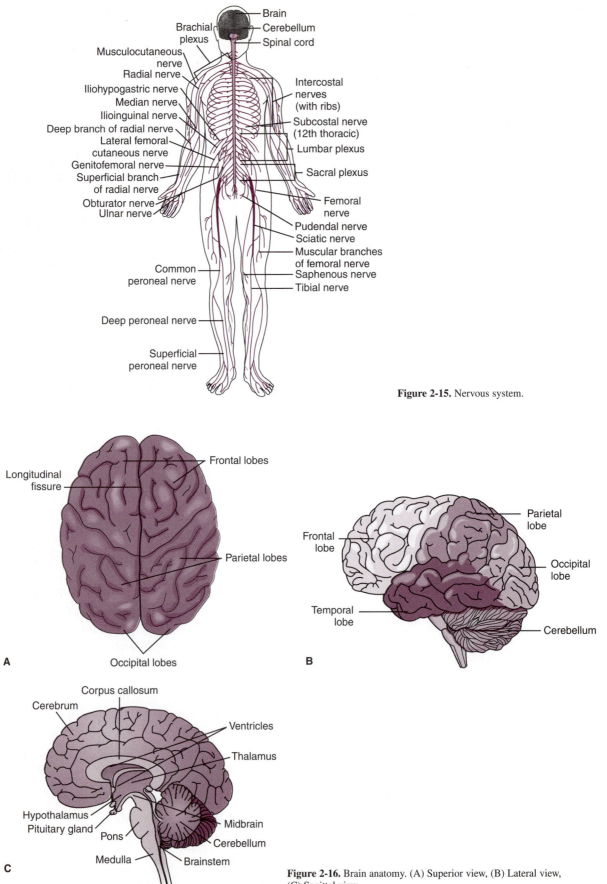

Brain
Brachial plexus
Cerebellum
Spinal cord
Musculocutaneous nerve
Radial nerve
Iliohypogastric nerve
Median nerve
Ilioinguinal nerve
Deep branch of radial nerve
Lateral femoral cutaneous nerve
Genitofemoral nerve
Superficial branch of radial nerve
Obturator nerve
Ulnar nerve
Intercostal nerves (with ribs)
Subcostal nerve (12th thoracic)
Lumbar plexus
Sacral plexus
Femoral nerve
Pudendal nerve
Sciatic nerve
Muscular branches of femoral nerve
Saphenous nerve
Tibial nerve
Common peroneal nerve
Deep peroneal nerve
Superficial peroneal nerve

Figure 2-15. Nervous system.

Longitudinal fissure
Frontal lobes
Parietal lobes
Occipital lobes

A

Frontal lobe
Parietal lobe
Temporal lobe
Occipital lobe
Cerebellum

B

Corpus callosum
Cerebrum
Ventricles
Thalamus
Hypothalamus
Pituitary gland
Pons
Midbrain
Cerebellum
Medulla
Brainstem

C

Figure 2-16. Brain anatomy. (A) Superior view, (B) Lateral view, (C) Sagittal view.

Common Diseases of the Nervous System

Alzheimer's disease: A progressive degenerative brain disease that alters the brain, causing impaired memory, thinking, and behavior.

Cerebral palsy: Loss or deficiency of motor control caused by brain damage before birth or during infancy.

Epilepsy: A disorder of the central nervous system in which abnormal electrical activity in the brain causes seizures and blackouts.

Meningitis: An inflammation of the membranes that surround the brain (meninges).

Multiple sclerosis: A slowly progressive disease of the brain and spinal cord resulting in difficulties with coordination and speech, impaired mobility, and disability.

Common Abbreviations Related to the Nervous System

ANS: <u>A</u>utonomic <u>N</u>ervous <u>S</u>ystem

CNS: <u>C</u>entral <u>N</u>ervous <u>S</u>ystem

CP- <u>C</u>erebral <u>P</u>alsy

EEG: <u>E</u>lectro<u>e</u>ncephalo<u>g</u>ram

PNS: <u>P</u>eripheral <u>N</u>ervous <u>S</u>ystem

Organs of Sense

The organs of sense include sight and hearing and are listed as a subsection of the nervous system. The eyes and ears receive and process signals, which are interpreted in the central nervous system.

■ The eye provides the sense of sight (Fig. 2.17). The eye is located in the bony orbit, or socket, formed by various bones. There are three layers to the eyeball: the retina (innermost), choroid (middle), and sclera (outermost). Additionally, the eye is separated into the anterior and posterior segments. The anterior segment includes the cornea, conjunctiva, iris, ciliary body, and chorid. The posterior segment includes the vitreous, retina, and optic nerve. The accessory structures include the eyelids, eyelashes, and lacrimal system. There are also six ocular muscles that work in opposition to move the eye in multiple directions.

■ The ear provides the sense of hearing (Fig. 2.18). The ear is divided into the outer ear (external ear, consisting of the pinna and auditory canal), middle ear (tympanic cavity, including three bones: malleus, incus, and stapes), and inner ear (cochlea, labyrinth). The outer ear captures the sound and sends it through to the middle ear. The middle ear transforms the sound waves and sends signals to the auditory sensory cells located in the inner ear. Once in the inner ear, the information is sent to the auditory nerve, which delivers the information to the brain.

Anatomical Terms Related to the Eye

Choroid: The middle layer of the eye consisting of blood vessels that furnish nourishment to other parts of the eye.

Conjunctiva: The mucous membrane that covers the eyeball and the undersurface of the eyelid.

Optic nerve: The cable that connects the eye to the brain.

Retina: A thin membrane covering the back of the eyeball that converts optical images to electrical impulses, which are sent along the optic nerve to the brain.

Sclera: The white of the eye that serves as a protective outer layer for the eye.

Common Ophthalmological Diseases

Blepharitis: Inflammation of the eyelids.

Cataract: A clouding of the natural lens of the eye.

Chalazion: A sebaceous cyst of the eyelid.

Nystagmus: Rapid involuntary movements of the eye.

Strabismus: Also known as "crossed eyes"; this is the abnormal alignment of one or both eyes.

Common Ophthalmological Abbreviations

OD: Right eye

OL: Left eye

OKN: <u>O</u>pto<u>k</u>inetic <u>n</u>ystagmus

OU: Both eyes

VA: <u>V</u>isual <u>A</u>cuity

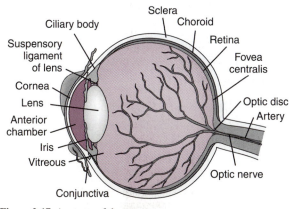

Figure 2-17. Anatomy of the eye.

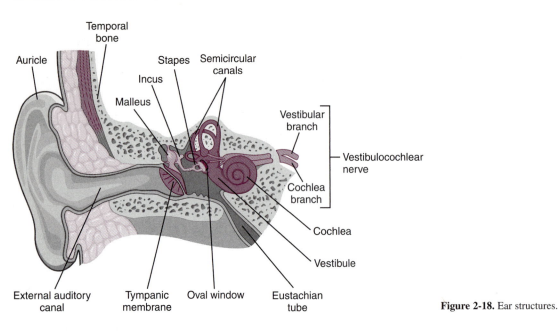

Figure 2-18. Ear structures.

Anatomical Terms Related to the Ear

Cochlea: A snail-shaped tube in the inner ear that contains the organ of Corti (the sensory organ of hearing).

Eustachian tube: One of a pair of tubes that connects the middle ear to the nasopharnyx, allowing for the passage of air.

Malleus: A hammer-shaped bone in the middle ear that transmits the sound vibration from the eardrum to the incus (one of three tiny bones in the inner ear).

Tympanic membrane: The membrane in the ear that vibrates to sound.

Vestibule: The central cavity of the ear (the middle part of the inner ear).

Common Otological Diseases

Acoustic neuroma: A slow-growing benign tumor located in the hearing canal.

Ménière's disease: A disorder of the inner ear causing vertigo, tinnitus, and hearing loss.

Otitis externa: Inflammation of the external ear.

Otitis media: Inflammation of the middle ear; this is most common in children.

Tinnitus: A noise that originates within the ear, such as a ringing in the ear.

Common Otological Abbreviations

AD: Right ear

Al: Left ear

AU: Both ears

MD: **M**énière's **D**isease

OM: **O**titis **M**edia

Hemic System

This system consists of red blood cells, white blood cells and platelets. The hemic system fights infections, carries oxygen and helps to control bleeding.

Medical Terminology Related to the Hemic System

Plasma: The clear yellowish fluid portion of the blood in which the red blood cells, white blood cells, and plates are suspended.

Platelets: A minute disc-shaped element in the blood that assists with blood clotting.

Red blood cells: The most common type of blood cells, which are responsible for carrying oxygen to the body tissues.

Serum: The clear liquid that can be separated from clotted blood. It differs from plasma, as the clear liquid is obtained after the blood has been allowed to clot and the clot has been removed.

White blood cells: There are several types of white blood cells. The primary function of white blood cells (leukocytes) is to fight infection.

Common Diseases of the Hemic System

Hemophilia: A hereditary disorder whereby the blood does not clot normally, resulting in uncontrolled bleeding.

Leukemia: Malignant neoplasm of the blood-forming tissue (bone marrow), causing the abnormal development of white blood cells.

Sepsis: An infection in the blood caused by the spread of bacteria or toxins via the bloodstream.

Sickle cell disease: A genetic disorder whereby the blood cells form a crescent shape that results in chronic anemia.

Thalassemia: An inherited form of anemia resulting in the inability to create enough hemoglobin (the red blood cell protein that carries oxygen to the body).

Common Abbreviations Related to the Hemic System

CBC: **C**omplete **B**lood **C**ount

PA: **P**ernicious **A**nemia

RBC: **R**ed **B**lood **C**ell

SCD: **S**ickle **C**ell **D**isease

WBC: **W**hite **B**lood **C**ell

Immune System

The immune system comprises special cells, proteins, tissues, and organs. The immune system acts as a defense against germs and microorganisms.

Medical Terminology Related to the Immune System

Antibodies: Proteins made by the body to neutralize or destroy foreign substances (antigens).

Immunodeficiency: The inability of the immune system to fight off infectious diseases.

Interferon: Proteins released by cells to stimulate the immune response.

Lymphocyte: A type of white blood cell that produces antibodies.

Monocyte: Large circulating white blood cells formed in the bone marrow that fight against fungi and bacteria.

Common Diseases of the Immune System

Allergies: An overreaction of the immune system to a substance or allergen.

Anaphylaxis: A severe and rapid allergic reaction that can become life threatening.

Autoimmune disease: A disease caused when the body's own immune system acts against itself.

Human immunodeficiency virus: A virus that causes failure of the immune system by infecting and destroying helper T cells of the immune system.

Rheumatoid arthritis: An autoimmune disease that causes chronic inflammation of the joints.

Common Abbreviations Related to the Immune System

HIV: **H**uman **I**mmunodeficiency **V**irus

IBD: **I**nflammatory **B**owel **D**isease

RA: **R**heumatoid **A**rthritis

SCID: **S**evere **C**ombined **I**mmunodeficiency **D**isease (Disorder)

SLE: **S**ystemic **L**upus **E**rythematosus

Some Current Procedure Terminology (CPT) books include illustrations and anatomical diagrams; this depends on the version or type of CPT book you have. This is one reason why you should carefully select the version or type of coding books you purchase. Many of these features are not included in the standard version of the coding books. If your book does not include any anatomical illustrations, you can always sketch them into your book on the blank pages closest to the CPT code descriptors for that particular organ system.

If you are coding, you should have by now taken a course on anatomy and medical terminology or at least have read some books on the subject, as the coding process is based on a good foundation of anatomy and medical terminology. There are many good books and flashcards on the market that make it fun and easy to learn (see "Learn More About It" at the end of this chapter). There are even anatomy coloring books. When was the last time you picked up your crayons?

Medical Terminology

Medicine has a language of its own. Most medical terms are over 2,000 years old and have Greek and Latin origins. You can learn the medical language by memorization or by learning the word parts, or elements, that form the medical term. By far, learning the prefix, suffix, and root words is a much easier way to learn medical terminology.

The key to understanding a medical term is to break it down into parts and consider how the parts fit together. Each part gives a special meaning to the entire word; therefore, if you translate each part separately and then recombine the parts, you will have the meaning of the word.

For example: let's look at a non-medical word: *Unmentionable.*

The prefix (an element placed at the beginning of a word to change its meaning) in this word is "un"; the root word (main body of the word) is "mention"; and the suffix (an element attached to the end of a word to change its meaning) is "able": un-**mention**-able

Here the root word is "mention"; the suffix **able** means "susceptible, capable, or worthy of a specific action." The word now changes to mean capable of being mentioned. The meaning of the prefix **un** is "not" or "the opposite of." The meaning of the word now changes to "that which is not to be mentioned" or "not fit to be mentioned."

Let's apply the same process to a medical term. Let's look at the medical term *electrocardiogram.*

Here the root is *cardio,* meaning "heart." The prefix is *electro,* meaning "pertaining to electricity," and the suffix is *gram,* meaning "recording or study." When we combine all the parts of the word (prefix + root + suffix), we have the meaning of electrocardiogram, a recording of the electrical current of the heart: electro-**cardio**-gram

Once again, some versions of CPT books include some basic prefixes and suffixes, although most do not include root words. If your version does not include this information, you can copy in the following common prefixes, suffixes, and roots.

Common Prefixes

Prefix	Meaning	Example
A(n)-	Absence, without	Anuria (lack of urine output)
Ambi-	Around, all sides	Ambidextrous (using both hands)
Bi-	Two	Bilateral (both sides)
Brady-	Slow	Bradycardia (slow heart rhythm)
Dys-	Difficult, painful	Dysuria (painful urination)
Eu-	Good, normal	Eucapnia (normal amounts of carbon dioxide in the blood)
Ex-	Out of	Exfoliate (peeling of layers)
Hetero	Different	Heterogeneous
Homo	Same	Homogeneous
Hyper-	Above, beyond, excessive	Hypernatremia (excess sodium)
Hypo-	Low, decrease, deficient, below	Hypothyroidism (underactive thyroid gland)
Intra-	Within, into	Intramuscular (into the muscle)
Litho	Stone, calculus	Lithotripsy (crushing of stones)
Mal-	Bad, abnormal	Malformation (abnormally formed)
Mega-	Great, large	Megacolon (enlarged colon)
Micr(o)-	Small	Micromyelia (small spinal cord)
Mono-	One	Monogenic (relating to one gene)
Olig(o)-	Few, little	Oligopnea (few breaths)
Poly-	Much, many	Polyuria (excessive urine)
Pseudo-	False	Pseudocyst (accumulation of fluid resembling a true cyst)
Tachy-	Rapid	Tachycardia (rapid heart beat)
Trans-	Across, through	Transdermal (through the skin)

A root can be part of a word or a whole word. In medical terminology, roots can refer to a procedure, a disease, or a body part/organ system. As well, two or more roots can be combined to form one word; for example, "cardiovascular." Here we see the roots *cardio* and *vascular* being combined to form one word referring to both the heart (cardio) and the blood vessels (vascular).

Common Roots

Root	Meaning	Example
Abdomin(o)	Abdomen	Abdominoperineal (abdomen and perineal area)
Aden(o)	Gland	Adenoma (glandular tumor)
Angi(o)	Lymph or blood vessel	Angioma (tumor of the blood vessels)
Ankyl	Crooked, bent, fusion	Ankylosis (bent or crooked joint)
Bili	Bile	Bilirubin (yellow pigment in bile)
Blephar(o)	Eyelid	Blepharoplasty (repair of the eyelid)
Brachi(o)	Arm	Brachioplasty (cosmetic surgery on the arm)
Carcin(o)	Cancer	Carcinoma (malignant growth)
Cardi(o)	Heart	Cardiomyopathy (a disease of the heart muscle)
Cephal(o)	Head	Cephalometer (a device used to measure the head)
Cerebr(o)	Cerebrum	Cerebropathy (disease of the brain)
Cervic(i)(o)	Neck	Cervicalgia (pain in the neck)
Chol(e)	Bile	Cholecystitis (inflammation of the gallbladder)
Chondr(o)	Cartilage	Chondritis (inflammation of cartlilage)
Cyst(i)(o)	Bladder	Cystoscopy (endoscopy of the bladder)
Derm	Skin	Dermatology (the study of the skin)
Gastro	Stomach	Gastroenterologist (a physician who specializes in diseases of the stomach and the intestinal tract)
Heme(a)(o)	Blood	Hematoma (swelling filled with blood)
Hepat(o)	Liver	Hepatitis (inflammation of the liver)
Lith(os)	Stone	Cholelithiasis (gallstones)
Myel(o)	Marrow, spinal cord	Myelogram (x-ray of the spinal cord)
Nephr(o)	Kidney	Nephrectomy (surgical removal of a kidney)
Neuro	Nerve	Neurology (the study of the nervous system)
Oss, Oste(o)	Bone	Osteoporosis (loss of bone tissue)
Pharyng(o)	Pharynx	Pharyngitis (inflammation of the pharynx)
Pleur(o)	Pleura, rib, side	Pleuralgia (pain in the side)
Pnea	Breathing	Dyspnea (difficulty breathing)
Pyel(o)	Renal pelvis	Pyelogram (radiograph of the renal pelvis)
Rhin(o)	Nose	Rhinorrhea (runny nose)
Sten	Narrowing	Stenosis (narrowing of a body canal or passage)
Thorac(o)	Chest	Thoracentesis (insertion of a needle into the chest wall)
Thromb(o)	Clot	Thombogenic (likely to produce a blood clot)

Common Suffixes

Suffix	Meaning	Example
-Algia	Pain	Neuralgia (nerve pain)
-Centesis	Puncture a cavity to remove fluid	Amniocentesis (extraction of amniotic fluid)
-Ectomy	Surgical removal	Splenectomy (removal of spleen)
-Itis	Inflammation	Appendicitis (inflammation of the appendix)
-Lysis	Destruction, breakdown	Hemolysis (destruction of red blood cells)
-Oma	Tumor	Fibroma (fibrous tumor)
-Opathy	Disease of	Arthropathy (disease of a joint)
-Oplasty	Surgical repair	Rhinoplasty (surgical repair of the nose)
-Orrhagia	Hemorrhage	Menorrhagia (prolonged menstruation)
-Orrhaphy	Surgical repair/suture	Herniorrhaphy (surgical repair of a hernia)
-Ostomy	A new permanent opening	Colostomy (opening from the colon to the surface of the body)
-Otomy	Cutting into (incision)	Tracheotomy (cutting an opening into the trachea)
-Otripsy	Crushing, destroying	Lithotripsy (crushing of kidney stones)
-Paresis	Weakness	Hemiparesis (weakness on one side of the body)
-Plasia	Growth	Dysplasia (abnormal tissue growth)
-Plegia	Paralysis	Paraplegia (paralysis of lower body)
-Poiesis	Production	Hematopoiesis (production of blood cells)
-Rrhea	Fluid discharge	Rhinorrhea (runny nose)
-Scope	Observe	Endoscope (tool for observing the interior of the body)
-Taxis	Movement	Ataxia (lack of coordination)
-Tripsy	Crushing	Lithotripsy (crushing of stones)
-Trophy	Growth	Hypertrophy (overgrowth)

The medical profession also has its own medical terminology for directions and positions. Some of the directions and positions are described with the use of prefixes and others are described with words themselves. Listed below are some of the common terms for directions and positions.

Directions and Positions

Prefix	Meaning	Example
Ab-	Away from	Abduction (movement of limbs away from the midline of the body)
Ad-	Toward	Adduction (moving of a body part toward the center of the body)
Ante-	Before, in front of	Anterior (front of body)
Ecto-, exo-	Outside, abnormal place or position	Ectogenous (origination outside a body or structure); exomphalos (an umbilical protrusion)
Endo-	Within	Endopelvis (within the pelvis)

Directions and Positions—cont'd

Prefix	Meaning	Example
Epi-	Upon	Epigastric
Infra-	Below, under	Inframandibular (below the lower jaw)
Ipsi-	Same	Ipsilateral (on the same side of the body)
Meta-	After, beyond, transformation	Metastasis (movement from one part of the body to another)
Peri-	Surrounding	Pericorneal (around the cornea)
Retro-	Behind, back	Retrouterine (behind the uterus)
Supra-	Above, upon	Supraorbital (above the orbit)
Trans-	Across, through	Transvaginal (through the vagina)

Directions and Positions

Word	Meaning
Anterior or ventral	Near or at the front of the body
Posterior or dorsal	Near or at the back of the body
Superior	Above
Inferior	Below
Lateral	Side
Distal	Furthest from origin
Proximal	Nearest to origin
Medial	Middle
Supine	Lying face upward
Prone	Lying face downward
Sagittal	Vertical body plane that divides the body into right and left
Transverse	Horizontal body plane that divides the body into top and bottom sections
Coronal	Vertical body plane that divides the body into front and back sections

Learn More About It

The more you read the more you know. Increase your knowledge with the following resources.

Recommended Web Sites

Inner Body: Your Guide to Human Anatomy Online

http://www.innerbody.com/htm/body.html

The Clinician's Ultimate Reference (Medical Abbreviations)

http://www.globalrph.com/abbrev.htm

Recommended Books

Netter's Anatomy Coloring Book

by John T. Hansen, PhD.; WB Saunders

Medical Terminology Systems: A Body Systems Approach, 6th ed.

by Barbara A. Gylys and Mary Ellen Wedding; F.A. Davis

Pocket Anatomy and Physiology

by Shirley A. Jones; F.A. Davis

STOP-LOOK-HIGHLIGHT

If your version of the CPT book includes an Illustrated Anatomical and Procedural Review, you should review the anatomical diagrams and supplement the prefixes, roots, suffixes, positions, and directions with those listed above by writing them into your CPT book for future reference.

If your CPT book does not include the Illustrated Anatomical and Procedural Review, you can write in the prefixes, roots, suffixes, positions, and directions given in this chapter. You can also sketch in some of the anatomical diagrams illustrated in this book. *It is important to remember that most versions of CPT list common medical abbreviations on the back flap of the book.*

TAKE THE CODING CHALLENGE

1. The largest organ system is:
   a. Lymphatic
   b. Cardiovascular
   c. Integumentary
   d. Musculoskeletal

2. The functions of the endocrine system include:
   a. Growth and development, tissue function, temperature regulation, and regulation of mood
   b. Growth and development, tissue function, metabolism, and regulation of mood
   c. Growth and development, tissue function, filtering of blood, and regulation of mood
   d. Growth and development, tissue function, temperature regulations, and reproduction.

3. Which organ system(s) provide(s) the body with protection and/or a defense system?
   a. Integumentary
   b. Immune
   c. Lymphatic
   d. All of the above

4. The suffix "-ectomy" refers to:
   a. A surgical removal
   b. A surgical repair
   c. Cutting into
   d. Incision

5. A patient diagnosed with cholelithiasis has the following condition:
   a. Kidney stones
   b. Gallstones
   c. An inflammation of the bile ducts
   d. An inflammation of the colon

6. A patient with a rapid heartbeat has:
   a. Hypercardia
   b. Megacardia
   c. Cardiopathy
   d. Tachycardia

7. Mary Franklin presented for a chest x-ray. The x-ray was taken with the patient in the lateral position. Define "lateral":
   a. Near or at the front of the body
   b. Lying face upward
   c. Side
   d. Above

8. The radiologist performed an ultrasound of the thyroid with multiple transverse images. Define "transverse":
   a. Vertically from right to left
   b. Vertically from front to back
   c. Horizontally from top to bottom
   d. None of the above

9. The foot is located _____ to the knee.
   a. Anterior
   b. Posterior
   c. Superior
   d. Distal

10. An *ectopic pregnancy* refers to a pregnancy:
    a. That occurs outside the womb
    b. With a fluid discharge
    c. With an abnormal growth
    d. That is weak

Answers and Rationales

1. The correct answer is **c.**, the integumentray system is the largest organ system. Although the lymphatic, cardiovascular, and musculoskeletal systems have lymph nodes, bones, veins, and arteries throughout the body, the skin encompasses the entire body, making it the largest organ system.

2. The correct answer is **b.**, growth and development, tissue function, metabolism, and regulation of mood; **a.** is incorrect because the integumentary system provides temperature regulation; **c.** is incorrect because the filtering of the blood is a function of the lymphatic system; **d.** is incorrect because, although the endocrine system plays a part in reproduction, the temperature regulation is a function of the integumentary system.

3. The correct answer is **d.**, all of the above. The integumentary system provides protection for the body, the immune system acts as a defense against germs and microorganisms, and the lymphatic system fights infections.

4. The correct answer is **a.**, a surgical removal; **b.** is incorrect because the suffix for a surgical repair is "-oplasty"; **c.** is incorrect because the suffix for cutting into is "-otomy"; **d.** is incorrect because the suffix for an incision is "-tomy."

5. The correct answer is **b.**, gallstones. If we break up the word into parts, it is easy to determine the correct answer. The prefix is "chole-" (bile), the root is "lithos" (stone), and the suffix is "-iasis" (formation or presence); **a.** is incorrect because the correct terminology for a kidney stone is *calculus of kidney;* **c.** is incorrect because the correct medical term for an inflammation of the bile duct is *cholangitis;* **d.** is incorrect because the

correct medical term for inflammation of the colon is *colitis.*

6. The correct answer is **d.**, tachycardia. Once again, if we breakdown the word, we see the prefix is "tachy-" (rapid); **a.** is incorrect because *hypercardia* is not a medical term; **b.** is incorrect because megacardia is an abnormal enlargement of the heart, better known as cardiomegaly; **c.** is incorrect because *cardiopathy* defines diseases of the heart.

7. The correct answer is **c.**, side; **a.** is incorrect because the term used to define "near or at the front of the body" is *anterior;* **b.** is incorrect because the term used to describe "lying face upward" is *supine;* **d.** is incorrect because the term used to describe "above" is *superior.*

8. The correct answer is **c.**, horizontally from top to bottom, or transverse; **a.** is incorrect because "vertically from right to left" refers to *sagittal;* **b.** is incorrect because "vertically from front to back" refers to *coronal.*

9. The correct answer is **d.**, *distal* refers to furthest from center; **a.** is incorrect because *anterior* refers to near or at the front of the body; **b.** is incorrect because *posterior* refers to near or at the back of the body; **c.** is incorrect because *superior* refers to above.

10. The correct answer is **a.**, an ectopic pregnancy occurs outside of the womb. The word *ectopic* means abnormal place or position. We can get a clue from the prefix "ecto-," which means abnormally placed or an abnormal position; **b.** is incorrect because the suffix for a fluid discharge is "-rrhea" and is not present in the term *ectopic pregnancy;* **c.** is incorrect because the suffix for growth is "-plasia," which is not present in the term; **d.** is incorrect because the suffix for weak is "-paresis," which is not present in the term.

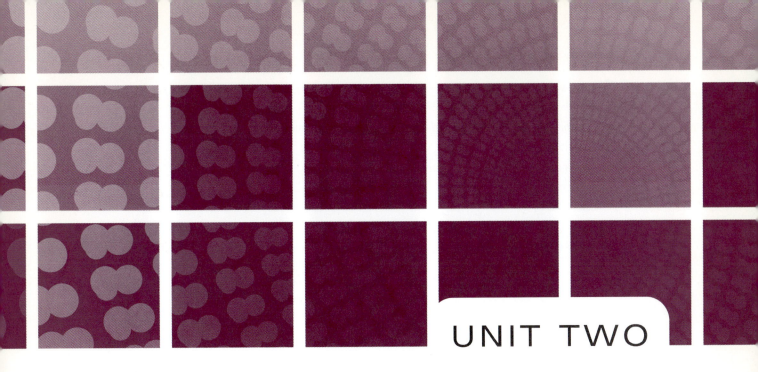

UNIT TWO

Coding Systems

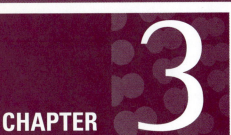

CHAPTER 3

Using the ICD-9-CM: An Overview

Diagnostic coding dates back to 17th-century England when the London Bills of Mortality were used to collect statistical data. In 1937, the collection of this information progressed into the International Causes of Death. In 1948, the World Health Organization (WHO) published a statistical listing called the International Classification of Diseases (ICD) used to track both morbidity and mortality. *The International Classification of Diseases, 9th Revision, Clinical Modification (ICD-9-CM)* is a modification of the WHO's ICD. The term *clinical* is used to highlight the modification's intent to serve as a useful tool to classify the following:

- Morbidity data for indexing medical records
- Medical care review
- Ambulatory and other medical care programs
- Basic health descriptions

The Many Uses of ICD-9-CM Today

Statistical Purposes: ICD-9-CM is present in our day-to-day lives. When we hear on the news about the number of cases of H1N1 virus (swine flu), this is an example of ICD-9-CM being used for statistical purposes. The number of cases (data) is derived from the number of times the H1N1 ICD-9-CM code was reported. Use of ICD-9-CM for statistical purposes assists in the following:

- Predicting health-care trends
- Monitoring and planning for future health-care expenses and needs

Payment of Health-Care Claims: ICD-9-CM codes are an integral part of facilitating payment of claims.

- In all cases, physician or health-care provider services (CPT codes) must be supported by the medical necessity for the service (ICD-9-CM). For example, strep throat (ICD-9-CM code 034.0) provides medical necessity for the service of a throat culture (CPT code 87070). Back pain would not provide medical necessity for a health-care provider to perform a throat culture. Medicare defines medical necessity as *"the determination that a service or procedure rendered is reasonable and necessary for the diagnosis or treatment of an illness or injury."* Therefore, it is important for the ICD-9-CM code to provide the medical necessity for the performance of a service.

- In some cases, the ICD-9-CM code alerts the insurance carrier that it is the correct payer of service. Certain "E codes" convey to the insurance carrier how an accident or injury occurred. These codes clearly identify if the claim should be reimbursed by workers' compensation, no-fault insurance, or the patient's private health insurance policy. For example, a patient with a fractured wrist could have fractured it on the job (E849.2 Place of occurrence, mine and quarry), in a motor vehicle accident (E813.0 Motor vehicle collision with other vehicle, injuring driver of motor vehicle other than motorcycle), or at home (E849.0 Place of occurrence, home).

Which Version of the ICD-9-CM Should You Use?

There are many versions of the ICD-9-CM (ICD-9-CM, Volumes 1 and 2 for Physicians, ICD-9-CM, Volumes 1, 2, and 3 for Hospitals, ICD-9-CM for Home Health Care, etc.). For the Certified Professional Coder and for the purposes of physician outpatient coding, we will review ICD-9-CM, Volumes 1 and 2 for Physicians.

- Volume I, Diseases tabular listing, provides instructional notes and detailed information (e.g., fourth and fifth digits, indicators of primary diagnosis codes, etc.).
- Volume II, Diseases alphabetical index, is an index that enables the coder to locate terms quickly for verification in the tabular list.

To ensure accurate and correct coding, the diagnosis code should always be selected from the tabular list.

KEY CODING TIP

Before we review the ICD-9-CM manual, let's take time to put tabs on various sections so we can locate them quickly as needed. Sticky notes work, but index dividers, available at any office supply or stationery store, work better. (Note: The page numbers will vary depending on the version of ICD-9-CM manual you have.) With sticky notes or index tabs, mark the following sections of the ICD-9-CM manual:

- Tag the page with the heading "ICD-9-CM Official Conventions" (located in the first few pages of the manual), and call this section **"Conventions."**
- Tag the page with the heading "Coding Guidelines" (also located in the front of the manual, a few pages after conventions), and call this section **"Coding Guidelines."**
- The next section to tag is located in the Volume 2 "Index to Diseases." Look up the word "Hypertension," and call this section **"Hypertension Table."**
- Also in the Volume 2 "Index to Diseases," look up the word "neoplasm," and call this section **"Neoplasm Table."**
- In the Volume 2 index, in Section 2 (which follows the "Index to Diseases") under the heading "Alphabetic Index to Poisoning and External Causes of Adverse Effects of Drugs and Other Chemical Substances," tag this page, and call this section **"Drugs and Chemicals."**
- In the Volume 2 index under Section 3, under the heading "Alphabetic Index to External Causes of

KEY CODING TIP—cont'd
Injury and Poisoning (E Code)," tag this page, and call this section **"External Causes."**
■ In the back of the manual in Volume 1, look up the diagnosis code "V01," tag this page, and call this section **"V Codes."**
■ Immediately at the end of the V Code section are the E Codes. Tag this page, and call this section **"E Codes."**

KEY CODING TIP
Additional fifth-digit codes (subclassification) are generally located in shaded boxes under the three-digit category code. Some shaded boxes contain more information than just the fifth digit. For example, Chapter 13, "Diseases of the Musculoskeletal System and Connective Tissue" (710–739) includes a shaded box (see Fig. 3.1) containing not just the fifth-digit information but also a description of the shoulder region, upper arm, and so on.

Other shaded boxes in Chapter 13 contain only general information, such as the fifth-digit code and location (see Fig. 3.2).

How the ICD-9-CM Is Organized

Now that your manual is properly indexed, let's take a look at how it is organized. The manual is divided into two sections. Volume 1 is called the Tabular List of Diseases, and Volume 2 is called the Alphabetical Index. It is interesting to note that in the ICD-9-CM manual, *Volume 2 comes before Volume 1.* Some versions of the ICD-9-CM manual include Volume 3, which provides ICD-9-CM codes that describe procedures. Procedure codes have a maximum of four digits: two in the category and one or two more following the decimal point (e.g., 45.23 Colonoscopy). The manual is further divided into two Supplementary Classifications: V codes and E codes. The manual also includes the following Appendices:

■ Appendix A, Morphology of Neoplasms
■ Appendix C, Classification of Drugs by American Hospital Formulary Service List Number and Their ICD-9-CM Equivalents
■ Appendix D, Classification of Industrial Accidents According to Agency
■ Appendix E, List of Three-Digit Categories

(Note: Appendix B, Glossary of Mental Disorders, was officially deleted October 1, 2004.)

The diagnosis codes in the Tabular List of Diseases (Volume 1) are classified by category, subcategory, and subclassification:

	Example
Category (three digits)	493 Asthma
Subcategory (four digits)	493.0 Extrinsic asthma
Subclassification (five digits)	493.01 Extrinsic asthma with status asthmaticus

The following fifth-digit subclassification is for use with categories 711–712, 715–716, 718–719, and 730:

0 site unspecified
1 shoulder region
   Acromioclavicular joint(s)
   Clavicle
   Glenohumeral joint(s)
   Scapula
   Sternoclavicular joint(s)
2 upper arm
   Elbow joint
   Humerus
3 forearm
   Radius
   Ulna
   Wrist joint
4 hand
   Carpus
   Metacarpus
   Phalanges (fingers)
5 pelvic region and thigh
   Buttock
   Femur
   Hip (joint)

6 lower leg
   Fibula
   Knee joint
   Patella
   Tibia
7 ankle and foot
   Ankle joint
   Digits (toes)
   Metatarsus
   Phalanges, foot
   Tarsus
   Other joints in foot
8 other specified sites
   Head
   Neck
   Ribs
   Skull
   Trunk
   Vertebral column
9 multiple sites

Figure 3-1. Fifth-digit codes (subclassification).

The following fifth-digit subclassification is for use with category 711; valid digits are in [brackets] under each code. See list at beginning of chapter for definitions.

0 site unspecified
1 shoulder region
2 upper arm
3 forearm
4 hand
5 pelvic region and thigh
6 lower leg
7 ankle and foot
8 other specified sites
9 multiple sites

Figure 3-2. Fifth-digit codes, general information.

ICD-9-CM Official Conventions

Now that we know how the manual is organized, let's take a look at the coding conventions. Open your manual to the section you indexed called "Conventions." The first page of the section should say "ICD-9-CM Official Conventions." This section defines the various footnotes, symbols, instructional notes, and conventions. **This is the section you will come to when you are asked questions on your exam regarding any of the coding conventions, their meaning, and how and when they are used.**

Official Government Symbols

The section mark, §, is the official government symbol. This symbol is used in the Tabular List; it precedes a code, and it denotes a footnote on the page.

Conventions Used in the Tabular List

In addition to government symbols and footnotes, the ICD-9-CM utilizes abbreviations, symbols, and punctuation called "conventions."

NEC, **N**ot **E**lsewhere **C**lassifiable—This abbreviation is used when the ICD-9-CM system does not provide a code specific for the patient's condition. The terminology "not elsewhere classifiable" will be included in the code description.

For example: Upon radiologic examination, a patient is diagnosed with "calcification of the lung." There is no specific code to define calcification of the lung; therefore, we must use a code that is not elsewhere classified, in this case, 518.89 Other diseases of lung, not elsewhere classified. To summarize, NEC codes are used when *the physician lists a diagnosis for which there is no specific code in the ICD-9-CM*.

NOS, **N**ot **O**therwise **S**pecified—This abbreviation is used only when the coder does not have sufficient information to code to a more specific four- or five-digit code. In other words, the ICD-9-CM manual *does* have a specific code to describe the patient's diagnosis; however, the *physician did not provide enough information for the coder to select a specific code,* and the coder therefore has no alternative but to use the code for "not otherwise specified."

For example: The physician diagnosis is asthma. There are many types of asthma: extrinsic, intrinsic, chronic obstructive, and others. In this case, the coder does not have enough information to select a specific type of asthma and therefore must select the code for unspecified asthma, 493.90 Asthma, unspecified, unspecified status.

> **KEY CODING TIP**
> Many of the ICD-9-CM codes that are NEC or NOS end in 8, 9, and sometimes 0. These codes are usually nonspecific and are sometimes referred to as "dump" codes.

[ ] **Brackets**—Brackets enclose synonyms, alternative terminology, or explanatory phrases and also indicate valid fifth digits for the code. If we look up the ICD-9-CM code 493.2 Chronic obstructive asthma, we see that it is followed by explanatory details:

493.2 Chronic Obstructive Asthma

[0-2] Asthma with chronic obstructive pulmonary disease [COPD]

This example shows the brackets being used in two ways. First, enclosed in the brackets are the numbers 0–2, which indicates that numbers 0, 1, and 2 are all valid fifth-digit choices for this code. Next, the abbreviation COPD is enclosed in brackets, and in this case, the brackets are being used to describe the alternative terminology for chronic obstructive pulmonary disease.

[ ] **Slanted brackets**—These are used in the Alphabetical Index to indicate mandatory multiple coding. Both codes must be coded, in the order they are listed, to fully describe the patient's condition. If we look up Amyloidosis with lung involvement in the Alphabetical Index, we find:

Amyloidosis

With lung involvement 277.39 *[517.8]*

The slanted brackets indicate *mandatory* multiple coding, so we first look up code 277.39 in the Tabular List to confirm it is the correct code. However, when we do this, we notice there is no mention of a secondary code or mandatory multiple coding. Now we look up code 517.8, as prompted by the slanted brackets, and we see the following code description:

517.8 Lung involvement in other diseases classified elsewhere
Code first underlying disease as:
Amyloidosis (277.30–277.39)

It is only when we looked up the secondary code that we are alerted to the mandatory multiple coding ("code first underlying disease"). It is therefore important when looking up codes in the Alphabetical Index to pay close attention to any coding convention corresponding to the code.

( ) **Parentheses**—Parentheses enclose supplementary words called "nonessential modifiers." Nonessential modifiers are words that may be present in the description of the disease but do not affect the code assignment. Parentheses can be found in both the Alphabetical Index and the Tabular List. For example:

217 Benign neoplasm of breast

Breast (male) (female)

Enclosed in parentheses are the words "male" and "female," which provide additional information. However, because the diagnosis is benign neoplasm of the breast, the supplemental words male and female would not change the code assignment.

: Colons—Colons are used after an incomplete term that needs one or more modifiers (additional terms) to make it assignable to a given category. Colons are used in the Tabular List. For example:

276.2 Acidosis

Acidosis:

NOS

lactic

metabolic

respiratory

Notice the modifiers—NOS, lactic, metabolic, and respiratory—all appear after the colon. These modifiers (whichever ones are appropriate) must be present in the provider's documentation to select ICD-9-CM code 276.2.

} Braces—A brace encloses a series of terms, each of which is modified by the statement appearing to the right of the brace. For example:

vertically center brace and "of lips" with Abscess, Cellulitis, Fistula, and Hypertrophy

528.5 Diseases of the lips

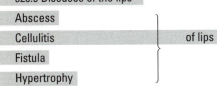

Abscess

Cellulitis   of lips

Fistula

Hypertrophy

Essential Modifiers—Essential modifiers are subterms that are listed below the main terms. They are indented two spaces and are usually in alphabetical order (with the exception of *with* or *without*). Each modifier clarifies the previous one and describes essential differences in site, etiology, and symptoms. *Essential modifiers will change your code selection.* For example:

—Weight

• Gain (abnormal) (excessive) 783.1

—During pregnancy 646.1X

» Insufficient 646.8X

You can see that each time the term is modified, the code selection changes.

Non-Essential Modifiers—Nonessential modifiers are subterms that are listed immediately after the main term and are enclosed in parentheses. They serve as examples to help translate written terminology into numeric codes, and they *do not change the code assignment.* For example:

Wound, open (by cutting or piercing instrument) (by firearm) (cut) (dissection) (incised) (laceration) (penetration) (perforating) (puncture) (with initial hemorrhage, not internal) 879.8

In this case, the ICD-9-CM code 879.8 can identify an open wound by any means indicated in the parentheses.

Other Conventions

Boldface—All codes and titles in the Tabular List are printed in boldface type.

Italics—All exclusion notes and codes that should not be used as primary diagnosis codes are printed in italicized type.

Instructional Notes in the Tabular List

The following instructional notes appear only in the Tabular List of Diseases.

KEY CODING TIP

The fact that some instructional notes appear only in the Tabular List of Diseases is an important reason that diagnosis codes should be selected only from the Tabular List (Volume 1) and not from the Alphabetical Index (Volume 2).

Includes—The "includes" notes clarify, further define, or provide examples that can apply to the chapter, subchapter, category, subcategory, or subclassification.

Let's take a look at a few examples.

| INCLUDES | **Chapter 15. Certain Conditions Originating in the Perinatal Period (760–779),** conditions which have their origin in the perinatal period, before birth through the first 28 days after birth, even though death or morbidity occurs later.

In this case the *"includes"* note *applies to all codes in the chapter.*

Organic Psychotic Conditions (290–294)

| INCLUDES | Psychotic organic brain syndrome

In this case the *""includes"* note *applies only to 290–294* (section).

600 Hyperplasia of prostate

| INCLUDES | enlarged prostate

In this case, the *"includes"* note *applies only to 600* (category).

Excludes—The *"excludes"* notes are the exact opposite of *includes*. They indicate **what is not** classified to the chapter, subchapter, category, subcategory, or specific subclassification. Excludes notes are italicized.

KEY CODING TIP

The "excludes" note may also provide the location of the excluded diagnosis.

045 Acute poliomyelitis

EXCLUDES Late effects of acute poliomyelitis (138)

As this example shows, when we look up the code for acute poliomyelitis, we not only see that it excludes late effects of poliomyletis but we are also given the code for the late effects.

Use Additional Code—This note prompts the coder to use an additional code to provide more complete information about the diagnosis *only if the information is available* to the coder (documented in the patient's medical record by the service provider). The additional diagnosis or a range of diagnosis codes will be provided. For example:

562 Diverticula of intestine

Use additional code to identify any associated:

Peritonitis (567.0–567.9)

If the documentation in the patient note supports the additional diagnosis, we *first code the diverticula of intestine, 562.XX followed by the correct code for the peritonitis.*

Code First Underlying Disease—This instructional note is a sequencing rule and most often applies to the etiology/manifestation convention. The instructional note, the code, and its descriptor appear in the Tabular List in italics. This note instructs the coder to sequence the underlying disease first. For example:

711.6X Arthropathy associated with mycoses

Code first underlying disease (110.0–118)

In this case, *the underlying disease is sequenced first,* 110.0–118, followed by the arthropathy associated with mycoses, 711.6X.

Code, if applicable, any causal condition first—This note alerts the coder to code any causal condition (if known) first; if no causal condition is known, the code may be used as the principal diagnosis.

788.2 Retention of urine

Code, if applicable, any causal condition first, such as:

Hyperplasia of prostate (600.0–600.9 with fifth digit 1)

For this scenario, if the cause of the retention of urine was the hypertrophy (benign) of prostate with urinary obstruction and other lower urinary tract symptoms (LUTS), we code this first (600.01), followed by retention of urine (788.2). *If we do not know the cause of the retention of urine, we can code the retention of urine as the principal diagnosis.*

Instructional Notes in the Alphabetical Index

Omit code—This note alerts the coder there is no code to be assigned. The medical term should not be coded as a diagnosis. For example:

Metaplasia

Cervix—omit code

Cross References

There are three types of cross references: *see, see also,* and *see category.* The cross references for *see* and *see also* direct the coder to another main term in the index where the information necessary to code the condition, disease, and so on, can be located.

See—Used in Volume 2 to direct the coder to a more specific term under which the correct code can be found. For example:

Fracture, bursting—see Fracture, phalanx, hand, distal

See Also—Indicates where supplementary information is available that may provide another code. For example:

Bartholin's

Adenitis (*see also* Bartholinitis) 616.89

Keep in mind: When the word *see* is in italics, this notation indicates that the coder should preview the specified category prior to deciding on a code.

See Category—This note alerts the coder to reference the Tabular List to select the appropriate code.

See Condition—This note alerts the coder to refer to a main term for the condition. This note references nouns for anatomical sites or adjectival forms of disease. For example, if we look up *knee* or *phlegmonous,* we are prompted to "see condition":

Knee—see condition (noun)

Phlegmonous—see condition (adjective)

KEY CODING TIP

When looking up a diagnosis code in the Alphabetical Index, *always look up the condition and not the anatomical site or descriptive adjective.*

Additional Conventions

Symbols and Notations
New and Revised Text Symbols
Symbols used to indicate new and revised text are as follows:
● A bullet denotes the code is new.
▲ A triangle in the Tabular List indicates the code title is revised. A triangle in the Alphabetical Index indicates the code has changed.
►◄ These symbols indicate new or revised text and are found at the beginning and the end of the section that is revised.

Additional Digits Required
Special attention should be paid to this notation because it indicates whether a code requires an additional fourth and/or fifth digit to code to the highest degree of specificity. Failure to code to the highest degree of specificity will result in a claim denial.

√ 4th — This indicates the code requires an additional fourth digit.

√ 5th — This indicates the code requires an additional fifth digit.

√ — This symbol is found only in the Alphabetical Index and the Table of Drugs and Chemicals. It alerts the coder that additional digits are required. The coder *must* refer to the Tabular List to locate the appropriate additional digit(s).

Eponyms
Eponyms are procedures, diseases, or syndromes named after a person. They can be located in the Alphabetical Index in two ways: under their name or under the syndrome. For example:

Syndrome:

Klinefelter's Syndrome 758.7 *OR* Syndrome, Klinefelter's 758.7

Disease:

Creutzfeldt-Jacob Disease (CJD) 046.19 *OR* Disease, Creutzfeldt-Jacob (CJD) 046.19

Coding Guidelines: Some Basics

Multiple Coding
Always document the primary diagnosis code first. Comorbid conditions and complications should be documented only when they affect the treatment of the patient.

For example: A patient with colitis managed by prescription medication of Asacol presents to the physician

with an ear infection. The patient is diagnosed with otitis media, and as part of the treatment plan, the physician prescribes an antibiotic. However, because the patient is already on Asacol for the colitis, the physician must find an antibiotic that will not have an adverse effect with the Asacol. In this case, both the otitis media (primary diagnosis) and the colitis (secondary diagnosis, comorbid condition) are coded. If the patient with colitis was not on any medication and the colitis was in remission, the colitis need not be coded as a secondary diagnosis because it did not affect the patient's treatment plan nor was the patient treated for colitis.

In some instances, multiple coding is prompted by ICD-9-CM coding conventions (e.g., with the slanted brackets—see description of this convention given earlier in the chapter).

Acute vs. chronic—If the same condition is described as both acute and chronic and separate entries exist in the Alphabetical Index at the same indentation level, code both conditions and list the acute code first.

Rule Out—Although physicians often write "rule out" as a diagnosis, it is important to note there are no diagnosis codes for rule out in the ICD-9-CM manual. When no definitive diagnosis can be made, code the signs and symptoms.

For example: A patient with a cough, fever, and chest pain is sent for a chest x-ray to "rule out" pneumonia. Because "rule out pneumonia" does not exist and the pneumonia cannot be coded because there is no definitive diagnosis to indicate the patient has pneumonia, we code the signs and symptoms. In this case, *cough* or *chest pain* would provide medical necessity for the chest x-ray.

Late Effects—A late effect is a residual condition (a condition left behind) after an acute illness or injury. With late effects, the residual is coded first, followed by the code of the condition that caused the residual effect. There is no time limit on when a residual may be used. When coding late effects, look up "late" as a main term in the Alphabetical Index followed by the subterm for the causal condition.

For example: As a result of poliomyelitis, the patient might be left with paraplegia. In this case, the paraplegia (residual) is coded first, followed by the poliomyelitis (cause).

And—when the word "and" appears in the Tabular List, it is read as and/or. In other words, within a category (three digits), there are separate subcategories (fourth digit).

For example: Consider the code Category 681 Cellulitis and abscess of finger **and** toe. Subcategory 681.0 refers to cellulitis and abscess of **finger,** and subcategory 681.1

refers to cellulitis and abscess of **toe.** Although the category code groups the finger and toe together, the subcategory codes separately describe the finger and toe.

With—When the word "with" is present, the documentation must support both conditions for the code to be selected.

For example: To select the code *closed fracture of shaft of fibula* **with** *tibia* both the fibula and tibia would have closed fractures.

How to Locate and Assign Diagnosis Codes

Now that we know how the manual is organized and what each coding convention identifies, let's review how to look up the codes. Looking up a diagnosis code is the same as following a roadmap: you need to know your starting point (key word, condition), you need to follow the signs along the way (coding conventions), and you need to know where you want to end up (diagnosis code). Follow these steps, and you will always end up at the correct "destination."

1. Identify the reason for the visit, the sign or symptom or diagnosis to be coded. Remember, if you look up codes by the anatomical site or by descriptive adjectives, you will be directed to "see condition."

2. Locate the main entry term (key word) in the Alphabetical Index. You will always begin your search by first looking up the code in the Alphabetical Index (Volume 2) and then referencing back to the Tabular List (Volume 1) to make the code selection.

3. Read and interpret any instructional notes listed with the main term.

4. Review any modifiers. Remember, nonessential modifiers are in parentheses and do not affect your code selection.

5. Review and interpret abbreviations, cross references, symbols, and brackets.

6. Choose a code and look it up in the Tabular List for more specific coding information. Remember: **Never** select the code from the Alphabetical Index. The Tabular List will contain more information and conventions necessary for you to make the correct code assignment.

7. Once you are in the Tabular List, look to see if the code requires additional digits, and read all the *includes, excludes,* and additional notes and conventions before selecting the code.

Special Coding Scenarios

Although this is a review manual, a few more special coding scenarios are worth mentioning. Let's take a look.

The hypertension table is divided into three columns: "malignant," "benign," and "unspecified." Malignant hypertension runs a rapid course and, if untreated, can quickly cause organ damage. The term *accelerated* refers to malignant hypertension. *Benign hypertension* is high blood pressure that is not causing any problems. It is important to understand that a diagnosis of elevated blood pressure is not hypertension. For this reason, elevated blood pressure reading without a diagnosis of hypertension (796.2) is coded from the Signs and Symptoms chapter of the ICD-9-CM. Perhaps you or someone you know has been diagnosed with "White Coat Hypertension." This peculiar term simply refers to a patient's temporary rise in blood pressure in the doctor's office (patients are sometimes nervous when they see the "white coat"/doctor), and therefore should not be coded as hypertension.

Remember when using this table to watch for the words "due to" and "with" as you make your code selection.

Table of Drugs and Chemicals

The Table of Drugs and Chemicals contains an extensive list of drugs, industrial solvents, corrosive gases, noxious plants, pesticides and other toxic agents. This Table of Drugs and Chemicals is also divided into columns. The first column is used to code the substance involved in the poisoning. The next five columns are grouped under the heading "External Cause (E Code)" and identifies the circumstances under which the poisoning occurred.

E codes in the five columns are described:

Accidental poisoning codes (E850–E858)

–Accidental ingestion of drug

–Incorrect use in medical/surgical procedures

–Incorrect administration or ingestion of the drug

–Accidental overdose

Therapeutic uses codes (E930–E949)

–Adverse effect or reaction to a drug that was properly administered, either therapeutically or for prophylactic purposes

Suicide attempt codes (E950–E959)

–Effects of substances or drugs that were taken in an attempt to commit suicide or to inflict self-injury

Assault codes (E960–E969)

–Drugs or substances used in a crime of violence against another person with intent to cause injury or death

Undetermined codes (E980–E982)

Hypertension Table

Index to Diseases

Hypertension, hypertensive	Malignant	Benign	Unspecified
Hypertension, hypertensive (arterial) (arteriolar) (crisis) (degeneration) (disease) (essential) (fluctuating) (idiopathic) (intermittent) (labile) (low renin) (orthostatic) (paroxysmal) (primary) (systemic) (uncontrolled) (vascular)	401.0	401.1	401.9
with chronic kidney disease			
stage I through stage IV, or unspecified ●	403.00	403.10	403.90
stage V or end stage renal disease ●	403.01	403.11	403.91
heart involvement (conditions classifiable to 429.0–429.3, 429.8, 429.9 due to hypertension) (see also Hypertension, heart)	402.00	402.10	402.90
with kidney involvement — see Hypertension, cardiorenal			
renal involvement (only conditions classifiable to 585, 586, 587) (excludes conditions classifiable to 584) (see also Hypertension, kidney)	403.00	403.10	403.90
with heart failure — see Hypertension, cardiorenal	403.01	403.11	403.91
failure (and sclerosis) (see also Hypertension, kidney)	403.00	403.10	403.90
sclerosis without failure (see also Hypertension, kidney)	401.0	—	—
accelerated (see also Hypertension, by type, malignant)			
antepartum — see Hypertension, complicating pregnancy, childbirth, or the puerperium			
cardiorenal (disease)	404.00	404.10	404.90

Hypertension, hypertensive	Malignant	Benign	Unspecified
Hypertension, hypertensive — *continued*			
due to — *continued*			
renal (artery)			
aneurysm	405.01	405.11	405.91
anomaly	405.01	405.11	405.91
embolism	405.01	405.11	405.91
fibromuscular hyperplasia	405.01	405.11	405.91
occlusion	405.01	405.11	405.91
stenosis	405.01	405.11	405.91
thrombosis	405.01	405.11	405.91
encephalopathy	437.2	437.2	437.2
gestational (transient) NEC	—	—	642.3 ⊠
Goldblatt's	440.1	440.1	440.1
heart (disease) (conditions classifiable to 429.0–429.3, 429.8, 429.9 due to hypertension)	402.00	402.10	402.90
with heart failure	402.01	402.11	402.91
hypertensive kidney disease (conditions classifiable to 403) (see also Hypertension, cardiorenal)	404.00	404.10	404.90
renal sclerosis (see also Hypertension, cardiorenal)	404.00	404.10	404.90
intracranial, benign	—	348.2	—
intraocular	—	—	365.04
kidney	403.00	403.10	403.90

Republished with permission from *International Classification of Diseases, 9th Revision, Clinical Modification (ICD-9-CM) Expert for Physicians.* Eden Prairie, MN: Ingenix, p. 154.

Table of Drugs and Chemicals

Anorexic agents

	Poisoning	Accident	Therapeutic Use	Suicide Attempt	Assault	Undetermined
			External Cause (E-Code)			
Alkalinizing agents (medicinal)	963.3	E858.1	E933.3	E950.4	E962.0	E980.4
Alkalis, caustic	983.2	E864.2	—	E950.7	E962.1	E980.6
Alkalizing agents (medicinal)	963.3	E858.1	E933.3	E950.4	E962.0	E980.4
Alka-seltzer	965.1	E850.3	E935.3	E950.0	E962.0	E980.0
Alkavervir	972.6	E858.3	E942.6	E950.4	E962.0	E980.4
Allegron	969.0	E854.0	E939.0	E950.3	E962.0	E980.3
Alleve — Naproxen						
Allobarbital, allobarbitone	967.0	E851	E937.0	E950.1	E962.0	E980.1
Allopurinol	974.7	E858.5	E944.7	E950.4	E962.0	E980.4
Allylestrenol	962.2	E858.0	E932.2	E950.4	E962.0	E980.4
Allylisopropylacetylurea	967.8	E852.8	E937.8	E950.2	E962.0	E980.2
Allylisopropylmalonylurea	967.0	E851	E937.0	E950.1	E962.0	E980.1
Allyltribromide	967.3	E852.2	E937.3	E950.2	E962.0	E980.2
Aloe, aloes, aloin	973.1	E858.4	E943.1	E950.4	E962.0	E980.4
Alosetron	973.8	E858.4	E943.8	E950.4	E962.0	E980.4
Aloxidone	966.0	E855.0	E936.0	E950.4	E962.0	E980.4
Aloxiprin	965.1	E850.3	E935.3	E950.0	E962.0	E980.0
Alpha amylase	963.4	E858.1	E933.4	E950.4	E962.0	E980.4
Alphaprodine (hydrochloride)	965.09	E850.2	E935.2	E950.0	E962.0	E980.0

	Poisoning	Accident	Therapeutic Use	Suicide Attempt	Assault	Undetermined
			External Cause (E-Code)			
Ammoniated mercury	976.0	E858.7	E946.0	E950.4	E962.0	E980.4
Ammonium						
carbonate	963.2	E864.2	—	E950.7	E962.1	E980.6
chloride (acidifying agent)	963.2	E858.1	E933.2	E950.4	E962.0	E980.4
expectorant	975.5	E858.6	E945.5	E950.4	E962.0	E980.4
compounds (household) NEC	983.2	E861.4	—	E950.7	E962.1	E980.6
fumes (any usage)	987.8	E869.8	—	E952.8	E962.2	E982.8
industrial	983.2	E864.2	—	E950.7	E962.1	E980.6
ichthyosulfonate	976.4	E858.7	E946.4	E950.4	E962.0	E980.4
mandelate	961.9	E857	E931.9	E950.4	E962.0	E980.4
Amobarbital	967.0	E851	E937.0	E950.1	E962.0	E980.1
Amodiaquin(e)	961.4	E857	E931.4	E950.4	E962.0	E980.4
Amopyroquin(e)	961.4	E857	E931.4	E950.4	E962.0	E980.4
Amphenidone	969.5	E853.8	E939.5	E950.3	E962.0	E980.3
Amphetamine	969.7	E854.2	E939.7	E950.3	E962.0	E980.3
Amphomycin	960.8	E856	E930.8	E950.4	E962.0	E980.4
Amphotericin B	960.1	E856	E930.1	E950.4	E962.0	E980.4
topical	976.0	E858.7	E946.0	E950.4	E962.0	E980.4
Ampicillin	960.0	E856	E930.0	E950.4	E962.0	E980.4
Amprotropine	971.1	E855.4	E941.1	E950.4	E962.0	E980.4
Amygdalin	977.8	E858.8	E947.8	E950.4	E962.0	E980.4
Amyl						

Republished with permission from *International Classification of Diseases, 9th Revision, Clinical Modification (ICD-9-CM) Expert for Physicians*. Eden Prairie, MN: Ingenix, p. 313.

–Cause of poisoning or injury is undetermined to be intentional or accidental.

When coding poisoning or a reaction to improper use of medication, ***three codes are used:***

■ The first code indicates the **poisoning** (poisoning column).

■ The second code identifies the **manifestation (e.g., coma).**

■ The third code indicates **how the poison occurred** (E code).

For example: A patient received trimethobenzamide (Tigan) capsules for nausea and vomiting. At home, she misread the dosing requirements and accidently took an overdose of medication. Her husband came home, found his wife unconscious, and rushed her to the emergency room.

In this case, the following codes are selected:

963.0 Poisoning trimethobenzamide HCl

780.09 Unconscious
E858.1 Accidental poisoning by systemic agents

The first code identifies the poison (trimethobenzamide HCl), the second code identifies the manifestation or condition (unconscious), and the third code identifies how the poison occurred (by accident).

In cases of an adverse effect (the drug was properly prescribed and administered), we first code the reaction, followed by the appropriate code from category E930–E949 (Drugs, Medicinal and Biological Substances Causing Adverse Effects in Therapeutic Use).

For example: Two-month-old Marissa was vaccinated by the pediatrician for polio. Two hours after receiving the vaccine, Marissa developed a 102°F fever and went into convulsions. She was taken to the hospital emergency room where she was treated and diagnosed as having an adverse effect to the polio vaccine.

In this case, the following codes are selected:

780.39 Other convulsions

E949.5 Poliomyelitis vaccine causing adverse effect in therapeutic use

Neoplasms

The table on page 38 lists neoplasms alphabetically by location and is followed by six columns. The first three columns fall under the main column head "Malignant." The codes in these three columns identify cancerous tumors, which can be located at a primary site (the original site of cancer) or a secondary site (the location where the cancer has metastasized) or may be carcinoma in situ (malignancy that is confined to one site or is noninvasive). The next three columns identify neoplasms as being either *benign*

(noncancerous neoplasms), of *uncertain behavior* (tissues that begin to exhibit neoplastic behavior but cannot yet be categorized as either benign or malignant), or *unspecified* (neoplasms of an unspecified morphology and behavior).

When a neoplasm has spread to, invaded, or extended to a new location, the growth is considered to be secondary to the primary (original) site. When coding these cases, it is important to remember the following:

–Determine both the primary and secondary sites.

–**First code the site requiring patient care.**

–Determine the code for the primary neoplastic site and list it second if it still exists or is being treated.

–When information regarding the primary site is not available, use 199.1 Malignant neoplasm w/o specification of site, other.

If the neoplasm has been removed or is in remission, use the V code for personal history malignant neoplasm (V10–V19). (V codes are discussed in more detail later in this chapter.) If the patient is presenting for postoperative services such as chemotherapy (V58.1X), follow-up examination for radiotherapy (V67.1), or examination following chemotherapy (V67.2), report the preoperative diagnosis as the secondary diagnosis code and the reason for the visit (chemotherapy, etc.) as the primary diagnosis code.

Diagnosis Coding for Burns

ICD-9-CM categories 940–949 are used to code most burns. Two types of burns that are classified elsewhere are sunburns (692.71, 692.76, 692.77) and friction burns (see injury to be specific).

To ensure accurate code selection, the following information is required:

■ Body area(s) involved

■ Depth of the burn (1st, 2nd, 3rd, or 4th degree)

■ If there are multiple burn sites

■ Total body surface area (TBSA) involved if the burns are 2nd or 3rd degree

Keep the following coding categories in mind when selecting a diagnosis code:

940.X—Classifies burns involving the **eye and adnexa**

947.X—Classifies burns of **internal organs,** including burns from chemicals or due to inhaled (ingested) agents

941–945—Code categories grouped according to the site of the burn(s) and requiring fourth- and fifth-digit specificity

When coding from categories 941–946, the fourth digit indicates the severity (depth) of the burn, and the fifth digit provides greater detail concerning the anatomical site of the burns. Complications such as infections, associated injuries, and comorbid conditions (e.g., diabetes, alcoholism) should be coded in addition to the burn code(s) because these conditions may impact or delay the healing process.

The Neoplasm Table

Index to Diseases

	Malignant			Benign	Uncertain Behavior	Unspecified
	Primary	Secondary	Ca in situ			
Neoplasm, neoplastic — continued						
brain — continued						
tapetum	191.8	198.3	—	225.0	237.5	239.6
temporal lobe	191.2	198.3	—	225.0	237.5	239.6
thalamus	191.0	198.3	—	225.0	237.5	239.6
uncus	191.2	198.3	—	225.0	237.5	239.6
ventricle (floor)	191.5	198.3	—	225.0	237.5	239.6
branchial (cleft) (vestiges)	146.8	198.89	230.0	210.6	235.1	239.0
breast (connective tissue) (female) (glandular tissue) (soft parts)	174.9	198.81	233.0	217	238.3	239.3
areola	174.0	198.81	233.0	217	238.3	239.3
male	175.0	198.81	233.0	217	238.3	239.3
axillary tail	174.6	198.81	233.0	217	238.3	239.3
central portion	174.1	198.81	233.0	217	238.3	239.3
contiguous sites	174.8	—	—	—	—	—
ectopic sites	174.8	198.81	233.0	217	238.3	239.3
inner	174.8	198.81	233.0	217	238.3	239.3
lower	174.8	198.81	233.0	217	238.3	239.3
lower-inner quadrant	174.3	198.81	233.0	217	238.3	239.3
lower-outer quadrant	174.5	198.81	233.0	217	238.3	239.3
male	175.9	198.81	233.0	217	238.3	239.3
areola	175.0	198.81	233.0	217	238.3	239.3
ectopic tissue	175.9	198.81	233.0	217	238.3	239.3
nipple	175.0	198.81	233.0	217	238.3	239.3
mastectomy site	174.8	198.81	233.0	217	238.3	239.3

Neoplasm, cervix

	Malignant			Benign	Uncertain Behavior	Unspecified
	Primary	Secondary	Ca in situ			
Neoplasm, neoplastic — continued						
canthus (eye) (inner) (outer)	173.1	198.2	232.1	216.1	238.2	239.2
capillary — *see* Neoplasm, connective tissue						
caput coli	153.4	197.5	230.3	211.3	235.2	239.0
cardia (gastric)	151.0	197.8	230.2	211.1	235.2	239.0
cardiac orifice (stomach)	151.0	197.8	230.2	211.1	235.2	239.0
cardio-esophageal junction	151.0	197.8	230.2	211.1	235.2	239.0
carina (bronchus)	162.2	197.0	231.2	212.3	235.7	239.1
carotid (artery)	171.0	198.89	—	215.0	238.1	239.2
body	194.5	198.89	—	227.5	237.3	239.7
carpus (any bone)	170.5	198.5	—	213.5	238.0	239.2
cartilage (articular) (joint) NEC (*see also* Neoplasm, bone)	170.9	198.5	—	213.9	238.0	239.2
arytenoid	161.3	197.3	231.0	212.1	235.6	239.1
auricular	171.0	198.89	—	215.0	238.1	239.2
bronchi	162.2	197.3	—	212.3	235.7	239.1
connective tissue — *see* Neoplasm, connective tissue						
costal	170.3	198.5	—	213.3	238.0	239.2
cricoid	161.3	197.3	231.0	212.1	235.6	239.1
cuneiform	161.3	197.3	231.0	212.1	235.6	239.1
ear (external)	171.0	198.89	—	215.0	238.1	239.2
ensiform	170.3	198.5	—	213.3	238.0	239.2

Republished with permission from *International Classification of Diseases, 9th Revision, Clinical Modification (ICD-9-CM) Expert for Physicians.* Eden Prairie, MN: Ingenix, p. 205.

When coding multiple burn sites from the *same general area* of the body (same three-digit category) but with different degrees of severity, code only the burn with the highest severity.

For example: A patient suffers from 1st-degree burns on the elbow and shoulder (**943.**12) and also sustains 2nd-degree burns on the shoulder (**943.**25). Because both codes are from the same three-digit category (943), only the most severe burn (in this case, the 2nd-degree burn) is coded.

When coding multiple burn sites from *different general areas* of the body, list the burns separately with the most severe burn listed first. In addition, we must select a code from category 948.XX, which represents the extent of the body surface involved, or the *T*otal *B*ody *S*urface *A*rea (TBSA). The TBSA is calculated by using the Rule of Nines, which allots 9% to each of the following body surfaces (Fig. 3-3):

■ Head (anterior and posterior head and neck) = 9%

■ Each upper extremity (anterior and posterior shoulder, arm, forearm, and hand) = 18%

■ Front and back halves of each lower extremity (anterior and posterior thigh, leg, and foot) = 36%

■ Front and back of the body torso are 18% each (anterior and posterior trunk) = 36%

■ Genitalia or perineum is 1%

In category 948.XX, the fourth digit signifies the TBSA, while the fifth digit signifies TBSA with third-degree burns only.

V Codes

V codes are generally used in any of the following four instances:

■ A person who is not currently sick utilizes health services for a specific purpose (e.g., to receive a prophylactic vaccination).

■ A person with a known disease or injury, whether current or resolving, presents for treatment of disease/injury (e.g., chemotherapy).

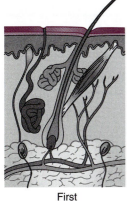 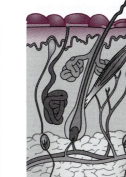 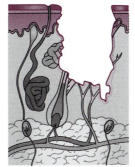 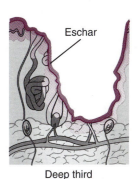

First (redness) Second (blistering) Third (full thickness) Deep third (deep necrosis)

A

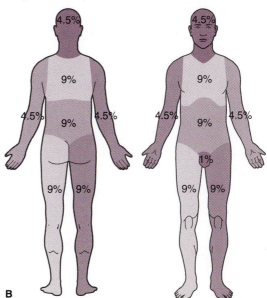

B

Figure 3-3. (A) Degrees of burns. **(B)** Rule of nines estimation of total body surface burned.

■ A circumstance or problem is present that influences a person's health status but is not in itself a current illness or injury (e.g., family history of breast cancer).

■ Birth status of newborns and outcome of delivery are reported.

V codes are divided into three classifications:

1. Problem-oriented (e.g., personal history of exposure to radiation [V15.3]).

2. Service-oriented (e.g., sterilization [V25.2]).

3. Fact-oriented (e.g., alcoholism within the family [V61.41]).

E Codes

E codes permit the classification of environmental events, circumstances, and other conditions as the cause of injury, poisoning, and other adverse effects. These codes are meant to be used in *conjunction* with an additional code from the main chapters of ICD-9-CM indicating the nature of the illness, injury, or condition. E codes are *never* used as *primary diagnosis codes.* E codes are used for statistical purposes, and they can also prevent claim denials by clearly identifying the appropriate payer of service.

For example: If you fractured your wrist by falling off a skateboard (E885.2) in the park (E849.4), your private health insurer would be responsible to pay the claim. If you fractured your wrist as a result of a motor vehicle accident (E816.1), no fault would be the insurer. If you fractured your wrist at work (E849.3) by using a lifting machine (E919.2), workers' compensation would be responsible to pay the claims.

Section 3 of the ICD-9-CM manual includes an alphabetical index to external causes of injury and poisoning. It is organized by main terms that describe the accident, circumstance, event, or specific agent that caused the injury or other adverse effect. Remember, this is an index, and once the code has been located in the index, it should be referenced in the Tabular List to assure accurate coding.

Let's Practice Coding

DIAGNOSTIC STATEMENT: *Left Ventricular aneurysm*

The key word (condition) is "aneurysm." In the **Alphabetical Index,** we look up aneurysm and then the subterm (ventricle); the corresponding code is 414.10. Now let's check for any instructional notes. This entry contains a cross-reference: "*see also* aneurysm, heart." When we look up "aneurysm, heart," we are provided with the same code, 414.10. Now we look up the code in the **Tabular List** to check for any additional notes or conventions. Once there, we can verify the code is at the highest degree of specificity (fifth digit) and accurately describes the diagnostic statement:

414.10 Aneurysm of heart (wall)
Aneurysm (arteriovenous):
mural
ventricular

Let's try another.

DIAGNOSTIC STATEMENT: *Nodular goiter with hyperthyroidism*

In the Alphabetical Index, we look up the key word (condition) "goiter" and then the subterm "nodular, with hyperthyroidism." The corresponding code is 242.3. Once again, the entry contains a cross reference—in this case, "see also Goiter, toxic," which results in the same code, 242.3. We also see the √ symbol, which means that additional digits are required. Now we look up the code in the Tabular List to check for any additional digits, notes, or conventions. We see that, as previously indicated in the Alphabetical Index, an additional fifth digit is required. We therefore look to the shaded box that is applicable to the category (242), which provides fifth digits for that category (Fig. 3-4). Because the diagnostic statement does not mention thyrotoxic crisis or storm, the fifth digit, "0," is the appropriate choice, resulting in a final code of 242.30

Now let's practice diagnosis coding for burns.

An adult patient suffered from 14% 2nd-degree burns on the chest (trunk area) and 15% 3rd-degree burns on the upper arms. In this case, to obtain the fourth digit in category 948, all of the TBSA is calculated:

■ 14% (2nd-degree burns) + 15% (3rd-degree burns) = 29% TBSA.
■ The fourth digit in the 948 category is therefore **"2"** (948.2), which identifies (20%–29% of body surface area

Let's Practice Coding—cont'd

To determine the fifth digit, we must identify the code for 15% of 3rd-degree burns on the arm.

■ The fifth digit is "1" (948.21), which identifies (10%–19% of body surface) with 3rd-degree burns.

This code (948.21) is used in addition to the codes for the burns. To correctly code this scenario, three codes are required:

■ 943.33: 3rd-degree burn of the upper arm.
■ 942.22: 2nd-degree burn of the chest wall.
■ 948.21: (10%–19% of body surface) with 3rd-degree burns.

Let's try another.

DIAGNOSTIC STATEMENT: *Chemotherapy for breast cancer*

In the Alphabetical Index, we look up the key words "encounter for," subterm "chemotherapy"; the corresponding code is V58.11. Now we look up the code in the **Tabular List** to check for any additional notes or conventions. Once there, we can verify the code is at the highest degree of specificity (fifth digit) and accurately describes the diagnostic statement. At first glance, it seems we are finished coding this diagnostic statement, but referencing the **Coding Guidelines** for "aftercare," we are instructed to list the code for the encounter for chemotherapy (V58.11) first, followed by the diagnosis code when a patient's encounter is solely to receive chemotherapy for the treatment of a neoplasm. Therefore, we report two codes: the code for the chemotherapy and the code for the breast cancer.

V58.11 Encounter for antineoplastic chemotherapy

174.9 Malignant neoplasm of breast (female), unspecified site

Let's practice coding for E codes.

DIAGNOSTIC STATEMENT: *Closed fracture of the medial malleolus due to a fall from a ladder while working at a warehouse*

In the Alphabetical Index, we look up the key word "fracture," subterm "malleolus (closed)," and subterm "medial (closed)"; the corresponding code is 824.0. Now we look up the code in the **Tabular List** to check for any additional notes or conventions. Once there, we can verify the code is at the highest degree of specificity (fourth digit) and accurately describes the fracture of the ankle (malleolus) at the correct location (medial). We now are required to code how and where the accident occurred. To correctly identify the appropriate E codes, we use the Alphabetical Index to External Causes of Injury and Poisoning. First we identify how the accident occurred by looking up the key word "fall," subterm "from, off," and subterm "ladder"; the corresponding code is E881.0. Next we identify the place of occurrence by also using the Alphabetical Index to External Causes of Injury and Poisoning. If we use the key words "place of occurrence of accident," we are directed to *see* Accident (to), occurring (at) (in). We then look up the key word "accident," subterm "occurring (at) (in)," and subterm "warehouse"; the corresponding code is E849.3. Now we look up both E codes in the **Tabular List** to check for any additional notes or conventions. Once there, we can verify the codes are at the highest degree of specificity. In this case three codes will be reported:

824.0 Closed fracture of medial malleolus

E881.0 Accidental fall from ladder

E849.3 Place of occurrence, industrial places and premises

Learn More About It

The more you read, the more you know. Increase your knowledge with the following resources.

The introduction of the ICD-9-CM manual includes a complete history of the ICD-9-CM.

The section that we indexed as "Guidelines" is a **must-read** section and a valuable tool to refer to when taking the exam. The guidelines take you through the complete ICD-9-CM, chapter by chapter, and teach you how to code and sequence various types of coding scenarios specific to each chapter.

Recommended Web Sites

CMS Diagnostic Codes for Providers

https://www.cms.gov/ICD9ProviderDiagnosticCodes/

Toxic nodular goiter, unspecified
Adenomatous goiter Nodular goiter Struma nodosa } Toxic or with hyperthyroidism
Any condition classifiable to 241.9 specified as toxic or with hyperthyroidism

The following fifth-digit subclassification is for use with categories 242: **0 without mention of thyrotoxic crisis or storm** **1 with mention of thyrotoxic crisis or storm**

Figure 3-4. Toxic nodular goiter ICD-9-CM code.

Free ICD-9-CM On-Line Look-Up

http://www.icd9data.com/

STOP – LOOK – HIGHLIGHT

If you have not done so already, take the time to insert the tab index dividers into your ICD-9-CM manual. This will enable you to quickly locate the coding conventions, guidelines, tables, and Index to External Causes.

■ On a blank area in the hypertension table, write the following:

- *Elevated blood pressure (796.2) is not coded as hypertension.*
- *Both essential hypertension and idiopathic hypertension are coded from category 401.*
- *Determine if the hypertension is malignant or benign, primary or secondary.*
- *If the hypertension accompanies both heart and renal disease, it is classifiable to category 404.*
- *Hypertension complicating pregnancy is coded from Chapter 11.*
- *Complications of pregnancy, childbirth, and the puerperium are coded from category 642.*
- *Hypertension affecting the fetus or newborn is coded as 760.0.*
- *If the hypertension is due to an underlying condition, look under "due to" or "secondary."*
- *The term* accelerated *means malignant.*

■ In Section 2, the Table of Drugs and Chemicals, write the following:

■ *Three codes are required to code poisoning:*

- *First, code the poison.*
- *Second, code the condition of the patient.*
- *Third, code the cause (E code).*

■ Look up code 948 (burns classified according to extent of body surface involved). At the bottom of the page, write the following:

■ *Coding Tips for Burns*

- *Determine the area involved.*
- *Determine the depth of the burn(s), 1st degree, 2nd degree, etc.*
- *Determine if multiple sites were involved.*
- *Calculate the TBSA (if applicable).*
- *If the burns are from the same three-digit category, code only the burn with the highest degree of severity.*

Vocabulary Words

On the bottom of the pages of the ICD-9-CM Official Conventions, write the following vocabulary words:

Etiology—The study of origination or causation.

Manifestation—An indication or presence of a sign or symptom associated with a disease or illness.

Morbidity—The rate of incidence of a disease

Mortality—The number of deaths in a given population.

Acronyms and Abbreviations

On the bottom of the pages of the ICD-9-CM Official Conventions, write the following abbreviations:

ICD-9-CM—International Classification of Diseases, 9th Revision, Clinical Modification

NEC—Not Elsewhere Classifiable

NOS—Not Otherwise Specified

TBSA—Total Body Surface Area

WHO—World Health Organization

TAKE THE CODING CHALLENGE

Assign the Appropriate Diagnosis Code

1. Hypertrophy of tonsils and adenoids

2. Dysphagia due to cerebrovascular disease

3. Chronic paranoid schizophrenia with acute exacerbation

4. Anemia in end-stage renal disease

5. Cardiac pacemaker status, without complications

Multiple Choice

1. Agranulocytosis is a disease of the
   _____ blood cells.
   a. Red
   b. White
   c. Both red and white
   d. Platelets

2. To properly code for poisoning, three codes are
   required to be sequenced as follows:
   a. The poison, the condition of the patient, the
      cause (E code)
   b. The condition of the patient, the poison, where
      the poisoning occurred (E code)
   c. The condition of the patient, the poison, the
      cause (E code)
   d. The cause (E code), the poison, the condition of
      the patient

3. When coding for multiple burns from different
   three-digit categories, you would:
   a. Code the burns in order of their severity
   b. Code the burns in order of their severity and a
      code from category 948
   c. Code only the burn with the highest degree of
      severity
   d. Code only the burn with the highest degree of
      severity and a code from category 948

4. A diagnosis code that is not otherwise specified
   (NOS) is used when:
   a. The physician lists a diagnosis code for which
      there is no specific code in the ICD-9-CM
   b. The physician did not provide enough informa-
      tion for the coder to select a specific code
   c. The code does not require any additional digits
   d. This code is nonspecific and should not be coded

5. Which of the following coding conventions appears
   in the Alphabetical Index and indicates mandatory
   multiple coding?
   a. Code first underlying disease
   b. Italicized type
   c. Essential modifiers
   d. Slanted brackets

6. Instructional notes appear:
   a. In the Coding Guidelines
   b. Only in the Alphabetical Index
   c. In both the Tabular List and the Alphabetical Index
   d. Only in the Tabular List

7. The patient is an 87-year-old female who fell out
   of bed at home. Upon hearing the noise, her
   daughter found her mother to be unconscious and
   rushed her to the emergency room where she was
   diagnosed with a subdural hematoma. Multiple
   MRIs revealed the hematoma was growing. The
   patient was taken to the operating room to have
   the hematoma evacuated. The correct diagnosis
   code(s) would be:
   a. 852.26, E849.0, E884.4
   b. 432.1, E849.0, E884.4
   c. E849.0, E884.4, 852.26
   d. 852.30, E849.0, E884.4

8. A patient presents to the radiology department
   for an x-ray of the right foot to rule out a fracture. Protocol: AP, lateral, and oblique views of
   the right foot. Findings: There is a mild acquired
   hallux valgus deformity of the first metatarsophalangeal joint space with early degenerative
   changes. The remaining osseous structures are
   intact. No fractures or dislocations are seen.
   There are no soft-tissue calcifications.
   Impression: Mild hallux valgus deformity. Mild
   degenerative changes first MP joint space. The
   correct codes would be:
   a. 735.0, 715.97
   b. 735.0, 715.98
   c. 755.66, 715.97
   d. 755.66, 715.98

9. While working in the kitchen, Diane accidently
   dropped a hot tea kettle and sustained 1st-degree
   burns on her right hand and 2nd-degree burns on
   her left hand. The correct diagnosis code(s) for the
   burns only would be:
   a. 944.20, 948.30
   b. 944.26
   c. 944.20
   d. 944.20, 948.30, E924.2

10. The correct code for an acute duodenal ulcer with
    perforation and bleeding would be:
    a. 532.20
    b. 532.10
    c. 532.31
    d. 532.21

ANSWERS AND RATIONALES

Assign the Appropriate Diagnostic Code

1. The correct answer is **474.10.** The main term (condition) in the Alphabetical Index is *Hypertrophy,* subterm *adenoids,* subterm *and tonsils,* which corresponds to code 474.10, OR *Hypertrophy,* subterm *tonsils,* subterm *and adenoids,* likewise corresponding to 474.10. This code is then confirmed in the Tabular List to be correct.

2. The correct answer is **438.12.** Looking at this diagnostic statement, we notice that the dysphagia is due to cerebrovascular disease and as such is considered a late effect. Therefore, the main term or condition is "Late" in the Alphabetical Index, followed by the subterm *effect,* subterm *cerebrovascular disease,* subterm *with,* and subterm *dysphagia,* which gives us code 438.12. This code is then confirmed in the Tabular List to be correct. Using *dysphagia* as the main term (key word) would have resulted in the incorrect diagnosis code 784.5, dysphagia that does not indicate this is a late effect. 437.9 Unspecified cerebrovascular disease would also be coded as the cause for the dysphagia.

3. The correct answer is **295.34.** In the Alphabetical Index, the main term (condition) is schizophrenia, subterm paranoid (type) (acute) 295.3. When we reference this code in the Tabular List, we can then select the appropriate fifth digit as 4, chronic with acute exacerbation.

4. The correct answer is **285.21.** In the Alphabetical Index, the main term (condition) is anemia, subterm "in," subterm end-stage renal disease, which corresponds to code 285.21. This code is then confirmed in the Tabular List to be correct.

5. The correct answer is **V45.01.** In the Alphabetical Index, the main term is "status (post)," subterm cardiac, subterm device, subterm pacemaker, resulting in V45.01. This code is then confirmed in the Tabular List to be correct.

Multiple Choice Answers

1. The correct answer is **b.** In this case, your ICD-9-CM manual serves as a medical dictionary. In the Alphabetical Index, look up the main term *Agranulocytosis,* which results in 288.09. When we go to confirm the code in the Tabular List, we notice that category 288 is for *diseases of white blood cells;* therefore, answers **a.** and **c.** are incorrect. Answer **d.** is incorrect, as platelets are not considered to be real cells: their main function is to stop the loss of blood from wounds.

2. The correct answer is **a.** The correct sequence is to first code the poison, second code the condition of the patient, and third code the cause—that is, how the poisoning occurred (E code). Answer **b.** is incorrect, as it is not necessary to code *where* the poisoning occurred. Answers **c.** and **d.** list the correct three codes but do not have the correct sequence.

3. The correct answer is **b.** When there are multiple burns from different three-digit categories (different general areas of the body), you sequence the burns in order of their severity and use a code to indicate the TBSA (948 burns classified according to extent of body surface involved). Answer **a.** is incorrect, as it does not include a code from category 948 (TBSA). Answer **c.** is incorrect: you would code only the burn with the highest degree of severity if the burns were from the *same* three-digit category (the same general area of the body). Answer **d.** is incorrect, as this answer states that you would list only one burn. However, you would list one burn only when the burns are in the same general area. When there are multiple burns from *different* three-digit categories, each burn should be listed separately.

4. The correct answer is **b.** A code that is not otherwise specified lacks sufficient documentation by the physician for the coder to select a more specific code. Answer **a.** refers to a code that is not elsewhere classifiable (the physician lists a diagnosis for which there *is* no specific code in the ICD-9-CM). Answer c. is incorrect, as codes that require additional digits are identified by a √ in the Alphabetical Index and with a √ fourth and/or √ fifth digit. Answer **d.** is incorrect, as nonspecific codes *can* be coded.

5. The correct answer is **d.** Slanted brackets appear in the Alphabetical Index and indicate mandatory multiple coding. Answer **a.** is incorrect because although "Code first underlying disease" refers to multiple coding, this is an instructional note that is located in the Tabular List. Answer **b.,** "Italicized type," is used for all exclusion notes and to identify codes that should not be used as primary diagnosis codes. Answer **c.** is incorrect, as essential modifiers change your code selection but do not refer to mandatory multiple coding.

6. The correct answer is **c.** Different instructional notes appear in both the Alphabetical Index and the Tabular List. That is why it is so important to always verify your code selection from the Alphabetical Index against the Tabular List. Answer **a.** is incorrect, as the Coding Guidelines are instructional notes on how to code from each chapter of the ICD-9-CM. Answer **b.** is incorrect, as different instructional notes appear in both the Alphabetical Index and Tabular List. Answer **d.** is incorrect, as different instructional notes appear in both the Alphabetical Index and the Tabular List.

7. The correct answer is **a.** The correct diagnosis codes are 852.26 Subdural hemorrhage following injury, without mention of open intracranial wound, loss of consciousness of unspecified duration; E849.0 Place of occurrence, home; and E884.4 Accidental fall from bed. Answer **b.** is incorrect: although the E codes are correct and 432.1 Subdural hemorrhage describes the condition, it does not include the loss of consciousness or the mention of an injury. Answer **c.** is incorrect, as the E codes were sequenced first; E codes are not primary diagnosis codes. Answer **d.** is incorrect: although the E codes are correct, 852.30 Subdural hemorrhage following injury, *with open intracranial wound,* state of consciousness unspecified, refers to an open wound. The diagnostic statement did not mention an open wound.

8. The correct answer is **a.** The correct diagnosis codes are 735.0 Hallux valgus (acquired) and 715.97 Osteoarthrosis, unspecified whether generalized or localized, ankle and foot. Tip: The osteoarthritis is coded as the impression states: "mild degeneration." Answer **b.** is incorrect, as 715.98 is not specific to the foot (osteoarthrosis, unspecified whether generalized or localized, *other specified sites*). Answers **c.** and **d.** are incorrect, as 755.66 refers to a *congenital* anomaly of toes (hallux valgus), and the diagnostic statement refers to an "acquired" deformity.

9. The correct answer is **c.** When there are multiple burns from the same three-digit category (in this case, 944 for hand), code only the burn with the highest severity. There is no documentation available to code the TBSA. Answer **a.** is incorrect, as there is no documentation available to code the TBSA (948.30 Burn [any degree] involving 30%–39% of body surface with third-degree burn of less than 10% or unspecified amount). Answer **b.** is incorrect, as 944.26 Blisters with epidermal loss due to burn (second degree) of *back of hand* refers specifically to the back of the hand, which was not mentioned in the diagnostic statement. Answer **d.** is incorrect, as the question requires the code only for the burn. This choice includes an E code and also the TBSA, which we were unable to code due to lack of documentation.

10. The correct answer is **a.** The correct diagnosis code is 532.20 Acute duodenal ulcer with hemorrhage and perforation, without mention of obstruction. Answer **b.** is incorrect, as 532.10 Acute duodenal ulcer with perforation, without mention of obstruction, does not include the bleeding (hemorrhage). Answer **c.** is incorrect, as 532.31 Acute duodenal ulcer *without mention of hemorrhage* or perforation, *with obstruction,* includes obstruction, which is not mentioned in the diagnostic statement and does not include the bleeding (hemorrhage). Answer **d.** is incorrect, as 532.21 Acute duodenal ulcer with hemorrhage, perforation, and *obstruction,* includes obstruction, which is not mentioned in the diagnostic statement.

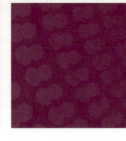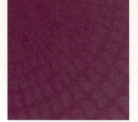

Introduction to ICD-10

Effective October 1, 2013, ICD-9-CM will be replaced with ICD-10-CM. There are many reasons for making this change:

- ICD-9-CM is running out of codes.
- ICD-10-CM codes are much more specific than those in ICD-9-CM.
- ICD-10-CM is currently used by most of the world to report morbidity and mortality statistics.
- ICD-10-CM can more accurately track patients with specific diseases and allow for development of programs for disease management.
- ICD-10-CM provides flexibility for the addition of codes.

ICD-10-CM Volumes 1 and 2 will replace ICD-9-CM Volumes 1 and 2. ICD-9-CM Volume 3 will be replaced by a separate manual called the ICD-10-PCS (Procedural Coding System).

It is important to note that this change affects only the diagnosis coding system and does not affect how we report Current Procedural Terminology (CPT) or Healthcare Common Procedural Coding System (HCPCS) codes.

The format of the ICD-10-CM manual is similar to that of ICD-9-CM; however, chapters have been added to ICD-10-CM, and other chapters have been reorganized. For example: the chapter on the nervous system no longer includes the sense organs. The eye and ear now have their own respective chapters.

ICD-10-CM includes many combination codes, which enable reporting of multiple diagnosis/symptoms with one code.

A notable difference between the ICD-9-CM and ICD-10-CM codes is the number of characters included in the codes. With the exception of V codes and E codes, which are alphanumeric, ICD-9-CM codes are five digits. ICD-10-CM codes are seven-character alphanumeric codes that provide a higher level of specificity than ICD-9-CM codes.

The new codes include laterality and identification of the type of encounter (e.g. initial, subsequent). Let's look at an example:

With ICD-9-CM, the code for acute mucoid otitis media is 381.02. When this code is crosswalked to ICD-10-CM, code selection increases to the following options:

- H65.111: Acute & subacute allergic otitis media right ear
- H65.112: Acute & subacute allergic otitis media left ear
- H65.113: Acute & subacute allergic otitis media bilateral
- H65.114: Acute & subacute allergic otitis media recurrent right ear
- H65.115: Acute & subacute allergic otitis media recurrent left ear
- H65.116: Acute & subacute allergic otitis media recurrent bilateral
- H65.117: Acute & subacute allergic otitis media recurrent unspecified ear
- H65.119: Acute & subacute allergic otitis media unspecified ear

As you can see, one ICD-9-CM can crosswalk into a number of ICD-10-CM codes. These codes also include laterality (right/left) and whether the illness is recurrent. A number of ICD-10-CM codes will require seven characters. For example: an abrasion of the right forearm, initial encounter, is coded as S50.811A. S50 represents the category (superficial injury of elbow and forearm), the additional digits 81 indicate an abrasion of the forearm, the additional digit 1 indicates the right forearm, and the seventh character A indicates this is the initial encounter.

Whereas the formatting of the codes looks different, the coding guidelines and conventions have remained the same for the most part. The guidelines include some updates and additional guidelines for the new chapters in ICD-10-CM.

A notable change regarding the coding conventions is the Excludes notes. ICD-10-CM includes two Excludes notes. Excludes 1 refers to "not coded here" and represents two conditions that cannot be reported together. Excludes 2 notes are not considered inclusive to a code; however, a patient may have both conditions at the same time and, if present, it is acceptable to report both the code and the excluded code together.

The transition to ICD-10-CM will affect many aspects of the physician/facility practice. One of the greatest challenges lies in the specificity of documentation recorded by the physician/provider in the patient's medical record. Without this level of specificity, the selection of an ICD-10-CM code required for the reporting of services may not be possible.

During this transition period, it is recommended that you learn more about the new coding system and what is required to move from ICD-9-CM to ICD-10-CM. There are many resources available to assist you.

Learn More About It

ICD10 Implementation

https://www.cms.gov/ICD10/

The Complete Official Draft Code Set

Ingenix

ISBN 978-1-60151-400-4

ICD-10-CM Mappings

Ingenix

ISBN 978-1-60151-475-2

Contexo/Media

Advanced Anatomy and Physiology for ICD-10-CM/PCD

ISBN: 978-1-58383-690-3

4

ICD-9-CM: Chapter-Specific Coding

Because this is a review book, we cover some of the more common diseases and illnesses and how to code them from each chapter of the ICD-9-CM Manual.

As discussed in Chapter 3, the ICD-9-CM includes a section called "Coding Guidelines." These guidelines are based on the coding and sequencing instructions in Volumes 1 and 2 and provide additional instructions on how to code for various illnesses and diseases on a chapter-by-chapter basis. The *Coding Guidelines* are a *must-read* for any coder.

Chapter 1, Infectious and Parasitic Diseases (001–139)

This chapter *includes* communicable and transmissible diseases (e.g., hepatitis, chickenpox) along with a few diseases of unknown but possibly infectious origin. It does *not* include certain *localized* infections. Localized infections are coded elsewhere—for example, influenza is coded from the respiratory section.

Intestinal Infectious Diseases
001–009

Intestinal Infectious Diseases are the first listed diseases. Because they affect the entire body, their codes are listed in this chapter and not the digestive system chapter. They include salmonella infections and food poisoning.

Category 009 includes infectious colitis, enteritis, gastroenteritis, and diarrhea. These same conditions are also listed in the digestive system chapter. The difference between the two is the word "infectious." The documentation must state "infectious" to code from this chapter.

Tuberculosis
010–018

Tuberculosis is an infectious bacterial disease that is transmitted through the air. It is caused by a bacterial infection that usually affects the lungs. The tuberculosis codes 010–018 require a fifth digit to identify how the tuberculosis was confirmed. Let's take a look:

011.1**3** Tuberculosis of lung, nodular, tubercle bacilli found (in sputum) *by microscopy*

The fifth digit *3* demonstrates tubercle bacilli found (in sputum) by microscopy.

011.3**5** Tuberculosis of bronchus, tubercle bacilli *not found by bacteriological examination, but tuberculosis confirmed histologically*

The fifth digit *5* demonstrates tubercle bacilli not found by bacteriological examination, but tuberculosis confirmed histologically.

In both cases, the codes identify how the tuberculosis was confirmed. When the method of confirmation is not documented, the fifth digit is "0 unspecified."

Zoonotic Bacterial Diseases

020–027

Zoonotic bacterial diseases, which are transmitted through animals, are also listed in Chapter 1. Interestingly, anthrax falls into this category. Anthrax is an infectious bacterial disease caused by the spore-forming bacterium *Bacillus anthracis*. It can occur in three forms: cutaneous (skin), inhalation, and gastrointestinal. It is usually transmitted by contact with infected animals or their discharge. All anthrax codes require a fourth digit to identify the route of introduction into the body.

Human Immunodeficiency Virus

The human immunodeficiency virus (HIV) attacks the body's immune system. When coding for this condition, there is much to consider before selecting the ICD-9-CM code.

First, only confirmed cases are coded. Documentation by the provider indicating a positive serology or culture for HIV or that the patient has an HIV-related illness would support confirmation.

For *patients who test positive for HIV* and *do not display any symptoms of the illness,* the code is *V08* Asymptomatic human immunodeficiency virus (HIV) infection status. As described in Chapter 18, one of the four instances in which V codes are assigned is when a person who is not currently sick utilizes health services for a specific purpose.

For *patients who are treated for any HIV-related illness* or *have been treated for any HIV-related illness* in the past, the code is *042* Human immunodeficiency virus (HIV). This code is listed in Chapter 1 of the ICD-9-CM book because HIV is an infectious disease.

Once a patient has developed an HIV-related illness, ICD-9-CM code 042 is always assigned thereafter.

For *patients with inconclusive HIV serology* (no definitive diagnosis), the code is *795.71* Nonspecific serologic evidence of human immunodeficiency virus (HIV). In this case, the code is selected from Chapter 16 of the ICD-9-CM book.

For *patients presenting for* an HIV test *(screening),* the code is V73.89 Special screening examination for other specified viral diseases. In this case, ICD-9-CM codes V69.8 Other problems related to lifestyle and V65.44 Human immunodeficiency virus (HIV) counseling may also be used in conjunction with the screening code (V73.89) if applicable.

Now that we know how to code the various stages of HIV, let's take a look at the sequencing.

■ If a patient is admitted for an HIV-related condition, the code 042 is used for the principal diagnosis, followed by diagnosis codes for any additional HIV-related conditions.

■ If a patient who has HIV (displays symptoms and illness associated with AIDS) is admitted for an

unrelated condition (e.g., injury), the diagnosis code for the *injury* is used for the principal diagnosis, followed by 042 and any additional HIV-related conditions.

Let's Try One Together

A known AIDS patient presented for treatment of pneumocystosis.

Following the guidelines, we know we must **first report the confirmed case of HIV infection** (042) supported by the documentation of "known AIDS." We then report the AIDS-related illness pneumocystosis (136.3).

Had a known AIDS patient presented for a fractured wrist, the fracture code would have been reported first, followed by the AIDS code (042).

Because there are a number of AIDS-related illnesses, it is a good idea to do a little research and create a list to reference when coding from this category. (Please remember you may not staple, tape, laminate, or keep sticky notes in your book when taking the exam.)

Chapter 2, Neoplasms (140–239)

Neoplasms are coded according to the Neoplasm Table provided in Chapter 2 of the ICD-9-CM book. Information on how to code for neoplasms is discussed in this book in Chapter 3.

Chapter 3, Endocrine, Nutritional and Metabolic Diseases, and Immunity Disorders (240–279)

KEY CODING TIP

For any condition or illness specific to the fetus and newborn, you will code from Chapters 14 and 15. For conditions relating to pregnancy, childbirth, and the puerperium, you will code from Chapter 11.

Diabetes

One of the most common and challenging illnesses to code is diabetes, the codes for which are listed under category 250.

When we look up category 250, we first see the Excludes note. Listed under the chapter heading is the *Excludes note,* which lets us know that endocrine and metabolic disturbances specific to the fetus and newborn are coded elsewhere. You are directed to codes 775.0–775.9 located in Chapter 15.

For example: Neonatal diabetes mellitus is an endocrine condition. Because the condition affects a neonate, it is coded as 775.1 and not from the endocrine chapter.

It is important to note that gestational diabetes (648.8X; a type of diabetes that occurs in some pregnant women and usually goes away after the pregnancy), hyperglycemia (790.29; elevated blood sugar), neonatal diabetes mellitus (775.1), nonclinical diabetes (790.29), and secondary diabetes (249.0–249.9) *are coded elsewhere.*

Fifth-digit subclassifications are required for all codes under category 250. The subclassifications are listed by Type (type I or type II) or as being controlled or uncontrolled, and as unspecified type or juvenile type. The term juvenile does not refer to the age of the patient. Most people with type I diabetes develop the condition before puberty; therefore, type I diabetes mellitus is also called juvenile diabetes.

If the specific type of diabetes mellitus (type I, type II) is not documented, type II is used as the default.

Additionally, in the subclassification for 250, we notice under type II diabetes:

■ We can use the additional digits 0 or 2 even if the patient requires insulin (typically, type I diabetes requires insulin).

■ We would use the additional code V58.67 for any associated long-term (current) use of insulin.

When associated conditions are documented, the code from category 250 should be sequenced first. You will find the corresponding secondary codes listed under each of the diabetes codes.

Let's Try One Together

Diagnostic Statement: Diabetes mellitus, juvenile onset with proliferative retinopathy

In the Alphabetical Index, we look up the main term **diabetes,** subterm **retinopathy.** This takes us to 250.5X *[362.01].* Then, according to the Tabular List, we assign the fifth-digit "1" to represent juvenile type not stated as uncontrolled. Additionally, listed beneath the code is the guidance to "Use additional code to identify manifestation as: diabetic: retinopathy (362.01–362.07)." We then look up the code selection in the code range presented and select 362.02, which represents proliferative diabetic retinopathy. Following the sequencing rule, we code as follows:

250.51 Diabetes with ophthalmic manifestations, type I [juvenile type], not stated as uncontrolled
362.02 Proliferative diabetic retinopathy

For insulin pump malfunctions, the following codes should be reported:

■ For an underdose of insulin due to mechanical pump failure, report 996.57 Mechanical complication due to insulin pump.

■ For an overdose of insulin due to a mechanical pump failure, report 996.57 Mechanical complication due to insulin pump *followed by* 962.3 Poisoning by insulins and antidiabetic agents.

Chapter 4, Diseases of the Blood and Blood-Forming Organs (280–289)

Included in this chapter are diseases of the blood (e.g., anemias, diseases of the white blood cells, purpura) and blood-forming organs, which include the bone marrow and spleen. Neoplastic blood disorders are located in Chapter 2.

Once again, we see that the chapter begins with an Excludes note reminding us that anemia complicating pregnancy or the puerperium is coded elsewhere with code 648.2.

Anemia

One of the major disorders of the blood, anemia, is coded from this chapter. With anemia, the capacity of the blood to transport oxygen to the tissues is reduced because of too little hemoglobin (the iron-containing substance in the red blood cells) or too few red blood cells.

In category 280 are codes for iron deficiency anemia, which can be caused by blood loss (280.0) or inadequate dietary iron intake (280.1).

Some anemias are hereditary. An area of confusion is sickle cell trait (282.5) and sickle cell anemia (282.6X). At first glance, these terms appear to describe the same conditions; however, they have very different meanings. With sickle cell anemia, the defective gene is inherited from both parents, whereas in sickle cell trait, the defective gene is inherited from only one parent. Another type of anemia is acute posthemorrhagic anemia (285.1), which is anemia due to *acute* blood loss. Care must be taken to read the Excludes note, which states that anemia due to *chronic* blood loss and blood loss anemia *NOS* are both coded with 280.0.

When we look up anemia in the Alphabetical Index, followed by the words "due to" and then "blood loss," we see that the word acute is an essential modifier, which leads us to code 285.1. Therefore, if the word acute is not used in the diagnostic statement, we would select 280.0 to report anemia due to blood loss.

Let's Try One Together

Diagnostic Statement: Iron deficiency anemia secondary to chronic blood loss

In the Alphabetical Index, we look up the main term **anemia** followed by **due to** and then **blood loss chronic.** This takes us to the correct code, 280.0 Iron deficiency anemia secondary to blood loss (chronic).
However, if we did not sequence our lookup order correctly, we would end up with a different code.

For example: If we were to look up the main term **anemia** followed by **deficiency** and then **iron,** we would be directed to 280.9 Unspecified iron deficiency anemia, which does not specifically define the iron deficiency anemia as being secondary to chronic blood loss.

This is an excellent example of the importance of confirming codes by looking them up in the Tabular List of the manual before making a code selection. Doing so verifies the code selection and specifically identifies the diagnosis, illness, or disease.

Chapter 5, Mental Disorders (290–319)

Although the ICD-9-CM includes a separate chapter for mental disorders, many behavioral health specialists utilize the DSM *(Diagnostic and Statistical Manual of Mental Disorders)* to code the diagnosis. The DSM is published by the American Psychiatric Association. The main difference between the ICD-9-CM and the DSM is that the DSM lists the diagnosis codes already coded out to the highest degree of specificity.

The ICD-9-CM chapter on mental disorders includes Psychoses, Neurotic Disorders, Personality Disorders and Other Nonpsychotic Mental Disorders, and Mental Retardation.

Psychoses
290–299

A psychosis is a severe mental disorder involving a highly distorted sense of reality or loss of the sense of reality.

For example: Schizophrenic Disorders (295) are characterized by abnormalities in perception and thought processes (hallucinations and delusions). The fourth digit describes the "type" of schizophrenia (e.g., disorganized, paranoid), and the fifth digit defines the period of time the patient experiences the symptoms (e.g., chronic, in remission).

Alcoholic Psychoses require careful thought when coding. Category 305 includes *"alcohol abuse,"* and

category 303 includes *"alcoholic intoxication,"* neither of which is a psychosis. To be considered a psychosis, specific symptoms such as delirium and withdrawal would be involved. The Excludes note directs you to category 303.0–303.9 for alcoholism without psychosis.

Organic Brain Syndromes
290–294

Organic brain syndrome describes a mental abnormality that has occurred as a result of physical damage to the brain tissue. Damage may be caused by disease, injury, or trauma, inherited physiology, chemical or hormonal abnormalities, or abnormal changes associated with the aging process.

For example: Both cerebrovascular disease, such as a stroke, and Alzheimer's disease, a neurodegenerative disease, are examples of organic brain syndrome, as both cause impairment to the brain.

Let's Try One Together

Diagnostic Statement: Multi-infarct dementia with depression

In this case, the depression is a mental illness that follows cerebral infarctions. In Volume 2, the main term is "dementia, multi-infarct (cerebrovascular)." We are instructed to "(see also Dementia, arteriosclerotic) 290.40." Staying in Volume 2, we look up the main term "dementia" and subterms "arteriosclerotic," "with," and then "depressed type." This takes us to 290.43 Vascular dementia, with depressed mood. When we confirm this code in Volume 1, we are instructed to "*use additional code to identify cerebral atherosclerosis* (437.0)." To correctly code this diagnostic statement, we report two ICD-9-CM codes, as follows:
290.43 Vascular dementia, with depressed mood
and
437.0 Cerebral atherosclerosis

Neurotic Disorders, Personality Disorders, and Other Nonpsychotic Mental Disorders
300–316

These comprise a functional mental disorder, less severe than psychosis, exhibited by anxiety or fear (e.g., anxiety, stress).

Personality Disorders are listed in the neurosis section under category 301. The best way to look up a personality disorder is to use the noun as the main term by first looking up "disorder" followed by "personality" and the specific manifestation.

For example: To look up Paranoid Personality Disorder, we use the main term "disorder" to begin the search in Volume 2. We next look up "personality" *(under which is a list of the various personality disorders)* and next look up "paranoid"; this takes us to 301.0 Paranoid personality disorder.

With psychogenic origins, the mental illness caused the physical symptoms or condition. Psychogenic origins are listed in category 306 if the condition does not include tissue damage (e.g., psychogenic paralysis) and in category 316 when the condition involves tissue damage (e.g., ulcers).

Let's Try One Together

Diagnostic Statement: Psychogenic torticollis

In Volume 2, we look up the main term "torticollis." We see that the condition may be classified either as a medical condition (congenital, spastic) or as psychogenic in origin. The subterm "psychogenic" leads us to the code assignment 306.0 Musculoskeletal malfunction arising from mental factors. We then confirm in Volume 1 that this is the correct code.

Mental Retardation

317–319

In this category, the level or degree of retardation determines the code. The level or degree of retardation is determined by the patient's IQ.

For example: An IQ of 20–34 is considered to be severe mental retardation, coded to 318.1. The IQ range is listed under each ICD-9-CM code in Volume 1.

Chapter 6, Diseases of the Nervous System and Sense Organs (320–389)

This chapter includes diseases of the central nervous system (CNS), the peripheral nervous system (PNS), and the eye and ear.

Bacterial Meningitis (320)

One of the common conditions located in this chapter is bacterial meningitis (category 320), which is a bacterial infection causing an inflammation of the membrane that covers the brain and spinal cord. Symptoms include headache, stiff neck, fever, and nausea.

The fourth digit identifies the type of bacteria; therefore, it is not necessary to double code with a code from category 041 (bacterial infection in conditions classified elsewhere and of unspecified site). In many cases, the meningitis is a complication of an underlying disease (e.g., typhoid fever, whooping cough). If this is the case, we follow the instructional note *"code first underlying disease"* and list the underlying condition first, followed by the meningitis.

For example: In Volume 1, we look up 320.7 Meningitis in other bacterial diseases. We are instructed to code first underlying disease. Then, a list of diseases along with either the ICD-9-CM code or the code range is provided. If the underlying condition was documented as typhoid fever, we would code the typhoid fever first, followed by the meningitis, as follows: 002.0 Typhoid fever and 320.7 Meningitis in other bacterial diseases classified elsewhere.

An Excludes note is also listed under 320.7 as a reminder that in some cases the meningitis will be coded as a complication in the infectious disease chapter. For example, meningococcal meningitis is coded as 036.0.

Epilepsy (345)

Epilepsy is a disorder of the CNS involving loss of consciousness and convulsions. One of the determining factors in selecting the correct code is whether the seizure was a petit mal seizure (minor seizure of a brief nature with possible short impairment of consciousness) or grand mal seizure (major seizure causing a loss of consciousness, followed by tonic [twitching] and clonic [relaxing] muscle contractions). The fifth digit (used only with certain fourth digits) in this category identifies whether intractable (difficult to manage) epilepsy is mentioned in the diagnosis.

Diseases of the Sense Organs

The ICD-9-CM book does not specify whether the disease of the organ of sense is in the right eye (OD), left eye (OS), right ear (AD), or left ear (AS). It does specify, however, whether the condition is monocular (one side) or unilateral; for example, 378.01 Monocular esotropia.

In category 369, blindness and low vision, the coder must describe the status of each eye (the better eye and the lesser eye).

For example: Code 369.0 identifies "profound vision impairment, both eyes," whereas adding the fifth digit "2" identifies the status of each eye: 369.02 Better eye: near-total vision impairment; lesser eye: not further specified.

The ICD-9-CM manual includes a table called Levels of Visual Impairment. It uses a number of visual acuity tests to assist in the determination of the level of impairment.

With hearing loss (389), the coder must determine if the cause was sensorineural (due to nerve damage), conduction (due to problems with the bones in the middle ear), or a combination of both. Subcategory 389.0 identifies conductive hearing loss, subcategory 389.1 identifies sensorineural hearing loss, and subcategory 389.2 identifies a combination of both.

Chapter 7, Diseases of the Circulatory System (390–459)

This chapter includes diseases of the heart and blood vessels. The hypertension table is reviewed in Chapter 3 of this book.

Ischemic heart disease is a condition in which the heart muscle is damaged or works inefficiently due to an obstruction or constriction of blood vessels serving the heart muscle. It is most often caused by atherosclerosis.

In category 410, the fourth digit identifies the site of the infarction (the death of tissue due to the blockage of the tissue's blood supply), and the fifth digit identifies the episode of care. Each episode of care is described in the fifth-digit subclassification box (Fig. 4-1).

If the myocardial infarct is stated as chronic or presenting with symptoms after 8 weeks from the date of infarction, it should be coded as 414.8 Other specified forms of chronic ischemic heart disease.

An old myocardial infarction is coded as 412 and is used when the patient had a myocardial infarct in the past but was unaware of it (it would be identified on an electrocardiogram) or when no symptoms are present. The main term is "infarction," and the subterms are "myocardium" and then "healed or old."

Also located in this chapter is the ICD-9-CM code to identify functional disturbances following cardiac surgery (429.4). This includes conditions such as cardiac insufficiency, pacemaker syndrome, and heart failure. It excludes cardiac failure in the immediate postoperative period (the time period from the surgery to the hospital discharge), which would be coded as 997.1.

Some situations require a full description of the patient's health status because it may affect the treatment of the patient. For example, it is important for a physician to indicate if a patient is the recipient of a heart donor or if there is a pacemaker in place. These "status codes" are located in the V code section, which is discussed in Chapter 3 of this book.

Let's Try One Together

Diagnostic Statement: Acute inferolateral myocardial infarction

In Volume 2, the main term is **infarct,** followed by the subterms **myocardium** and then **inferolateral.** This leads us to code 410.2, which requires an additional digit. Looking up 410.2 in Volume 1, we review our fifth-digit choices. Because the infarct is documented as acute, we assign the fifth digit "1" for the initial episode of care. Therefore, our final code selection is 410.21 Acute myocardial infarction of inferolateral wall, initial episode of care.

Chapter 8, Diseases of the Respiratory System (460–519)

This chapter includes conditions and disorders of the lungs, bronchus, larynx, nasal passages, and pharynx. It is important to read the instructional note at the beginning of this chapter, which states, "Use additional code to identify infectious organism." Carefully read the code descriptions, as some codes already include the organism, and in those cases there is no need to use the additional code.

For example: 482.2 Pneumonia due to Hemophilus influenzae (H. influenzae) does not require an additional code, as

---

The following fifth-digit subclassification is for use with category 410:

0 episode of care unspecified
Use when the source document does not contain sufficient information for the assignment of fifth-digit 1 or 2.
1 initial episode of care
Use fifth-digit 1 to designate the first episode of care (regardless of facility site) for a newly diagnosed myocardial infarction. The fifth-digit 1 is assigned regardless of the number of times a patient may be transferred during the initial episode of care.
2 subsequent episode of care
Use fifth-digit 2 to designate an episode of care following the initial episode when the patient is admitted for further observation, evaluation, or treatment for a myocardial infarction that has received initial treatment, but is still less than 8 weeks old.

Figure 4-1. Fifth-digit codes (subclassification).

the organism identified as *H. influenzae* is included in the code.

Before coding from Chapter 8, let's look at some of the terms frequently used to identify respiratory conditions.

First, it is important to understand the difference between *acute* and *chronic* respiratory disorders. An acute condition has a rapid onset and runs a severe but short course. A chronic condition is a long-lasting and recurrent condition. In some cases, a patient may experience an *acute exacerbation* (worsening or flare-up of the signs and symptoms of a condition). For example, a patient may have an acute exacerbation of *chronic* obstructive pulmonary disease. To code this disorder, we look up the main term "disease" and the subterm "pulmonary, obstructive diffuse (chronic)," then with exacerbation NEC (acute). The resulting code is 491.21 Obstructive chronic bronchitis, with (acute) exacerbation.

If the same condition is documented as being both acute (subacute) and chronic (e.g., acute and chronic sinusitis), and if separate subentries exist in the Alphabetical Index at the same indentation level (essential modifiers), we would code both conditions and list the acute (subacute) condition first. However, if either the acute or chronic condition is listed as an essential modifier, only the condition listed as an essential modifier should be reported.

For example: To determine if a patient with both acute and chronic sinusitis should be coded with one code or two, we first must determine if the words acute and chronic are both essential modifiers or if only one is listed as an essential modifier. When we look up the main term "sinusitis" in Volume 2, we see the following: Sinusitis (accessory) (nasal) (hyperplastic) (non-purulent) (purulent) (**chronic**) 473.9. *We can identify the word "chronic" as a nonessential modifier.* We now look to the subterms "**acute** 461.9," and we can identify the word "acute" as an essential modifier. Therefore, we report only the acute condition as 461.9 Acute sinusitis, unspecified.

Asthma (493)

Asthma is a common condition frequently coded from this chapter. Asthma may be caused by a number of factors (allergies, environment). The fourth digit describes the type of asthma (e.g., intrinsic, chronic obstructive), and the fifth digit describes the status as being either unspecified, with status asthmaticus (severe episode of asthma unresponsive to normal therapy) or with (acute) exacerbation. If the documentation supports both the exacerbation and the status asthmaticus, code only the status asthmaticus.

Let's Try One Together

Diagnostic Statement: Chronic obstructive asthma with status asthmaticus

In Volume 2, we look up the main term **asthma,** subterm **with chronic obstructive pulmonary disease.** This leads us to code 493.2. We note that this code is accompanied by a check mark (i.e., the code requires a fifth digit). Looking up code 493.2 in Volume 1, we review our fifth-digit choices and select **1, with status asthmaticus.** Our final code selection is therefore 493.21.

Chronic Obstructive Pulmonary Disease (COPD) (496)

COPD is a nonspecific code that usually includes asthma, chronic bronchitis, emphysema, or a combination thereof. If one of these *conditions is specifically documented* (e.g., asthma, chronic bronchitis), *code only the specific condition.*

Chapter 9, Diseases of the Digestive System (520–579)

This chapter includes codes for noninfectious enteritis and colitis, diseases of the pancreas, and hernias and ulcers.

Hernia

A hernia is a protrusion of an organ or the muscular wall of an organ through the cavity that normally contains it. Hernias can be located in various sites (e.g., hiatal, inguinal), and they may include obstruction. The terms *incarcerated* (constricted, unable to be returned), *strangulated* (blood supply is cut off), and *irreducible* (unable to be returned) all imply an obstruction. Additionally, a hernia may include gangrene, may be unilateral or bilateral, and may be recurrent. Clearly, there is a good deal to consider before selecting the correct code.

KEY CODING TIP
Before selecting a code for a hernia, you must:
- Identify the site of the hernia.
- Identify if there is an obstruction.
- Identify if there is gangrene.
- Identify if the hernia is unilateral or bilateral.
- Identify if the hernia is recurrent.

Let's Try One Together

Diagnostic Statement: Incarcerated right femoral hernia

The main term in Volume 2 is **hernia,** and the subterm is **femoral,** *with obstruction* (this is selected because the diagnostic statement includes the description of the hernia as "incarcerated"). The result is code 552.00. In Volume 1, we confirm the full code description: 552.00 Unilateral or unspecified femoral hernia with obstruction. This is the correct code because the diagnostic statement is "unspecified" whether the hernia is unilateral, recurrent, or bilateral.

Ulcers

Ulcers are sores or lesions of the lining of the mucous membranes usually caused by infection or inflammation. To properly code ulcers, we must know the site of the ulcer (gastric, jejunum), whether the condition is acute or chronic, and whether there is hemorrhage and/or perforation. Many "combination" codes identify these characteristics. For example:

534.2X Acute gastrojejunal ulcer with hemorrhage and perforation

534.3X Acute gastrojejunal ulcer without mention of hemorrhage or perforation

534.6X Chronic or unspecified gastrojejunal ulcer with hemorrhage and perforation

534.7X Chronic gastrojejunal ulcer without mention of hemorrhage or perforation

Care should be taken to select the code that accurately describes the ulcer and its characteristics.

A peptic ulcer is an unspecified ulcer and should be used only when a more specific code cannot be assigned.

Chapter 10, Diseases of the Genitourinary System (580–629)

Included in this chapter are diseases and conditions of the kidneys, ureters, urethra, urinary bladder, and the male and female genital organs.

Urinary tract infection (UTI), a common condition, is located in this chapter. It is important to note the code for UTI (599.0 Urinary tract infection, site not specified) is a nonspecific code. When possible (based on the documentation by the physician), the infective organism or the site should be identified.

The same is true for endometriosis, a condition in which the tissue that normally lines the uterus grows and functions in other areas of the body. Some of the common sites of endometriosis are the ovaries, fallopian tubes, and broad ligaments. When documented, report the site of the endometriosis and not the unspecified code (617.9).

Chapter 11, Complications of Pregnancy, Childbirth, and the Puerperium (630–679)

This chapter includes complications that occur during pregnancy, delivery, and the puerperium (the 6 weeks following childbirth). The codes in this chapter are to be used on the mother's record. The first page of the chapter shows a *fourth-digit box,* which *includes detailed information regarding the fourth digit* for categories 634–638; it is a valuable reference when coding. Additionally, many of the codes in this chapter require a fifth digit.

For example, in category 634 spontaneous abortion, the fourth digit identifies the complication:

634.0 Spontaneous abortion complicated by genital tract and pelvic infection

634.1 Spontaneous abortion complicated by delayed or excessive hemorrhage

634.2 Spontaneous abortion complicated by damage to pelvic organs or tissues

The fifth digit identifies the stage:

0 = Unspecified

1 = Incomplete

2 = Complete

Therefore, 634.02 identifies a complete spontaneous abortion complicated by genital tract and pelvic infection. The fourth digit "0" identifies the complication by genital tract and pelvic infection, and the fifth-digit "2" indicates it was a complete abortion.

Categories 640–649 identify complications directly related to the pregnancy. These codes are used to capture conditions prior to the pregnancy that are "currently" a complication of the pregnancy.

Let's Try One Together

Diagnostic Statement: Pregnancy complicated by diabetes mellitus

In Volume 2, we look up the main term **pregnancy,** subterm **complicated by,** and the condition **diabetes mellitus.** This leads us to 648.0. We note that this code is accompanied by a check mark indicating that an additional fifth digit is required. Looking up code 648.0 in Volume 1, we review our fifth-digit choices

continued

Let's Try One Together—cont'd

and select **0—unspecified as to episode of care or as not applicable,** as the diagnostic statement does not specify the episode of care. We also notice an instructional note: "Use additional code(s) to identify the condition," in this case the diabetes mellitus (250.00). Therefore, to correctly code this complication, we report:

648.00 Maternal diabetes mellitus, complicating pregnancy, childbirth, or the puerperium, unspecified as to episode of care

250.00 Diabetes mellitus without mention of complication, type II or unspecified type, not stated as uncontrolled

KEY CODING TIP

When coding complications of pregnancy, use the main term "pregnancy," subterm "complicated by," and then the complication.

KEY CODING TIP

Because many of the codes in this chapter require a fifth digit, carefully read the applicable fifth-digit choices by looking at the brackets underneath the diagnosis code, which will include the applicable fifth-digit code options. For example:

634.0
[0–2]

The delivery may be normal, reported with code 650, or may involve multiple gestation, as reported in category 651. Multiple gestation codes are used to report twin and triplet pregnancies as well as pregnancies in which there has been a loss of one or more fetuses with a retention of one or more fetuses.

Malpresentation codes (652) are used to report an abnormal position in the presentation of the fetus (e.g., breech, transverse). This category includes an instructional note to "code first any obstructed labor (660.0)."

Common V Codes Related to Pregnancy, Delivery, and the Puerperium

Outcome of Delivery

The outcome of the delivery is different from the delivery. The outcome of the delivery identifies if the baby was a single liveborn, twins, and so on. The outcome of delivery codes are located in the V27 category and are not found in this chapter.

Sterilization

Another common V code is V25.2 sterilization. In many cases, the mother elects to undergo sterilization during the hospital stay after the delivery.

Supervision of Pregnancy

Regular checkups during the antepartum period when there are no complications or problems are reported with either:

V22.0 Supervision of normal first pregnancy
V22.1 Supervision of other normal pregnancy

Supervision of a high-risk pregnancy is reported with a code from category V23 Supervision of high-risk pregnancy and requires additional digits to identify the reason for the high risk. For example, V23.2 Pregnancy with history of abortion identifies the pregnancy is high risk due to the patient's history of abortion.

Pregnancy as an incidental state (V22.2) is used as an additional code to show the patient is pregnant when being treated for a condition that does not affect the pregnancy, delivery, or puerperium.

There are also three V codes used during the postpartum period when there are no postpartum complications to report:

V24.0 Postpartum care and examination immediately after delivery
V24.1 Postpartum care and examination of lactating mother
V24.2 Routine postpartum follow-up

Chapter 12, Diseases of the Skin and Subcutaneous Tissue (680–709)

Included in this chapter are diseases and conditions of the skin, nails, sweat glands, hair, and hair follicles. This is one of the smaller chapters of the ICD-9-CM Manual.

Dermatitis is a common condition that is frequently coded. Category 692 Contact dermatitis and other eczema identifies substances the patient came in contact with, such as poison ivy and detergents. Category 693 is used when the dermatitis was caused by a substance that was taken internally, such as food and drugs.

Sunburn (692.71) is also included in this chapter and is not included with the more severe burns located in the injury and poisoning chapter.

Chapter 13, Diseases of the Musculoskeletal and Connective Tissue (710–739)

Included in this chapter are deformities; results of old injuries; and degeneration of the joints, muscles, tendons, ligaments, and bones. This chapter also includes some symptoms and residuals. It does *not* include traumatic fractures or injuries related to the musculoskeletal system, which are coded from Chapter 17.

The first page of Chapter 13 includes a fifth-digit box that contains detailed information regarding what is included in each anatomical site (Fig. 4-2).

These fifth digits are used with a number of categories throughout the chapter, but they are only shown in this level of detail on this page. For example, if we look at the box in Figure 4-2, we can identify that the fifth digit "3," fracture of the forearm, refers to the radius, ulna, and wrist joint. However, when we look at the fifth-digit box listed beneath category 711, we see the fifth digit 3 but are not provided with the level of detail given in the box.

Pathological fractures, breaks in the bone in an area weakened by an underlying disease or condition, are commonly caused by conditions such as osteoporosis and bone tumors. When locating the codes for pathological fractures, the main term should be **fracture,** followed by the subterm **pathological** *and then the site*. The key is to use the word **pathological** as the first subterm.

After reporting the code for the pathological fracture, we report the code that identifies the disease process responsible for the fracture.

Pathological fractures fall within the code range 733.1–733.19. These codes are used to *report a newly diagnosed pathological fracture* and are reported *while the patient is actively receiving care for the fracture,*

such as surgical care, emergency care, or evaluation and treatment by a new physician.

After the patient has **completed the active treatment** for the fracture and is being seen for **routine care during the healing or recovery phase,** an aftercare code should be reported—for example, cast change or removal, removal of internal or external fixation device, medication, and follow-up visits. The aftercare codes are V code subcategories: V54.0, V54.2, V54.8, and V54.9.

Let's Try One Together

Diagnostic Statement: Pathological fracture of neck of femur due to osteoporosis

In Volume 2, we look up the main term "fracture," subterm "pathologic, femur (neck)," resulting in 733.14. We confirm the code in the Volume 1. We are not done yet—we also must code the cause of the fracture, which is the osteoporosis. In Volume 2 we look up the main term "osteoporosis," and because we do not have any more specific information on the type of osteoporosis, we select the main term, osteoporosis (generalized) 733.00 and confirm the code selection in Volume 1. The result is:

733.14 Pathologic fracture of neck of femur

733.00 Osteoporosis unspecified

Sometimes fractures fail to heal or do not heal properly. Malunion (733.81) is the incomplete or faulty union of a fracture. Nonunion (733.82) is when the fracture fails to heal. When reporting either of these conditions, a late-effect code should also be reported to show the principal diagnosis is the result of a previous fracture.

Some common deformities reported from this chapter are knock-knees (genu valgum) and bowlegs (genu varus).

736.41 Genu valgum *(acquired)*

736.42 Genu varum *(acquired)*

Notice that the common factor for these two codes is the word "acquired." The deformities included in this chapter are acquired. Congenital deformities are coded from Chapter 14.

Spondylosis is abnormal wear on the cartilage and bones of the spine. The first factor to consider when coding spondylosis is the part of the spine involved: cervical, thoracic, or lumbar. Next we must identify whether myelopathy (spinal cord involvement) is present. In addition to the documentation specifically stating myelopathy, certain conditions such as paralysis and paresis also suggest spinal cord involvement.

The following fifth-digit subclassification is for use with categories 711–712, 715–716, 718–719, and 730:

0 site unspecified	**6 lower leg**
1 shoulder region	Fibula
Acromioclavicular joint(s)	Knee joint
Clavicle	Patella
Glenohumeral joint(s)	Tibia
Scapula	
Sternoclavicular joint(s)	**7 ankle and foot**
	Ankle joint
2 upper arm	Digits (toes)
Elbow joint	Metatarsus
Humerus	Phalanges, foot
	Tarsus
3 forearm	Other joints in foot
Radius	
Ulna	**8 other specified sites**
Wrist joint	Head
	Neck
4 hand	Ribs
Carpus	Skull
Metacarpus	Trunk
Phalanges (fingers)	Vertebral column
5 pelvic region and thigh	**9 multiple sites**
Buttock	
Femur	
Hip (joint)	

Figure 4-2. Fifth-digit codes (subclassification).

Chapter 14, Congenital Anomalies (740–759)

A congenital anomaly is something that is unusual or different at birth: it can be a deformity or an absence of or excess body part. Major abnormalities, such as cleft palate and cleft lip, affect the way a person looks and require medical and/or surgical treatment. A minor defect or abnormality, such as curvature of a toe, does not cause serious health or social problems. In some cases, the abnormality is not always discovered at birth but is identified later in life.

Codes from this chapter may be used throughout the life of the patient. Once a congenital anomaly has been corrected, a personal history code (V code) should be reported.

This is where prefixes come in handy. The prefixes "a-" and "an-" mean absence of, "macro-" means extremely large, "micro-" means extremely small, and "hypo-" means deficient.

It is also important to know some main terms relating to anomalies. "Accessory" refers to additional body parts, "atresia" refers to narrowing, and "ectopic" refers to out of place. Additionally, the main term "anomaly" or "defect" may be used when the code cannot be located under the specific terms.

One of the more common conditions in this chapter is the cleft palate and cleft lip. A cleft is a birth defect that occurs when the tissues of the lip and/or palate of the fetus do not fuse very early in pregnancy. When coding these conditions, we first need to identify if the condition involves cleft palate, cleft lip, or both. Then we must determine if the defect is unilateral or bilateral and whether it is complete or incomplete.

For example: A cleft palate with cleft lip, unilateral, incomplete is coded as 749.22 Unilateral cleft palate with cleft lip, incomplete.

Chapter 15, Certain Conditions Originating in the Perinatal Period (760–779)

The perinatal period is defined as before birth through the 28th day following birth. Codes from this chapter are *never reported on the mother's chart.* These codes are reported in the baby's chart with the exception of 779.9, stillbirth, which may be reported in the mother's chart because stillborns may not have their own chart. You may report a code from this chapter throughout the life of the patient as long as the condition is still present; for example, Erb's palsy (a condition affecting the nerves that control the muscles in the arm and hand).

To code premature birth (765), we must identify the weeks of gestation and the actual birth weight, which is identified by the fifth digit. Post-term births (extending past the 40-week gestation period) are coded with subcategories 766.21 for 40–42 weeks and 766.22 for gestation over the 42 weeks.

Category 760 refers to a maternal condition that caused an illness or death in the fetus. *These codes are to be reported only when the fetus is affected.* For example, an alcoholic mother whose condition affected the fetus is coded as 760.71 Noxious influences affecting fetus or newborn via placenta or breast milk, alcohol.

KEY CODING TIP
Begin looking up these codes in Volume 2 by condition, then look for the subterms "affecting fetus or newborn." *Make sure the code starts with a 700 number* (baby's chart) and not a 600 number, which would be coded in the mother's chart.

All newborns are assigned a V code (V30–V39) as a primary diagnosis code only once at the time of birth to indicate their birth status. Do not confuse this with the outcome of delivery codes (V27), which are reported in the mother's chart.

Chapter 16, Signs, Symptoms, and Ill-Defined Conditions (780–799)

Codes from this chapter are widely used by all physicians and providers of service. It is important to keep in mind that signs and symptoms are reported only when there is no definitive diagnosis.

For example: A patient who was sent for a chest x-ray to rule out pneumonia has a normal x-ray result. Because there is no rule-out diagnosis and the x-ray was normal, we would code the signs and symptoms that prompted the x-ray. In this case, the signs and symptoms of pneumonia, such as cough and fever, are reported.

A sign is any objective evidence of an illness or dysfunction apparent to a physician. A symptom is a change noticeable to the patient that prompts him or her to seek the advice of a physician.

Codes from this chapter may be used as primary diagnosis codes to identify the reason for the visit when no definitive diagnosis has been made. These codes may also be listed to convey additional information regarding the condition of the patient, when applicable.

Signs and symptoms are also located in other chapters of the ICD-9-CM Manual when they refer to a *specific* body system. For example, diarrhea (787.91) can be associated with a number of disorders and is located in the signs and symptoms chapter; however, functional diarrhea (564.5) is located in the digestive system chapter.

A number of diseases and conditions include signs and symptoms. When signs and symptoms are an inherent part of the disease or condition, they are not reported. For example, vomiting and diarrhea are an inherent part of ulcerative colitis. In this case, only the ulcerative colitis is reported.

Also included in this chapter are codes for nonspecific findings. In some cases, an abnormal result of a test is identified and requires further investigation before a definitive diagnosis can be made. Nonspecific findings can be made from blood tests, urinalysis, or radiological tests.

KEY CODING TIP

When looking up codes for nonspecific findings, use either of the main terms "abnormal" or "positive."

Let's Try One Together

Diagnostic Statement: Abnormal mammogram

In Volume 2, the main term is "abnormal," and the subterm is "mammogram." An alternative method of lookup is to use the main term "abnormal" and the subterms "radiologic examination, breast, mammogram." Either method will result in 793.80, which is confirmed in Volume 1.

Chapters 17, 18, and 19

Chapter 17, Injury and Poisoning (800–999); Chapter 18, Classification of Factors Influencing Health Status and Contact with Health Service (Supplemental V01–V91); and Chapter 19, Supplemental Classification of External Causes of Injury and Poisoning (E codes E800–E999) are reviewed in Chapter 3 of this book.

STOP-LOOK-HIGHLIGHT

The key to successfully passing the exam and selecting the correct code lies in your knowing how to use your coding book.

To help you navigate through your codebook and to make sure you have the most important information at your fingertips when you take the exam, highlight key text in the chapter guidelines and subheadings, and insert simple notes and coding tips directly into your codebooks.

When highlighting, use two different color highlighter pens: yellow for standard guidelines and global services and a second color for carve-outs and unique notes.

- In Chapter 1, Infectious and Parasitic Diseases (001–139)
  - Highlight the Includes note immediately after the heading: Includes: diseases generally recognized as communicable or transmissible as well as a few diseases of unknown but possible infectious origin.
  - In category 042 Human immunodeficiency virus (HIV) disease, highlight the Excludes note. Excludes: asymptomatic HIV infection status (V08), Exposure to HIV Virus (V01.79), Nonspecific serologic evidence of HIV (795.71).
- In Chapter 3, Endocrine, Nutritional and Metabolic Diseases, and Immunity Disorders (240–279)
  - Highlight the Excludes note immediately after the heading. Excludes: endocrine and metabolic disturbances specific to the fetus and newborn (775.0–775.9).
  - In category 250 Diabetes mellitus highlight the Excludes note. Excludes: gestational diabetes (648.8), hyperglycemia NOS (790.29), neonatal diabetes mellitus (775.1), nonclinical diabetes (720.29), secondary diabetes (249.0–249.9).
  - In red ink at the bottom of the page for diabetes (250), make a note indicating codes 250.4–250.8 require an additional code to indicate the manifestation.
- In Chapter 4, Diseases of the Blood and Blood-Forming Organs (280–289)
  - Highlight the Excludes note immediately after the heading. Excludes: anemia complicating pregnancy or the puerperium (648.2).
  - Highlight the Excludes note under 285.1 Acute posthemorrhagic anemia. Excludes: anemia due to chronic blood loss (280.0), blood loss anemia NOS (280.0).
- In Chapter 5, Mental Disorders (290–319)
  - In category 290 Dementias, highlight "code first the associated neurological condition."
  - In category 291 Alcohol induced mental disorders, highlight the Excludes note. Excludes: alcoholism without psychoses (303.0–303.9)

- In category 292 Drug-induced mental disorders, highlight "Use additional code for any associated drug dependence (304.0–304.9), Use additional E code to identify drug."

- In category 294.1 Dementia in conditions classified elsewhere, highlight "Code first any underlying physical condition as dementia in."

- In category 295 Schizophrenic disorders, in the fifth-digit box, next to fifth-digit 1 subchronic, write "> *6 months and <2 years"*; next to the fifth-digit 2 chronic, write "> *or = to 2 years"*; and next to the fifth-digit 5 in remission, write *"free of disease 5 years or greater."*

- In category 316 Psychic factors associated with diseases classified elsewhere, highlight underneath "Use additional code to identify the associated physical condition, as:".

- In Chapter 6, Diseases of the Nervous System and Sense Organs (320–389)

  - In category 320.7 Meningitis in other bacterial diseases classified elsewhere, highlight underneath "Code first underlying disease as:".

  - In category 326 Late effects of intracranial abscess or pyogenic infection, highlight "Use additional code to identify condition as: hydrocephalus (331.4), paralysis (342.0–342.9, 344.0–344.9)."

  - In category 342 hemiplegia and hemiparesis, highlight the last two sentences under the note, "The category is also for use in multiple coding to identify these types of hemiplegia resulting from any cause."

  - In category 344 Other paralytic syndromes, highlight the last two sentences under the note, "The category is also for use in multiple coding to identify these conditions resulting from any cause."

- In Chapter 7, Diseases of the Circulatory System (390–459)

  - In category 410 Acute myocardial infarction, in the fifth-digit box under the fifth-digit 2, highlight the last phrase.

  - In category 428 Heart failure, highlight underneath "Code, if applicable, heart failure due to hypertension first (402.0–402.9, with fifth digit 1 or 404.0–404.9 with fifth digit 1 or 3)".

  - In code 429.2 Cardiovascular disease, unspecified, highlight "Use additional code to identify presence of arteriosclerosis."

- In Chapter 8, Diseases of the Respiratory System (460–519)

  - In code 496 Chronic airway obstruction, not elsewhere classified, highlight the note "This code is not to be used with any code from categories 491–493."

  - In code 506 Respiratory conditions due to chemical fumes and vapors, highlight "Use additional E code to identify cause."

- In Chapter 9, Diseases of the Digestive System

  - Write the following key coding tip for hernias:

    - *Identify the site of the hernia.*

    - *Identify if there is an obstruction.*

    - *Identify if there is gangrene.*

    - *Identify if the hernia is unilateral or bilateral.*

    - *Identify if the hernia is recurrent.*

- In Chapter 11, Complications of Pregnancy, Childbirth, and the Puerperium

  - On the first page of the chapter, write *"the outcome of delivery is coded as V27.X."*

  - Under the heading Other Pregnancy with Abortive Outcome (634–639), highlight "The following fourth-digit subdivisions are for use with categories 634–638." Also underline in red the words "fourth-digit."

  - In 634 Spontaneous abortion, in the fifth-digit box next to 1 incomplete, write in the words *"retained placenta."*

  - In code 650 Normal delivery, highlight "Delivery requiring minimal or no assistance, with or without episiotomy, without fetal manipulation" and also highlight the last sentence "Use additional code to indicate outcome of delivery (V27.0)."

  - In code 657 Polyhydramnios, highlight the reminder "Use 0 as a fourth digit for this category."

  - In code 661 Abnormality of forces of labor, write *"Usually used in the labor room."*

  - In code 661.1 Secondary uterine inertia, write *"Usually used in the delivery room."*

  - On the last page of the chapter, you can write in some of the more commonly coded "V" codes reported in the mother's chart:

    - *V27.X Outcome of delivery*

    - *V22.0 Supervision of 1st normal pregnancy*

- *V22.1 Supervision of other normal pregnancy*
- *V22.2 Incidental state*
- *V25.2 Sterilization*
- *V24.0 Postpartum care and examination immediately after delivery*
- *V24.1 Postpartum care and examination of lactating mother*
- *V24.2 Routine postpartum care, follow-up*

- In Chapter 13, Diseases of the Musculoskeletal System and Connective Tissue (710–739)
- Place a tab on the first page of this chapter for quick and easy reference to the fifth-digit box for codes 711–712, 715–716, 718–719, and 730. This box includes the definition of the body regions used throughout the chapter (e.g., forearm includes the radius, ulna, and wrist joint).
- In Chapter 15, Certain Conditions Originating in the Perinatal Period (760–779)
- In code 779.9 Unspecified condition originating in the perinatal period, highlight the word "still-born" and write *"may be coded in the mother's chart."*
- On the last page of the chapter, write in the following reminders:
  - *All newborns will have a code from V30–V39 as their principal diagnosis.*
  - *In addition:*
    - *Report any clinically significant condition identified upon examination of the newborn.*
    - *Report any additional code from the perinatal chapter to show morbidity or mortality for the newborn.*
  - Remember, 700 codes = the baby's chart and 600 codes = the mother's chart.
- In Chapter 16, Symptoms, Signs, and Ill-Defined Conditions (780–799)
- In code 795.71 Nonspecific serologic evidence of human immunodeficiency virus (HIV), high-light the note underneath that states, "This code is only to be used when a test finding is reported as nonspecific. Asymptomatic positive findings are coded to V08. If any HIV infection symptoms or condition is present, see code 042. Negative findings are not coded."

Vocabulary Words

Infectious and Parasitic Diseases

Cholera–An acute intestinal infection caused by ingesting contaminated food or water.

Meningococcus–A bacterial infection that attacks the covering of the brain and spinal cord.

Mycosis–A fungal infection.

Streptococcus–A group of bacteria, commonly known as strep, that causes many illnesses, such as strep throat, pneumonia, and scarlet fever.

Tuberculosis–An infectious disease caused by mycobacteria, which usually affects the lungs, but it can also affect other areas, such as the liver, kidneys, stomach, bones, skin, breasts, brain, and spinal cord.

Endocrine, Nutritional, and Metabolic Diseases and Immunity Disorders

Crisis or storm–Refers to an acute exacerbation of all symptoms; usually related to thyroid conditions.

Diabetes mellitus–The inability to metabolize carbohydrates, proteins, and fats due to insufficient secretion of insulin.

Gestational diabetes–The elevation of blood glucose that begins during pregnancy and usually disappears following delivery.

Goiter–An abnormally enlarged thyroid gland.

Hyperglycemia–An unusually high concentration of sugar in the blood.

Hyperlipidemia–Abnormally high levels of lipids in the blood.

Diseases of the Blood and Blood-Forming Organs

Aplastic anemia–A condition in which bone marrow does not produce sufficient new cells to replenish blood cells.

Leukocytosis–An abnormal increase in the number of white blood cells.

Neutropenia–An abnormally low number of white blood cells.

Purpura–Red spots under the skin caused by the escape of blood from a vessel into the surrounding tissue.

Sickle cell disease–A genetic, lifelong blood disorder characterized by red blood cells that assume an abnormal, rigid sickle shape resulting in a severe form of anemia.

Mental Disorders

Agoraphobia–The fear of wide open or public spaces.

Bipolar–A form of depressive disease characterized by mood swings between great energy (manic) and clinical depression.

Dementia–The impairment of memory and other cognitive abilities due to damage or disease in the brain beyond what might be expected from normal aging.

Phobia–An irrational or obsessive fear or anxiety of certain situations, activities, things, or people.

Schizophrenia–A complex mental health disorder characterized by distortions of reality, disturbances of thought and language, and withdrawal from social contact.

Diseases of the Nervous System and Sense Organs

Bell's palsy–Paralysis of the facial nerve (cranial nerve VII) resulting in the inability to control facial muscles on the affected side. This condition may be temporary or permanent.

Encephalitis–An acute inflammation of the brain.

Esotropia–An eye that turns inward (crossed eyes).

Glaucoma–A disease of the optic nerve characterized by excessive fluid pressure within the eyeball.

Otitis media–inflammation of the middle ear.

Diseases of the Circulatory System

Angina–Severe constricting chest pain caused by insufficient blood flow to the heart muscle.

Atrial fibrillation–A rapid and irregular heart rate and rhythm.

Cerebrovascular accident–Another term for stroke, which occurs when a blood vessel to the brain is blocked.

Endocarditis–Inflammation of the intracardiac area (endocardium).

Myocardial infarction–Destruction of heart tissue due to reduced blood flow to the heart.

Diseases of the Respiratory System

Asbestosis–A chronic lung disease caused by inhaling asbestos particles.

Bronchospasm–A spasm of the bronchi due to constriction or squeezing of the surrounding muscles.

Emphysema–A chronic, irreversible disease of the lungs characterized by decreased respiratory function.

Pleurisy–Inflammation of the pleura of the lungs.

Siderosis–Fibrosis of the lungs caused by the inhalation of iron dust.

Diseases of the Digestive System

Cirrhosis–Hardened scar tissue that replaces normal liver tissue, impairing liver function.

Colitis–Inflammation of the colon characterized by abdominal pain, fever, and diarrhea with blood and mucus.

Diverticulitis–Inflammation of small, pouch-like sacs that protrude from the colon.

Diverticulosis–Small, pouch-like sacs protruding from the colon.

Volvulus–The abnormal twisting of the intestines, causing intestinal obstruction.

Diseases of the Genitourinary System

Endometriosis–Growth of endometrial tissue outside of the uterus.

Hematuria–Presence of blood in the urine.

Hydronephrosis–Accumulation of urine in the kidney due to a ureteral obstruction.

Leukorrhea–A white, viscid discharge from the vagina.

Peyronie's disease–Severe curvature of the erect penis due to fibrosis of the cavernous sheaths.

Complications of Pregnancy, Childbirth, and Puerperium

Breech presentation–The fetal presentation of buttocks or feet first.

Ectopic pregnancy–A pregnancy that takes place outside the uterine cavity.

Elderly primigravida–The first pregnancy in a woman who will be 35 years of age or older at the expected date of delivery.

Puerperium–The time following the expulsion of the placenta, during which a woman's body returns to its normal physical state, about 6 weeks.

Vertex presentation–The fetal presentation with the crown or top of the head first.

Diseases of the Skin and Subcutaneous Tissue

Cellulitis–A skin infection caused by bacteria characterized by fever, swelling, redness, and pain.

Dermatitis–Inflammation of the skin due to direct contact with an irritating substance or to an allergic reaction.

Furuncle–A painful, infected, pus-filled sore, also called a boil.

Pilonidal cyst–A hairy cyst near or on the natal cleft of the buttocks, which usually contains infected pus, hair, and skin debris.

Psoriasis–A chronic autoimmune disease that appears on the skin causing scaly patches of inflamed red skin, sometimes accompanied by painful joint swelling and stiffness.

Diseases of the Musculoskeletal System and Connective Tissue

Crepitation–A crackling sensation or sound produced by rubbing two fragments of a broken bone together.

Kyphosis–An abnormal curvature of the thoracic spine, causing a hunchback.

Lordosis–An excessive curvature of the spine, causing a hollow in the back, commonly called swayback.

Valgus–A condition that produces an outward curve at or below the knee area, commonly called knock-kneed.

Varus–A condition that produces an inward curve at or below the knee area, commonly called bowlegged.

Congenital Anomalies

Anencephalus–A lethal birth defect in which most of the brain is missing.

Down's syndrome–A genetic condition that causes delays in physical and intellectual development.

Hydrocephalus–An abnormal accumulation of cerebrospinal fluid in the cavities or ventricles of the brain.

Spina bifida–The failure of the baby's spine to develop completely, leaving the spinal cord exposed in that section.

Syndactyly–Partial or total webbing connecting two or more fingers or toes.

Conditions Originating in the Perinatal Period

Galactosemia–A condition in which the body cannot process galactose (a sugar), which makes up half of the sugar (called lactose) found in milk. In newborns, the condition can cause jaundice and other problems.

Perinatal period–The time period from 20 weeks' gestation through the 28th day following birth.

Signs and Symptoms

Ascites–An abnormal accumulation of fluid in the abdominal cavity.

Ataxia–An abnormal, asymmetric gait.

Dysphagia–Difficult or painful swallowing.

Dyspnea–Difficult or labored breathing.

Edema–Swelling due to an excess of fluid in the body tissues.

Acronyms and Abbreviations

Locate a blank area in your ICD-9-CM manual and write in these acronyms and abbreviations. You can usually find a large blank area in the front of the manual on the second page, which lists the ICD-9-CM Official Conventions.

AIDS–**A**cquired **I**mmuno**d**eficiency **S**yndrome

ASHD–**A**rterio**s**clerotic **H**eart **D**isease

CABG–**C**oronary **A**rtery **B**ypass **G**raft

CAD–**C**oronary **A**rtery **D**isease

CKD–**C**hronic **K**idney **D**isease

CNS–**C**entral **N**ervous **S**ystem

COPD–**C**hronic **O**bstructive **P**ulmonary **D**isease

DSM–*Diagnostic and Statistical Manual of Mental Disorders*

HIV–**H**uman **I**mmunodeficiency **V**irus

MI–**M**yocardial **I**nfarction

PID–**P**elvic **I**nflammatory **D**isease

SLE–**S**ystemic **L**upus **E**rythematosus

TIA–**T**ransient **I**schemic **A**ttack

URI–**U**pper **R**espiratory **I**nfection

UTI–**U**rinary **T**ract **I**nfection

TAKE THE CODING CHALLENGE

Assign the Appropriate Diagnosis Code

1. Food poisoning due to *Staphylococcus* organism

2. Hypoinsulinemia following total pancreatectomy

3. Thrombocytopenic purpura

4. Chronic paranoid schizophrenia with acute exacerbation

5. Traction detachment of retina with vitreoretinal organization

6. TIA

7. Common cold

8. Bilateral inguinal hernia, recurrent

9. Urolithiasis

10. False labor, 38 weeks, undelivered

11. Poison ivy

12. SLE

13. Drug withdrawal syndrome in the newborn

14. Change in bowel habits

Multiple Choice

1. The correct code for chickenpox is:
   a. 052.8
   b. 052.9
   c. 052.7
   d. 052.0

2. Mr. Jones presented to the clinic for results of his HIV test. He was found to be HIV positive. The correct diagnosis code is:
   a. V08
   b. 042
   c. V73.89
   d. 795.71

3. The endocrinologist recently diagnosed Mrs. Marks with a nontoxic multinodular goiter. The correct ICD-9-CM code is:
   a. 241
   b. 241.0
   c. 241.9
   d. 241.1

4. Adrenogenital disorders include disorders affecting:
   a. Males
   b. Females
   c. Both males and females
   d. Children under the age of 6

5. Mrs. Gibbs had been feeling weak and fatigued, which was accompanied by a loss of appetite. She was diagnosed with dimorphic anemia, which is coded as:
   a. 281.9
   b. 281.8
   c. 280.9
   d. 281.1

6. The correct code for sickle cell trait is:
   a. 282.41
   b. 282.42
   c. 282.5
   d. 282.60

7. Which of the following is a neurotic disorder?
   a. Schizophrenia
   b. Pedophilia
   c. Voyeurism
   d. Agoraphobia

8. Six-year-old Johnny developed diarrhea soon after his newborn brother was brought home. Johnny's mother took him to the doctor for a complete examination. The examination was negative, and it was determined there was no physical cause for the diarrhea. Johnny was diagnosed with psychogenic diarrhea. The correct code for psychogenic diarrhea is:
   a. 306.4
   b. 787.91
   c. 316
   d. 564.5

9. Acute allergic serous otitis media is coded as:
   a. 381.04
   b. 381.05
   c. 381.06
   d. 381.01

10. When coding proliferative diabetic retinopathy, what is sequenced first?
    a. The retinopathy
    b. The diabetes
    c. It makes no difference how they are reported.
    d. The code is based on how the physician sequenced the codes.

11. When coding for a myocardial infarction, which fifth digit indicates an MI that has received initial treatment but is still less than 8 weeks old?
    a. 0
    b. 1
    c. 2
    d. A fifth digit is not required.

12. ASHD of a transplanted heart is coded as:
    a. 414.04
    b. 414.05
    c. 414.06
    d. 414.01

13. Pneumonia due to the RSV (respiratory syncytial virus) is coded as:
    a. 480.1
    b. 486, 079.6
    c. 466.11
    d. 079.6, 486

14. Category 496 Chronic airway obstruction is not to be used:
    a. By itself
    b. With codes from category 491–493
    c. To describe nonspecific lung disease
    d. To describe obstructive lung disease

15. When coding for hernias, the coder must consider:
    a. The site, if there is an obstruction, if gangrene is present, and if the hernia is recurrent
    b. The site, if there is an obstruction, if gangrene is present, if the hernia is recurrent, and if the hernia is unilateral or bilateral
    c. The site, if gangrene is present, and if the hernia is recurrent
    d. The site, if there is an obstruction, if gangrene is present, if the hernia is recurrent, and the laterality of the hernia (right or left sided)

16. An acute peptic ulcer of the stomach with perforation is coded as:
    a. 533.10
    b. 531.50
    c. 531.10
    d. 531.11

17. Mr. Palmer was diagnosed with urinary retention due to hyperplasia of the prostate. Select the correct code(s).
    a. 600.01, 788.20
    b. 788.20
    c. 788.29
    d. 600.00, 788.20

18. Staghorn calculus is coded as:
    a. 593.2
    b. 592.9
    c. 592.1
    d. 592.0

19. Diagnosis codes reported in the maternal chart are reported with codes from which category of codes?
    a. 740–759
    b. 630–679, 760–779
    c. 630–679
    d. 760–779

20. V22.2 Pregnant state, incidental is reported:
    a. As a primary diagnosis
    b. For postpartum visits
    c. For antepartum visits
    d. As a secondary diagnosis

21. The ICD-9-CM code for sunburn is located in which chapter of the manual?
    a. Signs & Symptoms
    b. Injury & Poisoning
    c. Skin and Subcutaneous Tissue
    d. None of the above

22. Lichen planus, generalized is coded as:
    a. 697.0
    b. 697.1
    c. 697.8
    d. 697.9

23. The term malunion refers to:
    a. A bone that is not healing
    b. The faulty healing of a bone
    c. A broken bone
    d. A congenital disorder of the bone

24. Degenerative disk disease of the lumbar spine is coded as:
    a. 724.02
    b. 722.51
    c. 722.52
    d. 722.4

25. Congenital disorders are reported:
    a. Only at birth
    b. Only as a secondary diagnosis
    c. Throughout the life of the patient
    d. Only as a principal diagnosis

26. The congenital condition that describes the absence of a major portion of the brain is called:
    a. Hydronephrosis
    b. Hydrocephalus
    c. Anencephalus
    d. Anophthalmos

27. Signs and symptoms codes may be reported:
    a. As a primary diagnosis
    b. When there is no definitive diagnosis
    c. In place of "rule out"
    d. All of the above

28. Nonvisualization of gallbladder is coded as:
    a. 793.3
    b. 793.2
    c. 793.5
    d. 793.6

ANSWERS AND RATIONALES

Assign the Appropriate Diagnostic Code

1. The correct answer is **005.0.** The main term in Volume 2 is *poisoning,* subterm *food,* subterm *due to staphylococcus.* The code is then verified in Volume 1.

2. The correct answer is **251.3.** In Volume 2, the main term is *hypoinsulinemia, postsurgical* (as the patient had the pancreas removed), subterm *postpancreatectomy (complete) (partial).* The code is then verified in Volume 1.

3. The correct answer is **287.30.** In the Alphabetical Index, the main term is *purpura,* subterm *thrombocytopenic.* We are then directed to *see also Thrombocytopenia,* 287.30. If we follow the "see also," the main term is *thrombocytopenia,* and the subterm is *purpura,* 287.30. Either way we look up this code, we are referenced to the same code: 287.30. This code is further verified in Volume 1.

4. The correct answer is **295.34.** In the Alphabetical Index, the main term is *schizophrenia,* subterm *paranoid (type) (acute).* This leads us to 295.3; looking in the Tabular List, we select the fifth-digit "4" to identify the condition as chronic with an acute exacerbation.

5. The correct answer is **361.81.** In the Alphabetical Index, the main term is *detachment,* subterm *retina,* subterm *traction (with vitreoretinal organization),* resulting in 361.81. This code is then confirmed in the Tabular List to be correct.

6. The correct answer is **435.9.** TIA is the abbreviation for "transient ischemic attack." In the Alphabetical Index, the main term is *attack,* subterm *transient ischemic (TIA),* resulting in 435.9. This code is then confirmed in the Tabular List to be correct.

7. The correct answer is **460.** In the Alphabetical Index, the main term is *cold,* subterm *common (head),* resulting in 460. The common cold is also known as acute nasopharyngitis. This code is then confirmed in the Tabular List to be correct.

8. The correct answer is **550.93.** In the Alphabetical Index, the main term is *hernia,* subterm *inguinal,* resulting in 550.9. In the Tabular List, we select the fifth-digit "3," identifying the hernia as bilateral and recurrent.

9. The correct answer is **594.2.** In the Alphabetical Index, the main term is *urolithiasis,* resulting in 594.2. This code is then confirmed in the Tabular List to be correct. Urolithiasis is a stone or a blockage in the *urethra.* Be careful not to confuse this with **ureterolithiasis,** which is coded as 594.1.

10. The correct answer is **644.13.** In the Alphabetical Index, the main term is *pregnancy,* subterm *complicated by,* subterm *false labor (pains),* resulting in 644.1. In the Tabular List, we see our fifth-digit code selection is limited to either "0" or "3." We select the fifth-digit "3" to identify the antepartum status.

11. The correct answer is **692.6.** In the Alphabetical Index, the main term is *poison ivy, oak, sumac or other plant dermatitis,* resulting in 692.6. This code is then confirmed in the Tabular List to be correct. Note that the ICD-9-CM code remains the same for any of the causes (ivy, oak, etc.).

12. The correct answer is **710.0.** SLE is the abbreviation for "systemic lupus erythematosus." In the Alphabetical Index, the main term is *lupus,* subterm *erythematosus,* subterm *disseminated or systemic,* resulting in 710.0. This code is then confirmed in the Tabular List to be correct. Although localized lupus is a disease of the skin, it is categorized in the musculoskeletal system.

13. The correct answer is **779.5.** In the Alphabetical Index, the main term is *syndrome,* subterm *drug withdrawal, infant of dependent mother,* resulting in 779.5. This code is then confirmed in the Tabular List to be correct. You may also look up this code with the main term *withdrawal symptoms or syndrome,* subterm, *newborn, infant of dependent mother.*

14. The correct answer is **787.99.** In the Alphabetical Index, the main term is *change (of),* subterm *bowel habits,* resulting in 787.99. This code is then confirmed in the tabular list to be correct.

Multiple Choice Answers

1. The correct answer is **b.** When we look up chickenpox in the Alphabetical Index, we are directed to *see also Varicella 052.9.* In the Tabular List, the 052.9 code descriptor reads, "Varicella without mention of complication" and is identified as Chickenpox NOS, Varicella NOS, making this the correct choice. Answer **a.** is incorrect, as it describes chickenpox with unspecified complication. Answer **c.** is

incorrect, as it describes chickenpox with other specified complication. Answer **d.** is incorrect, as it describes postvaricella encephalitis.

2. The correct answer is **a.** According to the ICD-9-CM Coding Guidelines, V08 asymptomatic human immunodeficiency virus (HIV) infection is to be applied when the patient, without any documentation of symptoms, is listed as being HIV positive. Answer **b.** is incorrect, as it describes AIDS. Answer **c.** is incorrect, as it describes the screening examination, and Mr. Jones is presenting for the results of the screening test. Answer **d.** is incorrect, as it describes nonspecific serological evidence of human immunodeficiency virus (HIV). We have a definitive result: HIV positive.

3. The correct answer is **d.** Code 241.1 correctly describes the condition as nontoxic multinodular goiter. Answer **a.** is incorrect, as it is a three-digit category requiring a fourth-digit subcategory. Answer **b.** is incorrect, as it describes a nontoxic, *uninodular* goiter. Answer **c.** is incorrect, as it describes an *unspecified* nontoxic nodular goiter.

4. The correct answer is **c.** To obtain the information necessary to answer the question, we first look up the code. In the Alphabetical Index, the main term is *disorder,* subterm *adrenogenital,* resulting in 255.2. When we look up code 255.2 in the Tabular List and read the descriptor, we can see this disorder includes both males and females and makes no age distinction. Answer **a.** is incorrect, as the disorder includes females as well as males. Answer **b.** is incorrect, as the disorder includes males as well as females. Answer **d.** is incorrect, as the disorder does not make an age distinction.

5. The correct answer is **a.** 281.9 Unspecified deficiency anemia includes many types of anemias, including dimorphic. Dimorphic anemia is anemia due to two types of causes acting together (e.g., iron deficiency and vitamin B$_{12}$ deficiency). Answer **b.** is incorrect, as it describes anemia associated with other specified nutritional deficiency. Answer **c.** is incorrect, as it describes unspecified iron deficiency. Answer **d.** is incorrect, as it describes other vitamin B$_{12}$ deficiency anemia.

6. The correct answer is **c.** Code 282.5 represents sickle cell trait. Answer **a.** is incorrect, as it describes sickle cell. Answer **b.** is incorrect, as it describes sickle cell thalassemia without crisis. Answer **d.** is incorrect, as it describes sickle cell disease unspecified.

7. The correct answer is **d.** Agoraphobia is the fear of open spaces and is coded in the 300 category, which includes neurotic disorders. Answer **a.** is incorrect, as schizophrenia is a disorder with disturbances in thought and is classified according to the ICD-9-CM as a psychosis. Answer **b.** is incorrect, as it describes a condition of adults characterized by sexual activity with children and is classified as a sexual and gender identity disorder. Answer **c.** is incorrect, as it describes an uncontrollable impulse to observe others without their knowledge and is classified as other specified psychosexual disorders.

8. The correct answer is **a.** In this case, the diarrhea is classified as psychogenic (the mental condition—anxiety over the new baby—caused the physical symptoms). Additionally, when there is no tissue damage (the examination was negative), a code from category 306 would be assigned, in this case 306.4 for the psychogenic diarrhea. Answer **b.** is incorrect, as it describes diarrhea as a sign or symptom. Answer **c.** is incorrect, as this category encompasses psychogenic disorders that include tissue damage; we would also need two codes to appropriately report psychogenic illnesses with tissue damage. The first code would represent the psychogenic etiology, and the second code would represent the physiological manifestation. Answer **d.** is incorrect, as it describes functional diarrhea.

9. The correct answer is **a.** Answer **b.** is incorrect, as it describes acute allergic *mucoid* otitis media. Answer **c.** is incorrect, as it describes acute allergic *sanguinous* otitis media. Answer **d.** is incorrect, as it describes acute serous otitis media not described as allergic. Take care when reading the code descriptors to make sure you are making the right choice. In many cases, the words look the same and it is easy to choose the incorrect code.

10. The correct answer is **b.** When looking up the code for diabetic retinopathy (362.0) in the Tabular List, we are instructed to "code first diabetes (249.5, 250.5)." Answer **a.** is incorrect, as when looking up the code for diabetic retinopathy (362.0) in the Tabular List, we are instructed to "code first diabetes (249.5, 250.5)." Answer **c.** is incorrect; according to the ICD-9-CM Coding Guidelines, it does make a difference in sequencing of the codes. Answer **d.** is incorrect, as the ICD-9-CM Coding Guidelines provide clear guidance on how the codes should be sequenced. The physician may not always know or remember the correct sequencing

and may simply list diagnosis codes not necessarily in the correct order.

11. The correct answer is **c.** The fifth digit in the 410 category represents the episode of care. The note beneath the fifth digit "2" states, "Use fifth-digit 2 to designate an episode of care following the initial episode when the patient is admitted for further observation, evaluation, or treatment for a myocardial infarction that has received initial treatment, but is still less than 8 weeks old." Answer **a.** is incorrect, as the fifth-digit "0" is used when there is no sufficient information for the assignment of 1 or 2 as the fifth digit. Answer **b.** is incorrect, as the fifth-digit "1" is used to identify the first episode of care regardless of facility or site for a newly diagnosed MI. Answer **d.** is incorrect, as category 410 requires a fifth-digit subclassification.

12. The correct answer is **c.** The abbreviation ASHD stands for "arteriosclerotic heart disease." In some cases, patients who have a transplanted heart may also get ASHD in the new heart. Code 414.06 is the correct choice, as it describes ASHD of a native coronary artery of a transplanted heart. Answer **a.** is incorrect, as it describes ASHD of artery bypass graft. Answer **b.** is incorrect, as it describes ASHD of unspecified type of bypass graft. Answer **d.** is incorrect, as it describes ASHD of a native coronary artery.

13. The correct answer is **a.** Code 480.1 Pneumonia due to respiratory syncytial virus includes both the pneumonia and the cause as RVS; therefore, only one code is needed. Answer **b.** is incorrect, as it describes pneumonia, unspecified organism (486) and then codes the RSV (079.6): we do not report each condition separately when one code includes both conditions. Answer **c.** is incorrect, as it describes *acute bronchiolitis* due to RSV. Answer **d.** is incorrect, as we do not report each condition separately when one code includes both conditions.

14. The correct answer is **b.** The note under category 496 states, "This code is not to be used with any code from categories 491–493." Answer **a.** is incorrect, as this code may be used by itself if applicable. Answer **c.** is incorrect, as category 496 does include nonspecific lung disease. Answer **d.** is incorrect, as category 496 does include obstructive pulmonary disease.

15. The correct answer is **b.** Before selecting a hernia code, we must know the site, if there is an obstruction, if gangrene is present, if the hernia is recurrent,

and if the hernia is unilateral or bilateral. Answer **a.** is incorrect, as we need to know if the hernia is unilateral or bilateral. Answer **c.** is incorrect, as we need to know if there is an obstruction and if the hernia is unilateral or bilateral. Answer **d.** is incorrect, as we need to know if the hernia is unilateral or bilateral. The hernia codes do not specify laterality (right or left).

16. The correct answer is **c.** Category 531 Gastric ulcer includes a peptic stomach ulcer, the fourth-digit "1" identifies the ulcer as acute with perforation, and the fifth-digit "0" is selected because there is no mention of obstruction. Answer **a.** is incorrect, as it describes an acute peptic ulcer, *unspecified site,* with perforation, without mention of obstruction. Answer **b.** is incorrect as it describes a *chronic* or unspecified gastric ulcer with perforation, without mention of obstruction. Answer **d.** is incorrect, as it describes an acute gastric ulcer with perforation *and obstruction.*

17. The correct answer is **a.** The instructional note beneath Retention of urine (788.2) states, "Code, if applicable, any causal condition first, such as hyperplasia of prostate (600.0–600.9), with fifth-digit 1." Answer **b.** is incorrect, as it describes the retention of urine but not the cause, which is hyperplasia of the prostate. Answer **c.** is incorrect, as it describes o*ther specified* retention of urine and does not include the cause, which is hyperplasia of the prostate. Answer **d.** is incorrect, as code 600.00 describes hypertrophy (benign) of prostate *without urinary obstruction* and other lower urinary tract symptoms (LUTS).

18. The correct answer is **d.** Code 592.0 Calculus of kidney includes a staghorn calculus (a very large calculus or stone that fills the calyceal system and has the appearance of stag [deer] horns). Answer **a.** is incorrect, as it describes a kidney *cyst.* Answer **b.** is an unspecified urinary calculus. Answer **c.** is incorrect, as it describes a calculus of the ureter.

19. The correct answer is **c.** The category of codes 630–679 describes complications of pregnancy, childbirth, and the puerperium. Answer **a.** describes congenital anomalies. Answer **b.** codes only from category 630–679 and is reported in the maternal chart. Answer **d.** is incorrect, as it describes conditions originating in the perinatal period, which are reported in the baby's chart.

20. The correct answer is **d.** According to the V code diagnosis table located in the ICD-9-CM Coding

Guidelines, V22.2 is reported only as an additional diagnosis. We report this code as a secondary diagnosis when the pregnancy is in no way a complicating reason for the visit. Answer **a.** is incorrect; per the ICD-9-CM Coding Guidelines, V22.2 is never reported as a primary diagnosis. Answer **b.** is incorrect: postpartum visits are reported with a code from V24.0–V24.2. Answer **c.** is incorrect: antepartum visits are reported with the appropriate V code describing the type of pregnancy (e.g., V22.0 Supervision of normal first pregnancy).

21. The correct answer is **c.** According to the Excludes note under the burns category 940–949, sunburn is coded as 692.71, 692.76, or 692.77, all located in ICD-9-CM Chapter 12. Answer **a.** is incorrect, as sunburn is not classified as a sign or a symptom. Answer **b.** is incorrect, as this section includes burns from various anatomical locations at various degrees of burn. Answer **d.** is incorrect, as sunburns are located in Chapter 12.

22. The correct answer is **a.** Code 697.0 is used to report lichen planus, which is a pruritic skin disease. Answer **b.** is incorrect, as it describes lichen nitidus, a chronic, inflammatory, asymptomatic skin disorder. Answer **c.** is incorrect, as it describes other lichen, not elsewhere classified. Answer **d.** is incorrect, as it describes lichen, unspecified.

23. The correct answer is **b.** Answer **a.** is incorrect, as nonunion describes a bone that is not healing. Answer **c.** is incorrect, as malunion refers to the faulty healing of a bone, not a broken bone. Answer **d.** is incorrect, as malunion is not a congenital disorder.

24. The correct answer is **c.** Code 722.52 describes degeneration of lumbar or lumbosacral intervertebral disk. Answer **a.** is incorrect, as it describes lumbar spinal stenosis. Answer **b.** is incorrect, as it describes degeneration of the thoracic spine. Answer **d.** is incorrect, as it describes degeneration of the cervical spine.

25. The correct answer is **c.** Per the ICD-9-CM Coding Guidelines, codes from Chapter 14 may be used throughout the life of the patient. Answer **a.** is incorrect, as congenital codes may be reported throughout the life of the patient. Answer **b.** is incorrect; per the ICD-9-CM Coding Guidelines, a congenital anomaly may be the principal or first-listed diagnosis on a record or may be a secondary diagnosis. Answer **d.** is incorrect: per the ICD-9-CM Coding Guidelines, a congenital anomaly may be the principal or first-listed diagnosis on a record or may be a secondary diagnosis.

26. The correct answer is **c.** Anencephalus is the absence of a major portion of the brain. Answer **a.** is incorrect, as hydronephrosis is the accumulation of urine in the kidney because of an obstruction in the ureter. Answer **b.** is incorrect, as hydrocephalus (also called water on the brain) is an abnormal accumulation of cerebrospinal fluid (CSF) in the ventricles, or cavities, of the brain. Answer **d.** is incorrect, as anophthalmos is the congenital absence of the eyeball.

27. The correct answer is **d.** All of the above are correct. When there is no definitive diagnosis, we report the signs and symptoms. We do not want to tag a person with an illness or injury that has not been definitely diagnosed. Because there are no "rule-out" codes, we report the signs and symptoms of the illness or injury. Signs and symptoms codes are valid primary diagnosis codes.

28. The correct answer is **a.** 793.3 Nonspecific (abnormal) findings on radiological and other examination of body structure biliary tract correctly describes the nonvisualization of the gallbladder. Answer **b.** is incorrect, as it describes the nonspecific or abnormal finding of other intrathoracic organs. Answer **c.** is incorrect, as it describes a nonspecific or abnormal finding of the genitourinary organs. Answer **d.** is incorrect, as it describes a nonspecific or abnormal finding of the abdominal area, including the retroperitoneum.

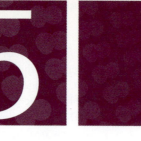

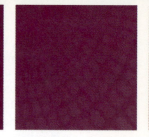

Healthcare Common Procedure Coding System

Healthcare Common Procedure Coding System (HCPCS) is a standardized coding system that was developed in the 1980s. HCPCS is a two-tier system. The first tier, developed by the American Medical Association (AMA), is the CPT coding system, which are Level I codes used by physicians and other health-care providers. The second tier was developed by the Centers for Medicare and Medicaid Services (CMS), and these HCPCS Level II codes are used to report products (e.g., durable medical equipment), supplies (e.g., bandages), and services (e.g., ambulance services) not identified in the CPT coding system. These Level II codes are alphanumeric, consisting of a single alphabet letter followed by four numbers.

Types of HCPCS Codes

The HCPCS codes are divided into types based on the purpose of the codes and who is responsible for maintaining the codes.

- **Permanent National Codes.** The national permanent Level II HCPCS codes are maintained by the HCPCS National Panel.

- **Dental Codes.** The codes that represent dental procedures and supplies are maintained by the American Dental Association (ADA). The dental codes are not included in the 2011 HCPCS Level II code set. The ADA holds the copyright and instructed CMS to remove them.

- **Miscellaneous Codes.** Miscellaneous or not otherwise classified codes are reported for products or services for which no national code exists. These codes are manually reviewed by the payer and require the submission of a full description of the product or service, the pricing information, and an explanation as to why the item or service is needed by the beneficiary.

- **Temporary National Codes.** Temporary codes are maintained by the CMS and members of the HCPCS National Panel. Because HCPCS codes are updated once a year (in January), these temporary codes allow payers to establish codes that are needed prior to the January update. The temporary codes include:

  - **G codes,** which identify professional health-care procedures and services for which there are no CPT codes available.

- **K codes,** which identify codes for supplies, durable medical equipment (DME), and drugs. Once these codes are approved for permanent inclusion in HCPCS, they become an A, E, or J code.
- **Q codes,** which identify services that are not usually assigned a CPT code (e.g., drugs, biologicals, casting supplies).
- **S codes,** used by Blue Cross/Blue Shield Association (BCBSA) and the Health Insurance Association of America (HIAA) to report drugs, services, and supplies for which no national codes exist but for which codes are needed by the private sector for the implementation of policies, programs, and/or for claim processing.
- ■ **Modifiers.** Like CPT modifiers, HCPCS modifiers provide additional information without changing the description of the code. Unlike CPT modifiers, HCPCS modifiers can be either two alphabetic (e.g., RT, right side) or alphanumeric (T2, Left foot third digit). These modifiers are discussed in more detail later in this chapter.

KEY CODING TIP
When billing Medicare, the appropriate HCPCS code, if one exists, takes precedence over a CPT code.

The HCPCS Codes—and When to Use Them

A Codes (Miscellaneous Services and Supplies). A codes represent transportation services (e.g., ambulance, rotary wing) and supplies related to ostomies, tracheostomies, and urologicals. DME deemed to be inexpensive (not priced higher than $150) and radiopharmaceutical agents are also found in the A section. A few examples of A codes are:

- A0225 Ambulance service, neonatal transport, base rate, emergency transport, one way
- A4361 Ostomy faceplate, each
- A4218 Sterile saline or water, metered dose dispenser, 10 ml
- A9500 Technetium Tc-99m sestamibi, diagnostic, per study dose, up to 40 millicuries

B Codes (Enteral and Parenteral Therapy). B codes represent enteral (nutrition delivered to the intestines via a tube) and parenteral (nutrition delivered by other means, e.g., intravenously) therapy supplies. These supplies include infusion pumps, formulas, feeding supplies, and nutritional solutions. Some examples of B codes are:

- B4034 Enteral feeding supply kit; syringe fed, per day
- B4103 Enteral formula, for pediatrics, used to replace fluids and electrolytes (e.g., clear liquids), 500 ml = 1 unit
- B4168 Parenteral nutrition solution; amino acid, 3.5% (500 ml = 1 unit) — home mix
- B9000 Enteral nutrition infusion pump — without alarm

C Codes (Outpatient PPS). C codes represent services provided under the Medicare Outpatient Prospective Payment System (OPPS). C codes represent drugs, biologicals, and devices eligible for transitional pass-through *payments for hospitals* and items classified in new technology *ambulatory payment classifications (APC) under OPPS. These codes are not used for services that are reimbursed under other Medicare payment systems.* Here are a few examples of C codes:

- C1750 Catheter, hemodialysis/peritoneal, long-term
- C9113 Injection, pantoprazole sodium, per vial
- C9725 Placement of endorectal intracavitary applicator for high intensity brachytherapy

D Codes (Dental Procedures). D codes represent dental services and procedures. A few examples of D codes are:

- D0120 Periodic oral evaluation—established patient
- D2710 Crown—resin-based composite (indirect)
- D7230 Removal of impacted tooth, partially bony

E Codes (DME). E codes represent a vast array of DME such as canes, crutches, walkers, wheelchairs, commodes, hospital beds, pacemakers, and fracture frames. For example:

- E0100 Cane, includes canes of all materials, adjustable or fixed, with tip
- E0143 Walker, folding, wheeled, adjustable or fixed height
- E0250 Hospital bed, fixed height, with any type side rails, with mattress
- E0610 Pacemaker monitor, self-contained (checks battery depletion, includes audible and visible check systems)

G Codes (Temporary Procedures and Professional Services). G codes are the first of four temporary code sets that identify professional health-care procedures and services for which no CPT codes are available. A few examples of G codes include:

- G0104 Colorectal cancer screening; flexible sigmoidoscopy
- G0109 Diabetes outpatient self-management training services, group session (2 or more), per 30 minutes

- G0101 Cervical or vaginal cancer screening; pelvic and clinical breast examination

H Codes (Alcohol and Drug Abuse Treatment Services). H codes are reported to state Medicaid agencies that are mandated by state law to establish separate codes for mental health services that include alcohol and drug treatment services. Let's look at a few examples:

- H0002 Behavioral health screening to determine eligibility for admission to treatment program
- H0007 Alcohol and/or drug services; crisis intervention (outpatient)
- H0032 Mental health service plan development by nonphysician

J Codes (Drugs Administered Other Than Oral Method). J codes represent drugs that cannot be self-administered or orally administered, such as chemotherapy drugs, inhalation solutions, and immunosuppressive drugs. To select the correct code, the following factors must be considered:

- The route of administration (e.g., subcutaneously, intravenously)
- The dose (e.g., 150 mg, 10 mg)

Appendix 1, Table of Drugs, lists the drug name, unit per, route of administration, and HCPCS code. Both the generic and brand names of the drugs are listed in alphabetical order, which enables you to quickly locate the correct drug. A few examples of J codes are:

- J0120 Injection, tetracycline, up to 250 mg
- J3360 Injection, diazepam, up to 5 mg
- J7609 Albuterol, inhalation solution, compounded product, administered through DME, unit dose, 1 mg

KEY CODING TIP

It is important to note that the J codes are dose-specific. When selecting the appropriate J code, pay close attention to the dose administered and dose amount in the code description.

For example: A patient receiving two nebulizer treatments may require two doses (2 mg) of albuterol. The HCPCS code for albuterol administered through DME is J7609 Albuterol, inhalation solution, compounded product, administered through DME, *unit dose, 1 mg.* The code describes one dose as 1 mg. However, the patient in this scenario received 2 mg. To be properly reimbursed for the cost of the drug, HCPCS code J7609 would be billed as two units listed as J7609 × 2.

K Codes (Temporary Codes for Supplies, DME, and Drugs). K codes are the second of four code sets that identify temporary codes for supplies, DME, and drugs. For example:

- K0899 Power mobility device, not coded by DME PDAC or does not meet criteria
- K0462 Temporary replacement for patient-owned equipment being repaired, any type

L Codes (Orthotics and Prosthetics). L codes represent orthotic and prosthetic procedures and devices, scoliosis equipment, orthopedic shoes, and prosthetic implants. For example:

- L0170 Cervical collar, molded to patient model
- L1900 Ankle-foot orthotic (AFO), spring wire, dorsiflexion assist calf band, custom fabricated
- L3215 Orthopedic footwear, ladies shoe, oxford, each

M Codes (Medical Services). M codes represent office services, cellular therapy, prolotherapy, intragastric hypothermia, IV chelation therapy, and fabric wrapping of an abdominal aneurysm. Most of the medical services are reported with CPT codes; currently, only six codes are listed in the M codes section.

P Codes (Pathology and Laboratory Services). Most of the pathology and laboratory services are reported with CPT codes; however, the P codes include some screening pathology and laboratory services and blood products. Examples include:

- P3000 Screening Papanicolaou smear, cervical or vaginal, up to 3 smears, by technician under physician supervision
- P9010 Blood (whole), for transfusion, per unit

Q Codes (Miscellaneous Temporary Codes). Q codes are the third of four temporary code sets. They represent many different services and supplies. Included in this section are cast supply codes. A few examples include:

- Q0510 Pharmacy supply fee for initial immunosuppressive drug(s), first month following transplant
- Q0495 Battery/power pack charger for use with electric or electric/pneumatic ventricular assist device, replacement only
- Q4003 Cast supplies, shoulder cast, adult (11 years +), plaster
- Q4025 Cast supplies, hip spica (one or both legs), adult (11 years +), plaster

R Codes (Diagnostic Radiology Services). Most radiology services are reported with CPT codes. Currently, three R codes are used to report the transportation of portable x-ray or electrocardiogram equipment to a patient's home, a nursing home, or other facility. The three codes are:

- R0070 Transportation of portable x-ray equipment and personnel to home or nursing home, per trip to facility or location, one patient seen
- R0075 Transportation of portable x-ray equipment and personnel to home or nursing home, per trip to facility or location, more than one patient seen
- R0076 Transportation of portable EKG to facility or location, per patient

S Codes (Temporary National Codes (Non-Medicare)). S codes are the last set of temporary code sets. They represent many of the local codes that were used by private payers that were phased out with the implementation of HIPAA legislation. Currently, BCBSA and HIAA use these codes for drugs, services, and supplies where no national codes exist. A few examples are:

- S0160 Dextroamphetamine sulfate, 5 mg
- S2060 Lobar lung transplantation
- S0274 Nurse practitioner visit at member's home, outside of a capitation arrangement
- S0515 Scleral lens, liquid bandage device, per lens

T Codes (National Codes for State Medicaid Agencies). T codes are used by Medicaid state agencies. They represent services and supplies that are not identified by any permanent HCPCS codes but are needed to administer the Medicaid program. For example:

- T1009 Child sitting services for children of the individual receiving alcohol and/or substance abuse services
- T1012 Alcohol and/or substance abuse services, skills development
- T2005 Nonemergency transportation; stretcher van

V Codes (Vision, Hearing, and Speech-Language Pathology Services and Supplies). Just as the heading states, these codes represent services and supplies associated with vision, hearing, and speech and language pathology. Let's look at a few examples:

- V2219 Bifocal seg width over 28 mm
- V5011 Fitting/orientation/checking of hearing aid
- V5362 Speech screening

Unlisted Codes. When you are unable to select the HCPCS code that accurately identifies the equipment, supply, and so on, the appropriate unlisted HCPCS code may be reported.

Modifiers

HCPCS modifiers, like CPT modifiers, are used to alert the insurance carrier that something is different about the procedure (or other service) that the CPT or HCPCS code is meant to report, without changing the description of the code itself. HCPCS modifiers can be either two alphabetic (e.g., RT, right side) or alphanumeric (T2, Left foot third digit).

Both CPT and HCPCS modifiers have the same function: to provide additional information about the service provided. HCPCS modifiers may be appended to either a CPT code or an HCPCS code. HCPCS modifiers can affect the reimbursement of the claim by providing information such as:

- Who provided the service: AH, Clinical psychologist.
- The anatomical location of the service provided: E2, Left lower eyelid.
- Additional information need to appropriately adjudicate the claim: GA, Advanced beneficiary notice (ABN) on file.

A complete list of HCPCS modifiers is given in Appendix 2 of the HCPCS book.

Modifiers Used With Anesthesia Services

These modifiers describe who performed the service, alert the carrier with regard to concurrent care cases, and identify monitored anesthesia care (MAC). (See Chapter 8 of the Manual for a list of HCPCS modifiers used with anesthesia services.)

Modifier QW—CLIA Waived Test

In 1988, Congress established the Clinical Laboratory Improvement Amendments (CLIA) to ensure quality standards for all patient laboratory testing with the exception of research. The law ensures the laboratory is qualified to handle laboratory tests with accuracy, reliability, and timeliness of patient test results. All laboratories in the United States handling human samples are required to become CLIA certified. A few simple tests have been designated as "CLIA Waived." Tests that fall under the CLIA Waived category may be performed without a CLIA certification.

This HCPCS modifier is appended to **laboratory tests** that have been designated CLIA Waived (certain laboratory tests may be provided in a physician office without a CLIA certification if the test has been designated as CLIA Waived).

Locating HCPCS Codes

Note: The **Introduction** of the HCPCS book is a mustread. It provides guidance on how to use the HCPCS book and how to locate codes, and it describes the various coding conventions. The index of the HCPCS book provides the starting point for locating codes.

Let's consider that we want to locate the code for blood tubing, venous for hemodialysis. To look up an HCPCS code, we use the index located in the front of the book and follow these few simple steps:

1. Identify the service, procedure, or supply the patient received. In this case, it is blood tubing, venous for hemodialysis.

2. Look up the key term (item, supply, or service) in the index. In this case, the key term is "tubing." When we look up in the index, we locate "Tube/tubing." Under Tube/tubing, we look for the word "blood" (the type of tubing), and we are presented with two options: A4750, A4755.

3. When we look up the codes, we get the full descriptions:

   a. A4750 Blood tubing, arterial *or* venous, for hemodialysis, each.

   b. A4755 Blood tubing, arterial **and** venous **combined,** for hemodialysis, each.

   At first glance, they both look alike, but take a careful look and you will notice the difference. HCPCS code A4750 describes the blood tubing as **either** arterial or venous. HCPCS code A4755 describes the blood tubing as both arterial and venous **combined.** Therefore, the correct code would be A4750.

4. Remember to look for any symbols, notes, or footnotes that provide definitions, guidelines, or coverage issues (e.g., non-covered by Medicare, female only, and so on).

5. Apply modifiers as applicable.

Let's Practice Coding

A patient with a broken leg was given a pair of wooden crutches before leaving the orthopedist's office. Select the correct code for the crutches, following the appropriate steps described previously.

Step 1. The key term is *crutches.* This identifies what the patient received (i.e., the supply).

Step 2. We look up *crutches* in the index and are presented with a number of choices. We can narrow our search by looking for the type of crutches, in this case, wooden. This leads us to HCPCS code E0112.

Step 3. We look up **HCPCS code** E0112 Crutches, underarm, wood, adjustable or fixed, pair, with pads, tips, and

handgrips. Doing this, we confirm this is the correct code. Do not be confused with HCPCS code E0113 Crutch, underarm, wood, adjustable or fixed, each, with pad, tip, and handgrip, as this code describes **"one"** crutch (as indicated by the word *each*), whereas our patient received a **"pair"** of crutches.

Learn More About It

The more you read, the more you know. Increase your knowledge with the following Web site:

CMS: An Overview of HCPCS. Remember to click on the links on the left.

http://www.cms.gov/medhcpcsgeninfo/

STOP-LOOK-HIGHLIGHT

The key to successfully passing the exam and selecting the correct code lies in your knowing how to use your coding book.

To help you navigate through your codebook, and to make sure you have the most important information at your fingertips when you take the exam, take the time to insert tab index dividers into your HCPCS book. This will enable you to quickly identify key areas of the book.

■ Place a divider tab on the first page of the index and label it "Index."

■ Place a divider tab on the first page of Appendix 1 and label it "Table of Drugs."

■ Place a divider tab on the first page of Appendix 2 and label it "Modifiers."

■ Place a divider tab on the first page of Appendix 3 and label it "Abbreviations & Acronyms."

Acronyms and Abbreviations

In your HCPCS book on a blank note page, write the following:

ABN–**A**dvanced **B**eneficiary **N**otice

ADA–**A**merican **D**ental **A**ssociation

APC–**A**mbulatory **P**ayment **C**lassification

BCBSA–**B**lue **C**ross/**B**lue **S**hield **A**ssociation

CLIA–**C**linical **L**aboratory **I**mprovement **A**mendments

DME–**D**urable **M**edical **E**quipment

DMEPOS–**D**urable **M**edical **E**quipment **P**rosthetics **O**rthotics and **S**upplies

HCPCS–**H**ealthcare **C**ommon **P**rocedure **C**oding **S**ystem

HIAA–**H**ealth **I**nsurance **A**ssociation of **A**merica
OPPS–**O**utpatient **P**rospective **P**ayment **S**ystem

TAKE THE CODING CHALLENGE

Assign the Appropriate HCPCS Code

1. Infusion, mitomycin, 40 mg

2. Alginate dressing, 36 sq inch pad

3. Wheelchair accessory tray

4. Trimming of dystrophic nails

5. Adult, long arm cast, fiberglass

Multiple Choice

1. Which HCPCS codes are used to report DME?
   a. E codes
   b. A codes
   c. K codes
   d. L codes

2. Mr. McGee received a new power pressure-reducing air mattress for his hospital bed. Select the correct code for the mattress.
   a. E0272
   b. E0373
   c. E0186
   d. E0277

3. There are _____ temporary code sets.
   a. one
   b. two
   c. three
   d. four

4. During a nebulizer treatment the physician administered 2 mg of albuterol. Select the correct code for the drug.
   a. J7620
   b. J7611
   c. J7613 × 2
   d. J7613

5. The physician performed a CLIA Waived laboratory test in his office on a Medicare patient. What HCPCS modifier would be appended to the laboratory test?
   a. GZ
   b. GY
   c. QQ
   d. QW

6. A patient with peripheral neuropathy was prescribed a pair of custom diabetic shoes. The shoes were molded from casts of the patient's feet. Select the correct HCPCS code.
   a. A5500
   b. A5501 × 2
   c. A5501
   d. A5506 × 2

7. While playing in her back yard, 6-year-old Melanie fell off her swing set and dislocated her ankle. The orthopedist performed a closed treatment of the ankle and applied a fiberglass short leg cast. Select the HCPCS code for the casting material(s).
   a. Q4045
   b. Q4046
   c. Q4047
   d. Q4048

8. A patient with advanced arthritis of the spine with limited mobility was prescribed a semi-electric hospital bed with mattress and rails. Select the correct HCPCS code(s).
   a. E0260
   b. E0261, E0272
   c. E0265
   d. E0266, E0272

9. A 68-year-old Medicare-established patient presented to the gynecologist for her preventive routine Pap test and breast examination. The physician sent the specimen to the laboratory for processing. Code for the services of the physician.
   a. 99397
   b. 99397, 99000
   c. G0101
   d. G0101, Q0091

10. Orthotic procedures and devices are reported:
   a. With both E codes and L codes
   b. With L codes only
   c. With A codes and L codes
   d. With G codes and L codes

Assign the Appropriate Diagnostic Code

1. The correct answer is **J9280.** We can locate the correct code by using Appendix 1, The Table of Drugs. When we look up mitomycin, we find J9280. Because the amount administered is 40 mg, we would report the code 8 times (J9280 ×8).

2. The correct answer is **A6197.** The key term is *dressing*. When we look up *dressing* in the Alphabetic Index, we are presented with the various types of dressing. Because we are looking for an alginate dressing, we are given the code range A6196–A6199. When we go to the A section of the HCPCS book and look at the codes our choices are:

   a. A6196 Alginate or other fiber gelling dressing, wound cover, sterile, pad size 16 sq in or less, each dressing

   b. A6197 Alginate or other fiber gelling dressing, wound cover, sterile, pad size more than 16 sq in but less than or equal to 48 sq in, each dressing

   c. A6198 Alginate or other fiber gelling dressing, wound cover, sterile, pad size more than 48 sq in, each dressing

   d. A6199 Alginate or other fiber gelling dressing, wound filler, sterile, per 6

   At first glance they all appear to be the same; the difference is in the size of the dressing. Because our dressing is a 36 sq inch pad, the correct code would be A6197, which lists the size as more than 16 sq inches but less than or equal to 48 sq inch, each dressing.

3. The correct answer is **E0950.** In the Alphabetic Index, the key term is *wheelchair*. It is further modified by the word *tray,* which is represented by HCPCS code E0950. When we look up E0950 in the E section, we can confirm this is the correct code: E0950 Wheelchair accessory, tray, each.

4. The correct answer is **G0127.** In the Alphabetic Index, the key term is *trimming* or *trim*. It is further modified by the word *nails,* which is represented by G0127.When we look up G0127 in the G section, we can confirm this is the correct code: G0127 Trimming of dystrophic nails, any number.

5. The correct answer is **Q4006.** In the Alphabetic Index, the key term is *cast.* It is further modified by the words *long arm,* which is represented by the code range Q4005–Q4008. When we look up the

code range in the Q section, we are presented with the following choices:

   a. Q4005 Cast supplies, long arm cast, adult (11 years +), plaster

   b. Q4006 Cast supplies, long arm cast, adult (11 years +), fiberglass

   c. Q4007 Cast supplies, long arm cast, pediatric (0–10 years), plaster

   d. Q4008 Cast supplies, long arm cast, pediatric (0–10 years), fiberglass

   Because we are looking for an adult cast, we can eliminate Q4007 and Q4008, as they both represent pediatric casts. We can then eliminate Q4005, which represents a plaster cast. This leaves us with the correct code: Q4006 Cast supplies, long arm cast, adult (11 years +), fiberglass.

Multiple Choice Answers

1. The correct answer is **a.** E codes are used to report DME. Answer **b.** is incorrect, as A codes are used to report miscellaneous services and supplies. Answer **c.** is incorrect, as K codes are *temporary* codes for supplies, DME, and drugs. Answer **d.** is incorrect, as L codes are used to report orthotics and prosthetics.

2. The correct answer is **d.** Although all of the codes listed represent mattresses, each code represents a different type of mattress. Answer **a.,** HCPCS code E0272, is incorrect, as it represents a foam rubber mattress. Answer **b.,** HCPCS code E0373, is incorrect, as it represents a nonpowered advanced pressure-reducing mattress, and answer **c.,** HCPCS code E0186, is incorrect, as it represents an air pressure mattress.

3. The correct answer is **d.** The four temporary code sets are G codes, K codes, Q codes, and S codes.

4. The correct answer is **c.** HCPCS code J7613 Albuterol, inhalation solution, FDA-approved final product, noncompounded, administered through DME, unit dose, 1 mg, would be coded two times, as the code represents 1 mg and the patient received 2 mg. Answer **a.** is incorrect, as J7620 includes *ipratropium bromide,* which was not administered to the patient. Answer **b.** is incorrect, as J7611 represents a concentrated form of albuterol, and answer **d.** is incorrect, as it represents only 1 mg of albuterol and the patient received 2 mg of the drug.

5. The correct answer is **d.** The QW modifier is reported to indicate a CLIA Waived test. Answer **a.** is incorrect, as the GZ modifier is used to report an item or service expected to be denied as not reasonable and necessary. Answer **b.** is incorrect, as the GY modifier is reported to indicate an item or service statutorily excluded, does not meet the definition of any Medicare benefit or, for non-Medicare insurers, is not a contract benefit. Answer **c.** is incorrect, as the QQ modifier is used to report a claim that was submitted without a written statement of intent.

6. The correct answer is **b.** HCPCS code A5501 ×2 For diabetics only, fitting (including follow-up), custom preparation and supply of shoe molded from cast(s) of patient's foot (custom molded shoe), *per shoe* is coded twice, as the patient received a *pair* of shoes and the HCPCS code A5501 represents only one shoe. Answer **c.** is incorrect, because although this is the correct HCPCS code, it represents only one shoe. Answer **a.** is incorrect, as HCPCS code A5500 represents one "off-the-shelf" diabetic shoe. Answer **d.** is incorrect because, although it represents a *pair* of shoes, the code A5506 represents off-the-shelf diabetic shoes "with offset heels."

7. The correct answer is **d.** HCPCS code Q4048 Cast supplies, short leg splint, pediatric (0–10 years), fiberglass. Answer **a.** is incorrect, as HCPCS code Q4045 represents a plaster adult cast for ages 11 and over. Answer **b.**, HCPCS code Q4046, is incorrect because, although it represents a fiberglass cast, it is for adults ages 11 and over. Answer **c.**, HCPCS code Q4047, is incorrect because, although the cast is for a pediatric patient, the cast described by this code is plaster.

8. The correct answer is **a.** HCPCS code E0260 Hospital bed, *semi-electric* (head and foot adjustment), with any type side rails, *with mattress.* In this case, the one HCPCS code is sufficient for both the appropriate type of bed and the mattress. Answer **d.** is incorrect, as HCPCS code E0266 represents a *total* electric bed without a mattress and HCPCS code E0272 represents a foam rubber mattress. Answer **b.** is incorrect because, while HCPCS code E0261 represents a semi-electric bed, it is without a mattress, and HCPCS code E0272 represents a foam rubber mattress. Answer **c.** is incorrect because, although HCPCS code E0265 represents a hospital bed with a mattress, the type of bed it describes is a *total* electric bed, whereas the patient in our scenario received a *semi*-electric bed.

9. The correct answer is **d.** When billing Medicare, the appropriate HCPCS code, if one exists, takes precedence over a CPT code, and therefore we can automatically eliminate answers **a.** and **b.**, both of which are CPT codes. Additionally, answer **d.** describes both the Pap test and breast examination (i.e., G0101 Cervical or vaginal cancer screening; pelvic and clinical breast examination) as well as the conveyance of the specimen for processing (i.e., Q0091 Screening Papanicolaou smear; obtaining, preparing and conveyance of cervical or vaginal smear to laboratory). Answer **c.** is incorrect, as it does not include obtaining and preparing the Pap smear for the laboratory.

10. The correct answer is **b.** Orthotic procedures and devices are reported with L codes. Answer **a.** is incorrect, as E codes are used to report DME. Answer **c.** is incorrect, as A codes are used to report miscellaneous services and supplies. Answer **d.** is incorrect, as G codes are used to report temporary procedures and professional services.

6

Current Procedural Terminology

Current Procedural Terminology (CPT) was developed by the American Medical Association (AMA) to translate medical, surgical, and diagnostic services into numeric data (codes). These data are used to process insurance claims, analyze information, and provide uniform communication among physicians, accreditation organizations, coders, and billers.

For example, an open treatment of patellar fracture, with internal fixation and/or partial or complete patellectomy and soft-tissue repair, can be communicated with just one CPT code, 27524. Despite the complexity of the description of the procedure/service, one code captures all of the aspects of that service. The CPT code enables us to communicate the service provided accurately and quickly.

Unlike ICD-9-CM codes, which describe *why* the provider performed the service, CPT codes describe *what* the provider did or what service was provided.

The codes, descriptions, and guidelines in CPT are utilized by physicians and other health-care providers, such as physical therapists, occupational therapists, audiologists, and social workers.

Codes listed in a specific section of the CPT manual do not limit the use of the code to the section in which it is listed. For example, CPT code 69210 Removal impacted cerumen (ear wax), 1 or both ears is located in the Auditory subsection of the Surgery section. However, the removal of ear wax may be performed by a pediatrician, family practice physician, nurse practitioner, or any other qualified physician or health-care provider and is not limited to a surgeon or an otolaryngologist (ear, nose, and throat) physician.

Types of CPT Codes

There are three types of CPT codes:

Category I Codes represent codes that have been approved by the AMA Editorial Panel. They are used by providers to report most of their services. To be assigned a Category I status, a CPT code must meet certain criteria: the procedure or service is approved by the Food and Drug Administration (FDA), the procedure or service is performed nationally by health-care providers, and the clinical efficacy of the procedure or service is proven.

Category II Codes represent tracking codes that are used for performance measurement. They simplify the collection and reporting of data at the time of service, precluding labor-intense chart review and record abstraction, and they make possible the collection of data regarding the quality of care provided by coding various services and test results that support nationally established performance measures. Because Category II codes describe services that are included in an evaluation and management service, they are not associated with a relative value unit (RVU). *Category II codes are optional* and may not be used as a substitute for a Category I code. Category II codes are easily identifiable: they consist of four numerals followed by the letter F (0001F-7025F).

Category III Codes represent temporary codes for emerging technology, services, and procedures. These include services or procedures that may not be commonly performed by many physicians and health-care providers or that are not FDA-approved and have not yet been proved for clinical efficacy. The reporting of CPT Category III codes enables researchers to track emerging technology, services, and procedures to validate widespread use and clinical efficacy. It is important to note that *if a Category III code exists that is applicable to the service you are reporting, it must be used instead of a Category I code.* These codes are easily identifiable because they are four numerals followed by the letter T (0016T-0207T).

KEY CODING TIP

When making your CPT code selection, you must select the code that *accurately* describes the service provided. It is *inappropriate to use* a code that *"comes close to"* or is *"approximate to"* the service provided. If you are unable to locate a specific code, the appropriate *unlisted* CPT code should be selected. Because medicine is a constantly evolving field, it is equally important to select codes from the current version of CPT.

How the CPT Codebook Is Organized

Sections of the CPT

The CPT is divided into six main sections: Evaluation and Management, Anesthesia, Surgery, Radiology, Pathology and Laboratory, and Medicine. With the exception of the Evaluation and Management section, which is the first section of the CPT codebook, the sections are presented in numeric order (i.e., based on the numeric ordering of the codes). These sections provide most of the CPT codes reported by physicians and nonphysician providers, as these codes are used to report various types of physician/nonphysician encounters (office visits, hospital visits), anesthesia services, surgical procedures, diagnostic and therapeutic procedures, and radiology and pathology services.

Each section begins with "Guidelines," which are a *must-read* because they provide coding guidance specific to that chapter. Notes pertaining to groups of codes or individual specific codes are also located throughout the CPT book before or after CPT codes.

Each section is further divided into subsections, subheadings, categories, and subcategories. Because the Surgery section is the largest of the CPT book, let's use it as our example.

The Surgery section is divided into subsections that begin immediately following the Surgery Guidelines.

Subsections include Integumentary System, Musculoskeletal System, Respiratory System, and Cardiovascular System, to name just a few (there are 19 subsections in in the Surgery section). We can always identify what subsection we are in by looking at the top of the page.

For example: Surgery/Nervous System

The section is **Surgery,** and the subsection is **Nervous System.** The subsection is further divided into subheadings, categories, and subcategories. Each division identifies anatomy, procedures, conditions, descriptions, or approaches. For example:

Nervous System ←——→ **Subsection**
Extracranial Nerves, Peripheral Nerves, and Autonomic Nervous System ←——→ **Subheading**
Introduction/Injection of Anesthetic Agent (Nerve Block), Diagnostic or Therapeutic ←—→ **Category**
Somatic Nerves ←————→ **Subcategory**

Format of CPT Codes

The formats of the CPT codes include standalone descriptions known as "standalone codes" and indented descriptions known as "indented codes." Standalone codes include the full description of the code. Some codes are indented to save space. With indented codes, the language before the semicolon of the previous nonindented CPT code (the "common part" of the code) is implied as part of the indented code. For example:

10120 Incision and removal of foreign body, subcutaneous tissues; simple
   10121 complicated

To get the full description of CPT code 10121, which is indented, we must read the portion of the previous nonindented CPT code 10120 up to the semicolon *and* the description of CPT code 10121. Therefore, the full description of CPT code 10121 would be: 10121 Incision and removal of foreign body, subcutaneous tissues; complicated.

Unlisted Procedure Codes

Unlisted codes represent new and emerging technologies, many procedures that are considered experimental, and services for which there is no Category I or Category III CPT code.

When reporting an unlisted procedure code, **documentation in the form of a special report** must be submitted. The report should include a description of the need for the procedure; the nature and extent of the procedure; and the effort, time, and any special equipment or technique necessary to provide the service. Unlisted procedure codes by body site are given in the Surgery Guidelines, and individual unlisted procedure codes can be found at the end of subsections or subheadings as appropriate. You can easily locate unlisted procedure codes in the CPT index by looking up "Unlisted Services and Procedures."

We discuss and practice locating these CPT codes later in the chapter.

Category II Codes

These two sections immediately follow the six main sections that provide the Category I codes. They are organized according to standard clinical documentation categories, such as Composite Measures, Patient Management, Patient History, Physical Examination, and Patient Safety.

Category III Codes

This section provides a list of Category III codes, the temporary codes used for emerging technology, services, and procedures that cannot be described by a nonspecific Category I unlisted code.

Appendixes

Appendix A is a complete list of modifiers. Modifiers provide additional information about the service provided without changing the description of the service. (See Chapter 7 of this textbook for a detailed discussion.)

Appendix B is a list of additions, deletions, and revisions to the CPT manual. When a code has been changed, the changed text is also listed in Appendix B.

Appendix C provides clinical vignettes or examples of many of the Evaluation and Management codes.

Appendix D is a list of the CPT add-on codes. These codes are identified by the plus (+) symbol.

Appendix E is a list of the CPT codes that are modifier 51 exempt. These codes are identified by a circle with a line through it.

Appendix F is a list of CPT codes that are modifier 63 exempt (procedures performed on infants less than 4 kg).

Appendix G is a list of CPT codes that include moderate conscious sedation. These codes are identified with a bull's-eye.

Appendix H is an alphabetical listing of clinical topics (alphabetical listing). Because this has become a continually expanding source of information linking to CPT Category II codes, this appendix has been removed from the CPT manual and can be accessed on the AMA Web site at www.ama.org/ go/cpt.

Appendix I is a list of Genetic Testing Code Modifiers. The modifiers in this appendix are reported with molecular laboratory procedures relating to genetic testing. These are two-character alphanumeric modifiers and are categorized by mutation (e.g., Neoplasia [Sarcoma], Neurologic, Non-Neoplastic). The *first* character is *numeric,* and it represents the *disease* category; the *second* character is *alpha,* and it represents the *gene* type.

For example: In modifier 3A, the number 3 represents non-neoplastic hematology/coagulation (the disease), and the letter A represents Factor V Leiden (the gene).

Appendix J is the Electrodiagnostic Medicine Listing of Sensory, Motor, and Mixed Nerves. This is an excellent resource when coding nerve conduction studies (NCS) and electromyograms (EMG). The appendix lists each sensory, motor, and mixed nerve with the appropriate NCS CPT code. It also includes a table that gives the reasonable maximum number of studies per diagnostic category necessary for a physician to arrive at a diagnosis in 90% of patients with that final diagnosis.

For example: If the patient has symptoms of carpal tunnel (unilateral), it is recommended the physician perform one needle EMG, three motor NCS, and four sensory NCS to confirm the diagnosis.

Appendix K is a list of Products Pending FDA Approval. These codes are identified by the flash symbol.

Appendix L is a list of the order of vascular families. The table makes the assumption the catheterization starting point is the aorta and lists the first-order, second-order, and third-order branches and beyond. If the vessel were to be accessed at another location, this categorization would be inaccurate. This table is helpful when coding catheterizations.

Appendix M is a summary of deleted codes and their descriptors and a crosswalk to the current code.

Appendix N is a summary of CPT codes that do not appear in numeric sequence within the CPT manual.

Index

The alphabetic index includes entries by procedure and anatomic site as well as procedures known by their eponyms and other designators. The first page of the index provides a quick reference for looking up a CPT code. We review the various methods of looking up a CPT code later in this chapter. It is important to note you should *never select a CPT code from the index:* you must *always look up the code in the main text* to determine if the code is accurate and to refer to any coding guidelines relating to the code.

Code Symbols

Just like the ICD-9-CM, the CPT uses signs and symbols throughout the book.

New Codes. New codes are identified by a bullet (•) located in front of the CPT code.

• **90460** Immunization administration through 18 years of age via any route of administration, with counseling by physician or other qualified health care professional; first vaccine/toxoid

Changed Codes. Codes whose descriptor has changed since the last edition are identified by a triangle (▲) in front of the code. Additions, deletions, and revisions to the code descriptor are all considered changes. See Appendix B for a complete list of changed codes.

▲ **64708** Neuroplasty, major peripheral nerve, arm or leg, open; other than specified

New or Revised Text. You can easily identify the changes in the code or the guidelines by looking for the text written between right and left triangles (▶◀).

See Appendix B for a complete list of revised text.

▶ (Report 64611 with modifier 52 if fewer than four salivary glands are injected) ◀

Add-on codes. Many procedures in the CPT are routinely carried out *in addition* to a primary procedure. These additional codes are called "add-on codes" and are identified by a plus sign (+) located in front of the code. You can also easily identify these codes by the terminology in their descriptor, such as, *"each additional"* or *"list separately in addition to primary procedure."* Add-on codes are *never reported alone* and are *always reported in addition to the primary procedure performed.* A complete list of add-on codes is given in Appendix D.

+ **15301** each additional 100 sq cm, or each additional 1% of body area of infants and children, or part thereof (list separately in addition to code for primary procedure)

Exemptions to modifier -51. Codes representing procedures that are exempt from modifier -51 (multiple procedures) are identified with a circle with a line through it (⊘). A complete list of procedures that are modifier -51 exempt is located in Appendix E.

⊘ **17004** Destruction (e.g., laser surgery, electrosurgery, cryosurgery, chemosurgery, surgical curettement), premalignant lesions (e.g., actinic keratoses), 15 or more lesions

Moderate Conscious Sedation. CPT codes that *include* moderate conscious sedation (described in Chapter 9) are identified with a bull's-eye (⊙). A list of CPT codes that include moderate conscious sedation is located in Appendix G.

⊙ **49440** Insertion of gastrostomy tube, percutaneous, under fluoroscopic guidance including contrast injection(s), image documentation and report

FDA approval pending. CPT codes that are pending FDA approval and have been assigned a CPT code are identified by a flash symbol (𝒩)

Reference. Many CPT codes include a reference to the *CPT Assistant, CPT Changes: An Insider's View,* or *Clinical Examples in Radiology* to further clarify the description of the code and the context in which the codes are to be reported. Such references are indicated with a circle around an arrow (➲). (These additional CPT resources are described later in this chapter.)

77080 Dual-energy X-ray absorptiometry (DXA), bone density study, 1 or more sites; axial skeleton (e.g., hips, pelvis, spine)

➲CPT Assistant Mar 07:7; CPT Changes: An Insider's View 2007

➲Clinical Examples in Radiology Fall 07:11

Reinstated or recycled codes. These codes are identified with a circle (○) in front of the code.

Out-of-numerical-sequence code. These codes are identified with a (#) in front of the code.

#21552 Excision, tumor, soft tissue of neck or anterior thorax, subcutaneous; 3 cm or greater

The term *Code is out of numerical sequence. See...* is placed numerically as an alert to direct the user to the location of the out-of-sequence code.

KEY CODING TIP
The inner front flap of your CPT book includes a quick guide to the symbols used in the CPT manual.

Symbols
▲ Revised code
• New code
▶◀ New or revised text
➲ Reference to *CPT Assistant, Clinical Examples in Radiology,* and *CPT Changes*
+ Add-on code
⊘ Exemptions to modifier 51
⊙ Moderate sedation
𝒩 Product pending FDA approval
○ Reinstated or recycled code
Out-of-numerical-sequence code

Locating CPT Codes

Located in the back of the CPT manual is an alphabetic index. Headings at the top right and top left corners of each page list the entries included on that page.

The code numbers appear in three different ways:

Single code choice:	Cyst	
	bladder	51500
Multiple code choices:	Cyst	
	brain	61515, 61524, 62162
Range of code choice:	Cyst	
	brachial	42810-42815

All code selections must be verified in the tabular section of CPT, even if there is only one code choice. Multiple code choices are separated by a comma; in this case, each code listed must be verified. In the case of a range of code choices (i.e., separated by a hyphen), you must verify each code within the given code range.

The index is organized by main terms followed by subterms. Before looking up a code, you must identify the main term. To do so, ask: "What procedure or service was performed?" Your answer will be your main term. For example, biopsy or colonoscopy; if you are unable to easily identify the main term, there are alternative ways to look up a CPT code. Let's take a look at these now:

1. Service or procedure; for example, arthroscopy, aspiration, excision, x-ray

2. Anatomic site; for example, brain, femur, cervix, eyelid

3. Condition or disease; for example, encephalitis, cyst, hypothermia, fracture

4. Synonym (words with similar meanings); for example, the word *wrist* is synonymous with the medical term *carpal bone.* If we look up the word wrist, we are directed to "see Arm, lower; Carpal bone." In this case, we can not only locate the correct CPT code by following the reference, we can also use the CPT to help identify the correct medical term.

5. Eponym (the person for whom something is named); for example, Abbe-Estlander procedure, Barr procedure, Bernstein test

6. Abbreviation; for example, CBC, CCU, CD4, ERCP

Let's Practice Coding

Locating a code by service or procedure

Let's look up the CPT code for **colonoscopy with polyp removal by snare technique.** We first identify the main term by the type of procedure performed, in this case, colonoscopy. In the CPT index, we look up colonoscopy (main term). Next, we consider what was done during the colonoscopy: removal of a polyp. We then look up "removal" as the subterm of "colonoscopy." We further modify the subterm with the word "polyp."

Colonoscopy ⟷ Main Term
Removal ⟷ Subterm
Polyp   45384-45385 ⟷ CPT code Range

Next, we look up and review our two choices in the tabular part of the CPT book before making our decision:

45384 Colonoscopy, flexible, proximal to splenic flexure; with removal of tumor(s), polyp(s), or other lesion(s) by hot biopsy forceps or bipolar cautery

45385 Colonoscopy, flexible, proximal to splenic flexure; with removal of tumor(s), polyp(s), or other lesion(s) *by snare technique*

At first glance, both codes appear to have a similar descriptor. However, when we look closer, we see that in **CPT code 45384** the polyp is removed by hot biopsy forceps or bipolar cautery, and in **CPT code 45385** the polyp is removed by snare technique, making 45385 our correct code choice.

Locating a code by anatomic site

We also can look up the procedure by the anatomic site, in this case, the *colon.*

Colon ⟷ Main term
Endoscopy ⟷ Subterm
Removal ⟷ Subterm
Polyp   44392, 45384-45385 ⟷ Multiple choice, code range

Let's Practice Coding—cont'd

We are presented with both a single choice and a code range.

44392 Colonoscopy *through stoma;* with removal of tumor(s), polyp(s), or other lesion(s) by hot biopsy forceps or bipolar cautery

45384 Colonoscopy, flexible, proximal to splenic flexure; with removal of tumor(s), polyp(s), or other lesion(s) by hot biopsy forceps or bipolar cautery

45385 Colonoscopy, flexible, proximal to splenic flexure; with removal of tumor(s), polyp(s), or other lesion(s) *by snare technique*

We are now presented with an additional CPT code (44392) to consider, which offers an additional approach, through stoma. With our patient, however, colonoscopy was not performed through stoma; furthermore, code 44392 again describes hot biopsy forceps or bipolar cautery. We select the code describing the polyp removal by snare technique, code 45385.

We also can find the correct code by beginning our search with the main term "removal," subterm "polyp," subterm "colon," which presents a code choice of 44392, 45385. Once we review the two choices, we can identify the correct code as 44385.

ANESTHESIA CODES: *An exception*

Anesthesia codes are very easily found by looking them up in the index under the main term "anesthesia" followed by the subterm of either the body area (e.g., abdomen, knee) or the procedure (e.g., embolectomy, hysterectomy). For additional information on how to locate anesthesia codes, please see Chapter 9.

KEY CODING TIP

Remember there are a number of ways you can look up a CPT code: by service or procedure, by anatomic site, by condition or disease, by synonym, or by eponym or abbreviation.

Learn More About It

The more you read, the more you know. Increase your knowledge with the following resources.

Additional CPT Resources

The *CPT Assistant* and *CPT Changes: An Insider's View* are published by the AMA. *Clinical Examples in Radiology* is published by both the AMA and the American College of Radiology.

The *CPT Assistant* is a newsletter containing in-depth information, coding tips, and vignettes for many of the CPT codes. It is a valuable resource for claims appeals and for validating code selections to auditors. *CPT Changes: An Insider's View* is published once a year, and it contains interpretations and rationales for every new, revised, and deleted CPT code and guideline change. *Clinical Examples in Radiology* is a newsletter that provides coding guidance specific to radiology coding scenarios.

Vocabulary Words

In your CPT book on a blank note page in the Introduction, write the following vocabulary words:

Classification–the distribution of things into classes or categories of the same type.

Nomenclature–a system of words used to name things in a particular discipline.

Relative Value Unit–quantifies the relative work, practice expense, and malpractice costs for physician services. RVUs are used in the calculation of a fee amount for physician services.

Acronyms and Abbreviations

In your CPT book on a blank note page in the Introduction, write the following acronyms and abbreviations:

AMA–**A**merican **M**edical **A**ssociation

CPT–**C**urrent **P**rocedural **T**erminology

RVU–**R**elative **V**alue **U**nit

TAKE THE CODING CHALLENGE

Assign the Appropriate CPT Code

1. Core needle biopsy of breast with imaging guidance

2. Incision and drainage of eyelid abscess

3. Insertion of intrauterine device (IUD)

_____

4. Diagnostic knee arthroscopy

_____

5. Unlisted procedure, arm

_____

Multiple Choice

1. Add-on codes are used:
a. As primary codes under certain circumstances
b. To identify the portion of a procedure that is usually considered bundled or inclusive to a primary procedure
c. To identify procedures that are usually carried out in addition to a primary procedure
d. To identify standalone codes

2. Which category of CPT codes represents codes that are used to collect and report data at the time of services for performance measurement?
a. Category I
b. Category II
c. Category III
d. All of the above

3. When looking up codes in the CPT index, the terms _proctosigmoidoscopy, cyst,_ and _eyelid_ would all be considered:
a. Cross references
b. Subheading
c. Main terms
d. Headings

4. A bull's-eye (☉) in front of a CPT code indicates:
a. Moderate conscious sedation is not included in the service.
b. Moderate conscious sedation was personally provided by an anesthesiologist.
c. Moderate conscious sedation is included in the service.
d. Moderate conscious sedation is performed by the physician who is providing the service.

5. A special report should be submitted when reporting an unlisted CPT code. The special report should include:
a. Effort, time, and special equipment
b. Need, service, and extent of procedure
c. Effort, need, and anatomic site
d. Time, effort, and the patient's condition

6. Select the correct CPT code for a flexible esophagoscopy, with removal of two tumor(s), by hot biopsy:
a. 43217
b. 43216
c. 43215
d. 43219

7. While playing in his backyard, 8-year-old John fell out of the tree he was climbing. When the tree branch snapped, a piece of tree branch landed in his eye. He was taken to the pediatrician and, upon examination, the foreign body was noted to be superficially located in the conjunctiva. The pediatrician removed the foreign body from John's external eye. Select the correct CPT code:
a. 65210
b. 65220
c. 65205
d. 65235

8. Select the correct CPT code for excision of a 1.2-cm malignant lesion of the scalp:
a. 11622
b. 11602
c. 11422
d. 11642

9. When there is no specific CPT code or Category III code to identify the service, you should:
a. Select the CPT code that comes closest to the service provided.
b. Select the CPT code that comes closest to the service provided and append the appropriate modifier.
c. Select an unlisted code.
d. Select the Category II code that best describes the service provided.

10. Experimental procedures and temporary codes for emerging technology services and procedures would be reported with:
a. An unlisted code
b. A Category III code
c. A Category I code with the appropriate modifier
d. An unlisted CPT code only if a Category III code is not available

ANSWERS AND RATIONALES

Assign the Appropriate CPT Code

1. The correct answer is 19102 Biopsy of breast; percutaneous, needle core, using imaging guidance. In the CPT index, you look up the main term, *biopsy,* subterm, *breast.* You are presented with a code range 19100-19103. Upon review and after you have verified the code in the tabular section of the CPT book, CPT code 19102 is the correct choice. You could also look up the code by anatomic site using *breast* as the main term and *biopsy* as the subterm; in this case, you are presented with the same code range.

2. The correct answer is 67700 Blepharotomy, drainage of abscess, eyelid. In the CPT index, you could use *abscess* as the main term, *eyelid* as the subterm, and *incision and drainage* as an additional subterm. You are presented with a single code, 67700, which when verified in the tabular section of the CPT book is determined to be the correct code. You could also look up the code by using *eyelid* as the main term, *abscess* as the subterm, and *incision and drainage* as an additional subterm, which leads to the same single code choice of 67700.

3. The correct answer is 58300 Insertion of intrauterine device (IUD). In the CPT index, if you look up *IUD* as a main term, you are directed to "see intrauterine device." When you look up *intrauterine device,* your subterm will be *insertion,* which will give you a single code of 58300. After verifying it in the tabular section of the CPT book, you would select it as the correct code.

4. The correct answer is 29870 Arthroscopy, knee, diagnostic, with or without synovial biopsy (separate procedure). In the CPT index, using the main term *arthroscopy,* subterm *diagnostic,* and additional subterm *knee,* you are presented with a single code, 29870, which when verified in the tabular section of the CPT book is correct. You could also use *knee* as the main term, *arthroscopy* as a subterm, and *diagnostic* as an additional subterm, which will also present you with one code, 29870. After verifying it in the tabular section of the CPT book, you would select it as the correct code.

5. The correct answer is 25999 Unlisted procedure, forearm or wrist. Using *unlisted services and procedures* and the subterm *arm,* you are presented with a single code, 25999. After verifying it in the tabular section of the CPT book, you would select it as the correct code. You can also locate this unlisted code by looking in the Surgery Guidelines under "unlisted service or procedure," which presents you with a list of all the unlisted CPT codes in the surgery section.

Multiple Choice Answers

1. The correct answer is **c.** Add-on codes are services that are usually carried out in addition to a primary service. Answer **a.** is incorrect, as add-on codes are never reported alone and therefore can never be primary codes. Answer **b.** is incorrect, as CPT codes that are usually inclusive to a primary procedure are listed as "separate procedure" codes (please refer to the Introduction to Surgery chapter). Answer **d.** is incorrect, as not all add-on codes include the full CPT code description.

2. The correct answer is **b.** Category II codes are supplemental tracking codes used for performance measurement and allow the collection of data at the time of service as opposed to record abstraction or chart review, and the use of these codes is optional. Category I codes are CPT codes approved by the AMA Editorial Panel and are used to report nationally recognized, FDA-approved services associated with a relative value unit. Category III codes are used to report new and emerging technology, and reporting these codes if one is available is mandatory.

3. The correct answer is **c.** All of these terms can be used as main terms when looking up CPT codes. Main terms may include (1) service or procedure; (2) anatomic site; (3) eponyms, synonyms, and abbreviations; and (4) condition or disease. *Proctosigmoidoscopy* is the procedure in this case; *cyst* is the disease or condition; and *eyelid* is the anatomic site. Answer **a.** is incorrect, as cross references in CPT will include the word "see." Answers **b.** and **d.** are incorrect, as subheadings and headings are located in the main body of the CPT and not in the index; subterms are located in the index.

4. The correct answer is **c.** A bull's-eye in front of a CPT code indicates moderate conscious sedation is included in the CPT code. Answer **a.** is incorrect, as you would not report moderate conscious sedation in addition to CPT codes identified with a bull's-eye. Answers **b.** and **d.** are incorrect, as the bull's-eye does not refer to "who" provided the service

5. The correct answer is **a.** Effort, time, and special equipment must be included in the special report. The full description of a special report and what is included in a special report is located in the surgery guidelines. Answers **b., c.,** and **d.** are incorrect; although the need, effort, time, and extent of the procedure should be included in the special report, the service, anatomic site, and patient's condition are detailed in the operative report.

6. The correct answer is **b.** 43216 Esophagoscopy, rigid or flexible; with removal of tumor(s), polyp(s), or other lesion(s) by hot biopsy forceps or bipolar cautery. Answer **a.** is incorrect, as CPT code 43217 Esophagoscopy, rigid or flexible; with removal of tumor(s), polyp(s), or other lesion(s) *by snare technique*, describes tumor removal by snare technique. Answer **c.** is incorrect: 43215 Esophagoscopy, rigid or flexible; with removal of *foreign body*, describes a foreign body removal. Answer **d.** is incorrect: 43219 Esophagoscopy, rigid or flexible; with *insertion of plastic tube or stent*, describes the insertion of a plastic tube or stent.

7. The correct answer is **c.** 65205 Removal of foreign body, external eye; conjunctival superficial. Answer **a.** is incorrect: 65210 Removal of foreign body, external eye; conjunctival *embedded* (includes concretions), subconjunctival, or scleral nonperforating, describes an embedded foreign body. Answer **b.** is incorrect: 65220 Removal of foreign body, external eye; *corneal, without slit lamp*, describes a foreign body removal from the cornea. Answer **d.** is incorrect: 65235 Removal of foreign body, *intraocular;* from anterior chamber of eye or lens, describes an intraocular foreign body removal.

8. The correct answer is **a.** 11622 Excision, malignant lesion including margins, scalp, neck, hands, feet, genitalia; excised diameter 1.1 to 2.0 cm. Answer **b.** is incorrect: 11602 Excision, malignant lesion including margins, *trunk, arms, or legs;* excised diameter 1.1 to 2.0 cm, describes a lesion located on the trunk, arms, or legs, not the scalp. Answer **c.** is incorrect: although the site and size of the lesion are correct in 11422 Excision, *benign* lesion including margins, except skin tag (unless listed elsewhere), scalp, neck, hands, feet, genitalia; excised diameter 1.1 to 2.0 cm, the lesion is benign, and you need to code for a malignant lesion. Answer **d.** is incorrect: in 11642 Excision, malignant lesion including margins, *face, ears, eyelids, nose, lips;* excised diameter 1.1 to 2.0 cm, the lesion is located on the face, ears, eyelids, nose, or lips, whereas the lesion you are coding is located on the scalp.

9. The correct answer is **c.** You would select an unlisted code. Answer **a.** is incorrect, as you would never select a code that comes close to or is almost the same as the service provided. Answer **b.** is incorrect, as there is no modifier to represent unlisted services. Answer **d.** is incorrect, as Category II codes are used to report performance measures.

10. The correct answer is **d.** You report any experimental procedure or temporary codes for emerging technology with an unlisted CPT code only if a Category III code is not available. Answer **a.** is incorrect, as you use the unlisted code only if a Category III code is not available. Answer **b.** is incorrect, as a Category III code is not available, you use the unlisted code. Answer **c.** is incorrect, as there is no modifier to report an unlisted service.

CHAPTER 7

CPT Modifiers

What Are Modifiers?

There are two types of modifiers: CPT modifiers (Level I) and HCPCS modifiers (Level II). This chapter focuses on the CPT modifiers only. The HCPCS modifiers are addressed in Chapter 5.

A CPT modifier is a two-position numeric code (with the exception of Anesthesia Physical Status modifiers, which are alphanumeric) that is added to the end of a CPT code, separated by a hyphen. Modifiers allow you to alert the insurance carrier, without changing the description of the CPT code itself, that something is *different* about the procedure (or other service) that the CPT code is meant to report.

For example, a patient may present to the physician for a core needle biopsy with imaging guidance of both breasts. The CPT code for the procedure is **19102 Biopsy of breast; percutaneous, needle core, using imaging guidance.** However, this code alone does not indicate that the service was provided bilaterally (on both breasts). The insurance carrier is alerted that the service was performed on both breasts by use of modifier 50–Bilateral procedure. The modifier is appended to the end of the CPT code as follows: 19102-50. As you can see, appending the modifier does not change the notification that a core needle breast biopsy was performed; the modifier merely provides the insurance carrier with additional information—that the service was performed on both breasts.

In some cases, it may be necessary to append more than one modifier to a single CPT code to accurately describe the service.

Some modifiers are appended only to specific types of CPT codes. For example, modifier 24–Unrelated Evaluation & Management (E/M) service by the same physician during a postoperative period would always be appended to an E/M code.

It is important to note, however, that not all CPT codes require modifiers.

Modifiers can increase or decrease your reimbursement; therefore, it is important to understand how and when to use them. They can also eliminate the appearance of duplicate billing and mitigate CCI (Correct Coding Initiative)[1] edits.

Because modifiers have an impact on reimbursement, modifier usage is often reviewed by many of the insurance carriers. Therefore, correct use of modifiers is important not only for correct payment but also for compliance purposes.

Appendix A in the CPT manual includes a complete list of Level I modifiers and some Level II modifiers (HCPCS).

The CPT Modifiers—and How to Use Them

Let's take a look at the different modifiers and their use.

Modifier 22–Increased Procedural Services

When the work required to provide a service is substantially greater than typically required, it may be identified by adding modifier 22 to the usual procedure code. Documentation must support the substantial additional work and the reason for the additional work (i.e., increased intensity, time, technical difficulty of procedure, severity of patient's condition, physical and mental effort required). **Note:** This modifier should not be appended to an E/M service.

What to Remember About Modifier 22

- Modifier 22 is used with procedure codes and *not* with E/M codes.

---

[1]The purpose of the CCI edits is to prevent improper payment when incorrect code combinations are reported.

- It is appended when the physician's skills involve:
  - Significant amount of increased time (e.g., extra work by the physician).
  - Significant amount of increased work (e.g., patient was morbidly obese).
  - Significantly complex procedures.
- It is used to report unusual procedural cases.
- It is used to report procedures complicated by extensive trauma.

Documenting Modifier 22

- Always submit the operative report/documentation and any additional laboratory and/or radiology reports that support the increased work or complexity of the procedure.
- The documentation should *clearly indicate the "increased work"* or the *"complexity of the procedure"* (any service provided that is above and beyond the work included in the CPT code descriptor).
- A letter requesting consideration for additional reimbursement should also be submitted with the documentation.
- Frequent use of this modifier will send a red flag to the carrier.

LET'S LOOK AT AN EXAMPLE

Dr. Fishman performed a myomectomy, with excision of fibroid tumors of the uterus, vaginal approach, on Mrs. Suderman. During the procedure, intraoperative bleeding began; the blood was direct, red, and brisk. Attempts were made to stop the bleeding with packing into the intrauterine environment. The packing was removed after watchful waiting for 10 minutes, but the bleeding continued. A second attempt was made with Monsel solution applied to the tip of the packing. After watchful waiting for an additional 10 minutes, the packing was removed and the bleeding stopped.

How to Code: Typically, patients undergoing this type of procedure do not encounter bleeding requiring packing. In this scenario, *the work of the physician was increased* by having to apply packing to the intrauterine cavity twice during the procedure. The time spent on the packing and waiting for the bleeding to stop also *increased the time* for this procedure. This service is reported by appending modifier 22 to the CPT code (58145-22). The operative report should also be submitted with the claim to clearly identify the increased work by the surgeon.

KEY CODING TIP
Because modifier 22 will result in additional reimbursement, its frequent use will send a red flag to the insurance carrier. Therefore, it is important the documentation supports the use of this modifier.

Modifier 23—Unusual Anesthesia

Occasionally, because of unusual circumstances, a procedure that usually requires either no anesthesia or local anesthesia must be done under general anesthesia. This circumstance may be reported by adding modifier 23 to the procedure code of the basic service.

What to Remember About Modifier 23

- Modifier 23 is used only with anesthesia service codes (00100-01999).
- It is used when services that typically require neither anesthesia nor local anesthesia are done under general anesthesia due to unusual circumstances.

LET'S LOOK AT AN EXAMPLE

A hyperactive child presents to the emergency room with headaches after falling from his bicycle and briefly losing consciousness. An MRI is ordered to determine the extent of the injury. The physician recommends general anesthesia to ensure the child will remain still during the procedure.

How To Code: General anesthesia is normally not administered for MRIs. However, due to the child's hyperactivity, general anesthesia was requested by the physician to ensure the procedure was completed without incident.

Modifier 24—Unrelated Evaluation and Management Service by the Same Physician During a Postoperative Period

The physician may need to indicate that an E/M service was performed during a postoperative period for one or more reasons unrelated to the original procedure. This circumstance may be reported by adding modifier 24 to the appropriate level of E/M service.

What to Remember About Modifier 24

- Modifier 24 is used only with E/M services.
- It is used when the E/M service provided is *unrelated* to the original procedure.

- It is used when the E/M service is provided by the *same physician* who previously performed the original procedure on the patient.
- It is used when the E/M service is provided during the *postoperative period* of the procedure.
- This modifier does not increase or decrease reimbursement. It does allow the E/M service to be reimbursed during the postoperative period, as it is unrelated to the surgical procedure.

LET'S LOOK AT AN EXAMPLE

On May 6, Mrs. Jones underwent arthroscopic knee surgery with meniscus repair, which carries a 90-day global period. On May 24, Mrs. Jones presented to the orthopedic surgeon who performed the knee surgery, complaining of pain and stiffness in her shoulder. The surgeon evaluated her shoulder, and she was diagnosed with calcifying tendinitis of shoulder.

How to Code: Because Mrs. Jones is an established patient presenting for the evaluation and management of a new medical problem, the code 99213 is applied. However, because this evaluation is occurring during the 90-day postoperative period of a previous, unrelated procedure, the orthopedic surgeon would append modifier 24 to the appropriate level of E/M to alert the carrier the visit was unrelated to the knee surgery (e.g., 99213-24). (The diagnosis code 726.11 Calcifying tendinitis of shoulder would also support the visit was unrelated to the knee surgery.)

KEY CODING TIP
The key words to look for in the documentation in order to append modifier 24 are *unrelated, same physician,* and *postoperative period.*

Modifier 25—Significant Separately Identifiable Evaluation and Management Service by the Same Physician on the Same Day of the Procedure or Other Service

It may be necessary to indicate that on the day a procedure or service identified by a CPT code was performed, the patient's condition required a significant, separately identifiable E/M service above and beyond the other service provided or beyond the usual preoperative and postoperative care associated with the procedure that was performed. A significant, separately identifiable E/M service is defined or substantiated by documentation that satisfies the relevant criteria for the respective

E/M service to be reported (see Evaluation and Management Service Guidelines for instructions on determining level of E/M service). The E/M service may be prompted by the symptom or condition for which the procedure and/or service was provided. As such, different diagnoses are not required for reporting of the E/M services on the same date. This circumstance may be reported by adding modifier 25 to the appropriate level of E/M service. **Note:** This modifier is not used to report an E/M service that resulted in a decision to perform surgery. See modifier 57. For significant, separately identifiable non-E/M services, see modifier 59.

What to Remember About Modifier 25

- *Modifier 25 is always appended to the code for E/M service, not to the code for the procedure.*
- It is *not* used when the E/M resulted in a decision to perform major surgery.
- It is *not* used to report an E/M visit by the same physician on the same day as a minor surgery or for endoscopy that is part of the global package (i.e., a single fee for all necessary services before, during, and after surgery; see also Chapter 10).
- Documentation must support both the E/M and the additional service or procedure (e.g., preventive visit and E/M, osteopathic manipulation and E/M).

Also keep in mind: The diagnosis can be either the same as or different from that of the condition for which the (other) procedure or service was performed. If the diagnosis is different, however, be sure to link the correct diagnosis to the correct CPT code.

KEY CODING TIP
Modifier 25 is always appended to the code for the E/M service, not to the code for the procedure.

LET'S LOOK AT AN EXAMPLE

A 28-year-old female presented to the doctor's office for follow-up of asthma and a refill of her prescription medication. The doctor performed a problem-focused history, an expanded problem-focused physical examination, and a moderate decision. During the examination, the doctor noted a splinter imbedded in the patient's hand. The doctor removed the splinter during the same office visit.

How to Code: In this scenario, modifier 25 is appended to the E/M visit to show it was a separately identifiable service from the splinter removal. The splinter removal is coded 10120 (Incision and removal of foreign body, subcutaneous tissues; simple). The E/M service is coded 99213.

continued

LET'S LOOK AT AN EXAMPLE—cont'd

The modifier is appended to the E/M code. With the diagnosis codes, the final coding is as follows: 99213-25 diagnosis 493.90 (Asthma, unspecified, unspecified status), 10120 diagnosis 914.6 (Hand(s) except finger(s) alone, superficial foreign body [splinter], without major open wound and without mention of infection).

Modifier 26—Professional Component

Certain procedures are a combination of a physician component and a technical component. When the physician component is reported separately, the service may be identified by adding modifier 26 to the usual procedure number.

The technical component represents the equipment, the technician, and supplies, while the professional component represents the skill of the physician in interpreting the test.

What to Remember About Modifier 26

- Modifier 26 is appended to the procedure/service.
- It represents the skill of the physician interpreting the test. When modifier 26 is used, it is appended to codes in the Surgery, Radiology, Pathology and Laboratory, and Medicine sections.
- It is *not* used if the physician is providing the global service (both the professional and technical components).

Note: The *technical* portion of the service, which includes the equipment, supplies, technician(s), and facility, is reported with the HCPCS modifier TC (technical component).

LET'S LOOK AT AN EXAMPLE

A 68-year-old female was diagnosed with colon cancer. As part of the patient's treatment plan, the physician ordered chemotherapy. The patient was sent to the operating room for an insertion of Port-a-Cath for chemotherapy. The procedure was performed under fluoroscopic guidance.

How to Code: In this scenario, because we are coding for the services of the physician, we would code 36571 (Insertion of peripherally inserted central venous access device, with subcutaneous port; age 5 years or older) and 77001-26 (Fluoroscopic guidance for central venous access device placement, replacement [catheter only or complete], or removal). Modifier 26 is appended to the fluoroscopic guidance to indicate the professional component of the service, namely, the use of fluoroscopic guidance throughout the procedure to guide the catheter placement and to check the positioning of the catheter tip.

Modifier 32—Mandated Services

Services related to *mandated* consultation and/or related services (e.g., third-party payer, governmental, legislative, or regulatory requirement) may be identified by adding modifier 32 to the basic procedure.

What to Remember About Modifier 32

- Modifier 32 may be used with codes in all sections of the CPT book.
- It is *not* used when a patient or family member requests a second opinion.
- It is *not* used to report a confirmatory consult.

LET'S LOOK AT AN EXAMPLE

Mr. Smith was detained at airport security upon arrival into the country for suspicion of drug trafficking. A radiological examination of the upper gastrointestinal tract was ordered by the judge for evidence of ingested drug packets.

How to Code: In this scenario, modifier 32 is appended to the radiological procedure to indicate the test (74240-32) was court ordered by the judge.

Modifier 47—Anesthesia by Surgeon

Regional or general anesthesia provided by the surgeon may be reported by adding modifier 47 to the basic service. (This does not include local anesthesia.) **Note:** Modifier 47 would not be used as a modifier for the anesthesia procedures.

What to Remember About Modifier 47

- To use modifier 47, anesthesia must have been provided by the surgeon performing the procedure.
- It is appended to the surgical code only.
- It is *not* appended to anesthesia codes.
- It is *not* used to report moderate conscious sedation.
- It is *not* used by an anesthesiologist.

KEY CODING TIP
Modifier 47 is *never* reported with an anesthesia code.

LET'S LOOK AT AN EXAMPLE

A 30-year-old woman with carpal tunnel syndrome underwent a neuroplasty to decompress a portion of median nerve to restore feeling to the hand. The surgeon administered a regional nerve block.

LET'S LOOK AT AN EXAMPLE—cont'd

How to Code: In this scenario, modifier 47 is appended to the CPT code for the neuroplasty (64721-47). The physician would also code for the nerve block: 64450 Injection, anesthetic agent; other peripheral nerve or branch.

Note: Refer to Chapter 9 for additional information about modifier 47.

Modifier 50—Bilateral Procedure

Unless otherwise identified in the listings, bilateral procedures that are performed at the same operative session should be identified by adding modifier 50 to the appropriate five-digit code.

What to Remember About Modifier 50

- Modifier 50 is used to report procedures performed on both sides of the body at the same operative session.
- It is used when the same procedure is performed on both paired organs (e.g., kidneys).
- It is not used with codes whose descriptors include "bilateral" or "unilateral."

LET'S LOOK AT AN EXAMPLE

A 55-year-old woman underwent bilateral needle core breast biopsies using imaging guidance (19102-50).

How to Code: CPT code 19102 (Biopsy of breast; percutaneous, needle core, using imaging guidance) refers to a unilateral procedure (performed on one breast only) unless otherwise specified—that is, by modifier 50. By appending modifier 50, you indicate that the procedure was performed on both breasts (bilaterally).

Modifier 51—Multiple Procedures

When multiple procedures other than E/M services, physical medicine and rehabilitation services, or provision of supplies (e.g., vaccines) are performed at the same session by the same provider, the primary procedure or service may be reported as listed. The additional procedure(s) or service(s) may be identified by appending modifier 51 to the additional procedure or service code(s). **Note:** This modifier should not be appended to designated "add-on" codes (see Appendix D of the CPT book).

What to Remember About Modifier 51

- Modifier 51 is used to report multiple surgical procedures performed at the same session.

- It is used to report a combination of medical and surgical procedures performed at the same session.
- It is appended to each additional procedure performed after the first procedure, with the exception of procedures designated as modifier 51 exempt.
- It is *not* used when two or more physicians each perform distinctly different, unrelated surgeries on the same patient at the same session (e.g., multiple trauma cases).
- It is *not* used with an add-on code (add-on codes, designated by the symbol +, are used to indicate procedures commonly performed in addition to the primary procedure and are listed in Appendix D of the CPT book).
- It is *not* used to report an *E/M service* and a procedure performed on the same day.
- It is *not* used with CPT codes listed as modifier 51 exempt (Appendix E of the CPT book). Modifier 51 exempt procedures are usually performed with other procedures, but they also may be standalone procedures and as such are not always performed with another procedure.
- It is *not* used with anesthesia CPT codes.

LET'S LOOK AT AN EXAMPLE

A 62-year-old man was diagnosed with a neoplasm of uncertain behavior of the liver. The surgeon performed a needle biopsy of the liver and ablation of the liver tumor by radiofrequency.

How to Code: Ablation of the liver tumor is coded 47380, and biopsy of the liver is coded 47100. In this scenario, because neither CPT code is modifier 51 exempt, it is appropriate to append modifier 51 to the second procedure to indicate multiple procedures were performed at the same operative session (47380, 47100-51). **Note:** When coding for multiple surgical procedures at the same operative session, the multiple surgical rule applies (see Chapter 10); therefore, the CPT code for the ablation of the liver tumor would be coded first because it is the higher paying procedure.

Modifier 52—Reduced Services

Under certain circumstances, a service or procedure is partially reduced or eliminated at the physician's discretion. Under these circumstances, the service provided can be identified by its usual procedure number and the addition of modifier 52, signifying that the service is reduced. This provides a means of reporting reduced services without disturbing the identification of the basic service. **Note:** For hospital outpatient reporting of a previously scheduled procedure/service that is partially reduced or canceled as a result of extenuating circumstances or those that threaten the well-being of the patient prior to or after administration of anesthesia, see modifiers 73 and 74 (see modifiers approved for ambulatory surgery center [ASC]/hospital outpatient use).

What to Remember About Modifier 52

- Modifier 52 is used to indicate that the service was not completed to the full extent of the CPT code descriptor.

- It is used when the service was *reduced or eliminated (only a portion of the procedure was performed) at the discretion of the physician.*

- It is *not* used for procedures that were terminated.

- The patient's record should include documentation explaining the circumstances surrounding the reduction in services.

- Documentation should be sent with the claim.

LET'S LOOK AT AN EXAMPLE

A 7-year-old child presented for his preventive visit. During the visit, the physician administered the age-appropriate vaccines and performed a hearing examination, urinalysis, and vision screening via the Snellen chart. After examining one eye, the physician discontinued the examination due to the child's disruptive behavior.

How to Code: In this scenario, modifier 52 is appended to the eye examination (99173-52) to indicate the service was reduced (only a portion of the examination was completed) and was discontinued at the request of the physician. You would also code for the other services provided (age-appropriate preventive visit, vaccines, vaccine administration, urinalysis, and hearing test).

Modifier 53—Discontinued Procedure

A physician may elect to terminate a surgical or diagnostic procedure because of extenuating circumstances or those that threaten the well-being of the patient. A surgical or diagnostic procedure that was started but discontinued may be reported by adding modifier 53 to the code reported by the physician for the discontinued procedure. **Note:** This modifier is not used to report the elective cancellation of a procedure prior to the patient's anesthesia induction and/or surgical preparation in the operating suite. For outpatient hospital/ASC reporting of a previously scheduled procedure/service that is partially reduced or canceled as a result of extenuating circumstances or those that threaten the well-being of the patient prior to or after administration of anesthesia, see modifiers 73 and 74 (see modifiers approved for ASC/hospital outpatient use).

What to Remember About Modifier 53

- Modifier 53 is used when a procedure was started but discontinued before completion *due to the patient's condition* (e.g., uncontrolled bleeding).

- It is used when a procedure was discontinued due to any situation that threatens the well-being of the patient.

- Documentation should be submitted with the claim to determine the correct reimbursement amount.

- It is *not* used with an E/M code.

- It is *not* used to report elective cancellations of a procedure before the patient's anesthesia induction and/or surgical preparation in the operating suite.

- It is *not* used to report laparoscopic or endoscopic procedures that were converted into open procedures.

- It is *not* used when a procedure is changed into a more extensive procedure.

LET'S LOOK AT AN EXAMPLE

While undergoing a colonoscopy for ablation of polyps by snare technique, the patient went into respiratory distress. The physician withdrew the scope and terminated the procedure.

How to Code: In this scenario, modifier 53 is appended to the CPT code for the colonoscopy (45383-53). In this case, the procedure was discontinued due to the patient's medical circumstances (respiratory distress).

Modifiers 54, 55, and 56

These three modifiers break out the surgical package.[2] In some cases, one physician performs the surgery (intraoperative; modifier 54) while another physician sees the patient for the preoperative visit (modifier 56) and/or the postoperative care (modifier 55).

KEY CODING TIP

If the physician is providing the complete (global) service, no modifier is appended.

Modifier 54—Surgical Care Only

When one physician performs a surgical procedure and another provides preoperative and/or postoperative management, surgical services may be identified by adding modifier 54 to the usual procedure number.

---

[2] The surgical package includes the preoperative visits, the intraoperative service, and the postoperative visits.

What to Remember About Modifier 54

■ Modifier 54 is reported with codes from the Surgery section (10021-69990).

■ Its use requires documentation of an agreement between two providers regarding the transfer of care for the patient.

■ It is used for major procedures. It is not used for minor surgical procedures (e.g., ear lavage).

Modifier 55—Postoperative Management Only

When one physician performs the postoperative management and another physician performs the surgical procedure, the postoperative component may be identified by adding modifier 55 to the usual procedure number.

What to Remember About Modifier 55

■ Modifier 55 is reported when a provider other than the operating surgeon provides the postoperative care.

Modifier 56—Preoperative Management Only

When one physician performs the preoperative care and evaluation and another physician performs the surgical procedure, the preoperative component may be identified by adding modifier 56 to the usual procedure number.

What to Remember About Modifier 56

■ Modifier 56 is reported when a provider other than the operating surgeon provides the preoperative service.

LET'S LOOK AT SOME EXAMPLES

Mary Jones was out of town visiting a friend when she slipped on a patch of ice and dislocated her shoulder. Mary went to the hospital and underwent an open treatment of acute shoulder dislocation (23660) performed by Dr. Williams. When Mary returned home, she received her follow-up care from her local orthopedist, Dr. Frank.

How to Code: In this scenario, Dr. Williams performed the surgery (intraoperative) portion of the surgical package. Dr. Williams reports his services with 23660-54. Dr. Frank provided the follow-up care (postoperative visits). Dr. Frank reports his service with 23660-55.

In another example, Roberta Smith, who lives in a rural area, is seen by her primary care physician for preoperative management for her scheduled laparoscopic cholecystomy to be performed the next day by the general surgeon who provides services to this area on a monthly schedule.

How to Code: In this case, the primary care physician codes 47562-56 and will be reimbursed for the preoperative portion of the surgical package. The general surgeon reports the same CPT code 47562 but appends modifier 54 to indicate he provided the surgical service.

Modifier 57—Decision for Surgery

An evaluation and management service that resulted in the initial decision to perform the surgery may be identified by adding modifier 57 to the appropriate level of E/M service.

What to Remember About Modifier 57

■ Modifier 57 is used when the surgery is scheduled for the same day as or next day after the E/M service.

■ It is always appended to the E/M code.

■ It is *not* used when the surgical procedure has a global period (i.e., the time following the surgical procedure; see Chapter 10) of 0–10 days (see modifier 25).

■ It does not increase the reimbursement fee but allows for both the E/M and procedure to be paid on the same day.

LET'S LOOK AT AN EXAMPLE

A 15-year-old boy fell while bike riding and later that day experienced pain and swelling in the leg. The patient was examined by the orthopedic surgeon at the request of the emergency room physician and was diagnosed with a tibial shaft fracture. At the same encounter, the orthopedic surgeon provided a closed treatment of the tibial shaft without manipulation.

How to Code: In this scenario, modifier 57 is appended to the evaluation and management service (in this case, Level II consultation visit, 99242) because the decision to provide the surgical service was made during the evaluation and management service: 99242-57, 27750 Closed treatment of tibial shaft fracture (with or without fibular fracture; without manipulation).

Modifier 58—Staged or Related Procedure or Service by the Same Physician During the Postoperative Period

It may be necessary to indicate that a procedure or service performed during the postoperative period was (a) planned or anticipated (staged); (b) more extensive than the original procedure; or (c) for therapy following a surgical procedure. This circumstance may be reported by adding modifier 58 to the staged or related procedure. **Note:** For treatment of a problem that requires a return to the operating/procedure room (e.g., unanticipated clinical condition), see modifier 78.

What to Remember About Modifier 58

■ Modifier 58 is used to report that an additional **related** surgery was required during the postoperative period of a previously completed surgery by the same physician.

■ It is used only during the global surgical period for the original procedure.

■ It is always appended to the procedure code for the second procedure performed during the postoperative period.

Also keep in mind: A new postoperative period begins when the next procedure in the staged procedure series is billed.

LET'S LOOK AT AN EXAMPLE

A patient had a breast lesion removed (19120). Two weeks later (less than the 90-day global period), the patient underwent the removal of the entire breast (19307).

How to Code: In this scenario, modifier 58 is appended to the CPT code for the second procedure—in this case, the mastectomy (removal of the entire breast)—to indicate that a more extensive procedure was necessary. CPT code 19120 is reported for the May 7 procedure, and CPT code 19307-58 is reported for the May 21 procedure. Modifier 58 is appended to the breast removal to indicate a more extensive procedure was required during the global period.

Modifier 59—Distinct Procedural Service

Under certain circumstances, it may be necessary to indicate that a procedure or service was distinct or independent from other non-E/M services performed on the same day. Modifier 59 is used to identify procedures/services, other than E/M services, that are not normally reported together but are appropriate under the circumstances. Documentation must support a different session, different procedure or surgery, different site or organ system, separate incision/excision, separate lesion, or separate injury (or area of injury in extensive injuries) not ordinarily encountered or performed on the same day by the same individual. However, when another already established modifier is appropriate, it should be used instead of modifier 59. Only if no more descriptive modifier is available, and the use of modifier 59 best explains the circumstances, should modifier 59 be used. **Note:** Modifier 59

should not be appended to an E/M service. To report a separate and distinct E/M service with a non-E/M service performed on the same date, see modifier 25.

What to Remember About Modifier 59

■ Modifier 59 is used to report a different session or patient encounter. For example, a patient received a bronchodilation (94060) at 9 a.m. Later that same day, the patient still had difficulty breathing and returned to the physician's office (different encounter) for a nebulizer treatment (94640). If the bronchodilation and the nebulizer are reported at the same encounter, they are considered bundled, whereas appending modifier 59 to the nebulizer treatment alerts the carrier the service was provided at a separate encounter and will be separately reimbursed.

■ It is used to report a different procedure/service performed on the same day. For example, a patient having a colonoscopy may have a polyp removed by snare technique and a biopsy taken (two separate procedures) at the same session.

■ It is used to report a different site or organ system.

■ It is used to report a separate incision/excision. For example, a patient may have two separate incisional biopsies performed on the same breast (same service, separate incisions on the same body area).

■ It is used to report a separate lesion. For example, a patient having 10 skin tags removed from his trunk may, at the same session, have a facial lesion biopsied. To ensure reimbursement for both services, modifier 59 is appended to the CPT code for the skin tags (11200).

■ It is used to report a separate injury.

■ It is appended to the code for the separate or distinct procedure.

■ It is *not* used if there is a more appropriate modifier (i.e., if there is *any* other appropriate modifier, that one should be used instead of modifier 59).

■ It is *not* used with E/M codes.

■ Use modifier 59 with caution because it allows the payment of multiple procedures that are usually considered bundled or inclusive to each other.

LET'S LOOK AT AN EXAMPLE

A patient with squamous cell carcinoma of the left parietal region of the scalp and an occipital lesion of the scalp was brought into the operating room for excision of the lesions. The occipital lesion was excised first and was done down to the fascia. The lesion was completely excised. The lesion on the left parietal region was also excised.

LET'S LOOK AT AN EXAMPLE—cont'd

How to Code: In this scenario, the procedure is coded 11626 (Excision, malignant lesion including margins, scalp, neck, hands, feet, genitalia; excised diameter over 4.0 cm) twice, with modifier 59 appended to the second CPT code (11626, 11626-59) to indicate that the procedure was performed on two separate lesions.

Modifier 62—Two Surgeons

When two surgeons work together as primary surgeons performing distinct parts of a procedure, each surgeon should report his or her distinct operative work by adding modifier 62 to the procedure code and any associated add-on codes for that procedure as long as both surgeons continue to work together as primary surgeons. Each surgeon should report the co-surgery once using the same procedure code. If additional procedures (including add-on procedures) are performed during the same surgical session, separate codes may also be reported with modifier 62 appended. **Note:** If a co-surgeon acts as an assistant in the performance of an additional procedure during the same surgical session, those services may be reported using a separate procedure code with modifier 80 or modifier 82 added as appropriate.

What to Remember About Modifier 62

■ Modifier 62 is used when two surgeons *work together as primary surgeons.* For example, for some complicated procedures (e.g., spine surgery), one surgeon may open and close, and the other surgeon may perform the procedure. Although the CPT code remains the same, each surgeon is providing a portion of the code.

■ Each surgeon will report the same CPT code with modifier 62 appended.

■ It is *not* used if the second surgeon is acting as an assistant. In this case, refer to assistant surgeon modifiers 80, 81, and 82.

■ The medical necessity for both surgeons should be clearly documented.

LET'S LOOK AT AN EXAMPLE

Two orthopedic surgeons are working together as primary surgeons to perform an arthrodesis (22612) and decompression (63047) on opposite sides of the midline of the lumbar spine.

How to Code: Because both surgeons are working as primary surgeons performing distinct parts of multiple reportable procedures, each surgeon would report the same CPT codes with modifier 62 appended. In this case, both surgeons would report 22612-62 and 63047-62.

Modifier 63—Procedure Performed on Infants Less Than 4 kg

Procedures performed on neonates and infants up to a present body weight of 4 kg may involve significantly increased complexity and physician work. This circumstance may be reported by adding modifier 63 to the procedure number. **Note:** Unless otherwise designated, this modifier may be appended only to procedures/services listed in the 20000-69990 code series. Modifier 63 should not be appended to any CPT codes listed in the Evaluation and Management Services, Anesthesia, Radiology, Pathology and Laboratory, or Medicine sections.

What to Remember About Modifier 63

■ Modifier 63 alerts the carrier of the increased complexity of the skill and work required because of the weight of the neonate/infant.

■ It is used to report procedures performed on infants weighing less than 4 kg.

■ It is *not* used with CPT codes that are modifier 63 exempt and are listed in Appendix F of the CPT book.

■ It is *not* used with codes in the Evaluation and Management Services, Anesthesia, Radiology, Pathology and Laboratory, and Medicine sections of the CPT book.

LET'S LOOK AT AN EXAMPLE

A 1-week-old infant weighing 3.2 kg received a push transfusion of blood.

How to Code: Because CPT code 36440 (Push transfusion, blood, 2 years or younger) is not modifier 63 exempt, and the weight of the infant is less than 4 kg, modifier 63 is appended to the CPT code: 36440-63.

Modifier 66—Surgical Team

Under some circumstances, highly complex procedures (requiring the concomitant services of several physicians, often of different specialties, plus other highly skilled, specially trained personnel and various types of complex equipment) are carried out under the "surgical team" concept. Such circumstances may be identified by each participating physician with the addition of modifier 66 to the basic procedure number used for reporting services.

What to Remember About Modifier 66

■ Modifier 66 is used when multiple surgeons of various specialties perform different portions of a highly complex procedure.

■ It is used only with codes from the Surgery section of the CPT book.

■ It must be supported by documentation indicating each surgeon's performance as a team member.

LET'S LOOK AT AN EXAMPLE

A 52-year-old male with peripheral vascular disease and a myocardial infarction three days ago underwent a heart transplant. Due to the complexity of the operation, a team of surgeons was required to perform the operation.

How to Code: Because a team of surgeons was required, each surgeon would report the same procedure code with modifier 66 appended (33945-66).

Another abdominal x-ray was taken to assure the lap band was still in place.

How to Code: In this scenario, the same service was provided to the same patient on the same day by the same physician. To ensure reimbursement for the two abdominal x-rays taken on the same day, modifier 76 is appended to the second abdominal x-ray (74010, 74010-76) to indicate this was a repeat procedure by the same physician and not a duplicate billing error. Also, because this service was provided in a hospital setting, but the physician is interpreting the test results (in this case, the x-ray), modifier 26 is appended to the codes for both abdominal x-rays to indicate the physician is coding for the professional component of the x-rays: 74010-26, 74010-76-26.

Modifier 76—Repeat Procedure or Service by Same Physician or Other Qualified Health Care Professional

It may be necessary to indicate that a procedure or service was repeated by the same physician or other qualified health-care professional subsequent to the original procedure or service. This circumstance may be reported by adding modifier 76 to the repeated procedure/service. Note: This modifier should not be appended to an E/M service.

What to Remember About Modifier 76

■ Use of modifier 76 alerts the carrier that the claim is not a duplicate.

■ It is used when:

The service is the same.

The *physician is the same.*

The patient is the same.

■ It is used when the service is provided on the same day or during the postoperative period.

■ It is appended to the repeated service (second CPT code).

■ It is *not* used for repeat clinical laboratory tests (in that case, use modifier 91).

■ Documentation must support medical necessity for providing the repeat procedure.

Modifier 77—Repeat Procedure by Another Physician or Other Qualified Health Care Professional

It may be necessary to indicate that a basic procedure or service was repeated by another physician or other qualified health-care professional subsequent to the original procedure or service. This circumstance may be reported by adding modifier 77 to the repeated procedure or service. Note: This modifier should not be appended to an E/M service.

What to Remember About Modifier 77

■ Modifier 77 is used when:

The service is the same.

The patient is the same.

The *physician is different.*

■ It is used when the service is provided on the same day or during the postoperative period.

■ It is always appended to the repeated service (second CPT code).

■ It is *not* used for repeat clinical laboratory tests—use modifier 91.

■ It must be supported by documentation in the chart.

LET'S LOOK AT AN EXAMPLE

A patient underwent gastric bypass surgery for gastric banding. After the surgery, an abdominal x-ray was taken to assess the placement of the band. Later that day, the patient began vomiting and complaining of stomach pains.

LET'S LOOK AT AN EXAMPLE

A patient with a malignant neoplasm of the lung and pleural effusion underwent a thoracentesis. Later that day, the thoracentesis needed to be repeated by another physician because the original physician was not available to perform the repeat procedure.

LET'S LOOK AT AN EXAMPLE—cont'd

How to Code: In this scenario, the physician who repeated the procedure would code the thoracentesis with modifier 77 appended (32421-77) to indicate that this was a repeat procedure by a different physician and not a duplicate billing error.

Modifier 78–Unplanned Return to the Operating/Procedure Room by the Same Physician or Other Qualified Health Care Professional Following Initial Procedure for a Related Procedure During the Postoperative Period

It may be necessary to indicate that another procedure was performed during the postoperative period of the initial procedure (unplanned procedure following initial procedure). When this procedure is related to the first and requires the use of an operating/procedure room, it may be reported by adding modifier 78 to the related procedure. (For repeat procedures, see modifier 76.)

What to Remember About Modifier 78

- Modifier 78 is used to report a procedure that is *related* to the initial surgery but is not a *repeat* procedure.
- It is used to report a procedure performed by the *same physician* who performed the initial procedure.
- It is used during the postoperative period of the initial procedure.
- It is appended to *all* related procedures performed (if more than one unplanned procedure is performed) and is not limited to the first unplanned procedure only.
- It is appended to the related, unplanned procedure and *not* to the initial procedure.

LET'S LOOK AT AN EXAMPLE

The physician repaired an abdominal aneurysm. The patient developed internal bleeding later in the day. The patient was returned to the operating room to correct the active bleeding sites.

How to Code: In this scenario, the physician would code for both the procedure (35082 Aneurysm repair) and the control of internal bleeding (35840). Modifier 78 is appended to the CPT code for the control of internal bleeding (35840-78) to indicate the second procedure was provided by the same physician for an *unplanned* return visit to the operating room for a *procedure related* to the initial procedure during the postoperative period.

Modifier 79–Unrelated Procedure or Service by the Same Physician During the Postoperative Period

The physician may need to indicate that the performance of a procedure or service during the postoperative period was unrelated to the original procedure. This circumstance may be reported by using modifier 79. (For repeat procedures on the same day, see modifier 76.)

What to Remember About Modifier 79

- Modifier 79 is used to report procedures that are *unrelated* to the initial surgery.
- It is used to report procedures performed by the *same physician* who performed the initial procedure.
- It is used to report procedures performed during the postoperative period of the initial procedure.
- It is appended to all unrelated procedures performed and is not limited to the first procedure only.

LET'S LOOK AT AN EXAMPLE

A patient underwent an excision of a tumor of the left ankle. At 40 days postoperative, the patient was rushed to the emergency room where he was diagnosed with a ruptured appendix. The patient was immediately taken to the operating room for an appendectomy.

How to Code: In this scenario, modifier 79 is appended to the CPT code for the appendectomy (44960-79) to indicate that the appendectomy was unrelated to the original procedure (excision of tumor, ankle) but happened to be performed by the same surgeon during the postoperative period of the original procedure.

Modifier 80–Assistant Surgeon

Surgical assistant services may be identified by adding modifier 80 to the usual procedure number(s).

What to Remember About Modifier 80

- Modifier 80 is used when the assistant surgeon is **assisting the primary surgeon for the entire procedure.**
- The operative report should clearly document the services of the assistant surgeon.
- The assistant surgeon reports the same CPT code reported by the surgeon.
- Only the assistant surgeon appends modifier 80 to the CPT code.

LET'S LOOK AT AN EXAMPLE

Dr. Smith assisted Dr. Jones (primary surgeon) during an inguinal hernia repair of a 54-year-old male patient. Dr. Smith assisted during the entire procedure.

How to Code: Dr. Jones (primary surgeon) submits CPT code 49521 (Repair recurrent inguinal hernia, any age; incarcerated or strangulated incarcerated or strangulated). Dr. Smith (assistant surgeon) submits the same CPT code with modifier 80 appended (49521-80) to indicate he was the assistant during the entire procedure.

Modifier 81—Minimum Assistant Surgeon

Minimum surgical assistant services are identified by adding modifier 81 to the usual procedure number.

What to Remember About Modifier 81

■ Modifier 81 is used when the assistant surgeon is *assisting the primary surgeon only for a portion of the procedure or for a limited amount of time.*

■ The assistant surgeon reports the same CPT code reported by the surgeon.

■ Only the assistant surgeon appends modifier 81 to the CPT code.

■ The operative report should clearly document the services of the assistant surgeon.

LET'S LOOK AT AN EXAMPLE

Dr. Smith assisted Dr. Jones (primary surgeon) during an inguinal hernia repair of a 54-year-old male patient. Dr. Smith assisted for a portion of the procedure.

How to Code: Dr. Jones (the primary surgeon) submits CPT code 49521 (Repair recurrent inguinal hernia, any age; incarcerated or strangulated). Dr. Smith (the assistant surgeon) submits the same CPT code but with modifier 81 appended (49521-81) to indicate that he assisted for only a portion of the procedure.

Modifier 82—Assistant Surgeon (When Qualified Resident Surgeon Not Available)

The unavailability of a qualified resident surgeon is a prerequisite for use of modifier 82 appended to the usual procedure code number(s).

What to Remember About Modifier 82

■ To use modifier 82, a qualified resident surgeon must have been unavailable.

LET'S LOOK AT AN EXAMPLE

Due to the unavailability of a qualified resident surgeon, Dr. Smith (an attending physician) was asked to assist Dr. Jones (primary surgeon) during an inguinal hernia repair of a 54-year-old male patient. Dr. Smith assisted during the entire procedure.

How to Code: Dr. Jones (primary surgeon) submits CPT code 49521 (Repair recurrent inguinal hernia, any age; incarcerated or strangulated). Dr. Smith (assistant surgeon) submits the same CPT code with modifier 82 appended (49521-82) to indicate he was the assistant due to the unavailability of a qualified resident surgeon.

Modifier 90—Reference (Outside) Laboratory

When laboratory procedures are performed by a party other than the treating or reporting physician, the procedure may be identified by adding modifier 90 to the usual procedure number.

What to Remember About Modifier 90

■ Modifier 90 is used when a physician who does not have an office laboratory has an arrangement with an outside laboratory by which the laboratory bills the physician and the physician in turn bills the patient or insurance carrier.

■ It is *not* used for Medicare patients. (The Centers for Medicare and Medicaid Services does not recognize use of this modifier.)

Note: Use of this modifier is carrier specific. Insurance carriers should be contacted to determine if they recognize use of modifier 90.

LET'S LOOK AT AN EXAMPLE

A patient presents to the primary care physician for a yearly preventive visit. During the encounter, the physician performs a venipuncture and sends the blood to an outside reference laboratory (with which he has an agreement) for analysis of a general health panel (80050).

How to Code: Because the physician has an agreement with the outside reference laboratory, the physician codes for the general health panel and appends modifier 90 (80050-90) to indicate to the insurance carrier the blood was analyzed by an outside reference laboratory (not a laboratory in the physician's office). The physician will be reimbursed by the insurance carrier, and the outside reference laboratory will be reimbursed by the physician.

Modifier 91—Repeat Clinical Diagnostic Laboratory Test

In the course of treatment of a patient, it may be necessary to repeat the same laboratory test on the same day to obtain subsequent (multiple) test results. Under these circumstances, the laboratory test performed can be identified by its usual procedure number and the addition of modifier 91. **Note:** This modifier may not be used when tests are rerun to confirm initial results; due to testing problems with specimens or equipment; or for any other reason when a normal, one-time, reportable result is all that is required. This modifier may not be used when other codes describe a series of test results (e.g., glucose tolerance tests, evocative/suppression testing). This modifier may be used only for laboratory tests performed more than once on the same day on the same patient.

What to Remember About Modifier 91

- Modifier 91 is used when a laboratory test needs to be repeated *on the same day* to obtain multiple test results.
- It is used when the laboratory test is the same (i.e., repeated) and performed on the same patient on the same day.
- It is *not* used to confirm an initial laboratory result.
- It is *not* used when a laboratory test needs to be repeated due to equipment failure or a spoiled specimen.
- It is *not* used when a CPT code describes a *series* of tests (e.g., glucose tolerance tests, evocative/ suppression testing).

LET'S LOOK AT AN EXAMPLE

A diabetic patient undergoes a glucose blood test that indicates a high glucose level. The patient is then treated with Glucophage (a drug used to treat high blood sugar) and monitored in the office. A glucose blood test is repeated later that day, and the results indicate a declining glucose level.

How to Code: In this scenario, CPT code 82962 (Glucose, blood by glucose monitoring device[s]) is reported twice, and modifier 91 is appended to the second code to indicate the test was repeated twice and was not a duplicate billing error (82962, 82962-91).

Modifier 92—Alternative Laboratory Platform Testing

When laboratory testing is being performed using a kit or transportable instrument that wholly or in part consists of a single-use, disposable analytical chamber, the service may be identified by adding modifier 92 to the usual laboratory procedure code (HIV testing, 86701-86703). The test does not require permanent dedicated space and therefore may be hand carried or transported to the vicinity of the patient for immediate testing at that site, although location of the testing is not in itself determinative of the use of this modifier.

What to Remember About Modifier 92

- Modifier 92 is used with only three CPT codes (HIV testing): 86701, 86702, 86703.
- It is used when the laboratory test is performed using a kit or transportable instrument that wholly or in part consists of a single-use, disposable analytical chamber.

LET'S LOOK AT AN EXAMPLE

A 23-year-old established female presented to her primary care physician for her annual preventive visit. Because the patient had had multiple sexual partners, she requested an HIV test. The physician performed a rapid HIV test (results of rapid testing are available in 5 to 30 minutes, allowing for the HIV testing, counseling, and referrals to be provided in one visit).

How to Code: In addition to the age-appropriate preventive visit (99395) CPT code, the HIV testing is coded with modifier 92 to indicate the test was performed using a kit (86703-92).

Modifier 99—Multiple Modifiers

Under certain circumstances, two or more modifiers may be necessary to completely delineate a service. In such situations, modifier 99 should be added to the basic procedure, and other applicable modifiers may be listed as part of the description of the service.

What to Remember About Modifier 99

- Modifier 99 is used when more than two modifiers are appended to a CPT code.
- It does not have an effect on reimbursement because it is for informational use only.

LET'S LOOK AT AN EXAMPLE

During the repair of bilateral ventral hernias, Dr. Michaels, the assistant surgeon, reported the service as unusual due to the additional time and difficulties encountered during the surgery.

How to Code: More than two modifiers are required to properly identify the services of Dr. Michaels, whose services are reported as 49560-80-50-22-99.

Learn More About It

The more you read, the more you know. Increase your knowledge with the following resources.

Recommended Books

Coding With Modifiers
Author: Deborah J. Grider
ISBN# 978-1-57947-889-6
Publisher: American Medical Association

Break Through the Modifier Maze
Product ID#: BTM10
Publisher: Decision Health

STOP-LOOK-HIGHLIGHT

In Appendix A, **highlight the following (remember to use two different color highlighters, yellow for standard guidelines and global services and an alternate color for carve-outs and unique notes):**

■ In the description of modifier 22, the fourth line down, highlight in yellow: "Documentation must support the substantial additional work and the reason for the additional work (i.e., increased intensity, time, technical difficulty of procedure, severity of patient's condition, physical and mental effort required)."
Using your alternate color highlighter, highlight: "**Note:** This modifier should not be appended to an E/M service."

■ In the description of modifier 25, the twelfth line down, highlight in yellow: "The E/M service may be prompted by the symptom or condition for which the procedure and/or service was provided. As such, different diagnoses are not required for reporting of the E/M services on the same date."
Using your alternate color highlighter, highlight: "**Note:** This modifier is not used to report an E/M service that resulted in a decision to perform surgery. See modifier 57. For significant, separately identifiable non-E/M services, see modifier 59."

■ In the description of modifier 59, the seventh line down, highlight in yellow: "Documentation must support a different session, different procedure or surgery, different site or organ system, separate incision/excision, separate lesion, or separate injury (or area of injury in extensive injuries) not ordinarily encountered or performed on the same day by the same individual."

Using your alternate color highlighter, highlight: "**Note:** Modifier 59 should not be appended to an E/M service. To report a separate and distinct E/M service with a non-E/M service performed on the same date, see modifier 25."

■ In the description of modifier 63, on the third line of the note, highlight using your alternate color highlighter: "Modifier 63 should not be appended to any CPT codes listed in the Evaluation and Management Services, Anesthesia, Radiology, Pathology/Laboratory, or Medicine sections."

■ In the description of modifier 91, highlight in yellow: "In the course of treatment of the patient it may be necessary to repeat the same laboratory test on the same day to obtain subsequent (multiple) test results."

■ Using your alternate color highlighter, highlight: "**Note:** This modifier may not be used when tests are rerun to confirm initial results; due to testing problems with specimens or equipment; or for any other reason when a normal one-time, reportable result is all that is required. This modifier may not be used when other codes describe a series of test results (e.g., glucose tolerance tests, evocative/suppression testing)."
In red ink at the end of the description for modifier 91, write in the following: *"This modifier is always appended to the second CPT code."*

TAKE THE CODING CHALLENGE

Assign the Appropriate Modifier

1. An assistant surgeon was present to assist for only a portion of the surgery.

   _____

2. A laboratory test was repeated due to equipment failure.

   _____

3. A patient was seen by an ophthalmologist who recommended a cornea transplant. The patient's HMO (insurance carrier) requested a second opinion.

   _____

4. Multiple surgical procedures (i.e., the additional procedures).

   _____

5. An E/M service during which a decision was made to schedule surgery for the next day.

   _____

Multiple Choice

1. An orthopedic surgeon performs a closed treatment of a Colles' fracture (90 days global). One month later, the same patient returns to the same physician's office complaining of pain and swelling in the ankle after falling from a skateboard. X-rays reveal an ankle fracture. The surgeon provides closed treatment of bimalleolar ankle fracture without manipulation. What modifier would be appended to closed treatment of the ankle fracture?
   a. 79
   b. 78
   c. 77
   d. 76

2. Modifier 58 is used when:
   a. Multiple procedures are performed.
   b. A physician who performs an initial procedure performs a related or staged procedure during the postoperative period of the initial procedure.
   c. A repeat procedure is performed by the same physician.
   d. A physician who performed an initial procedure returns the patient to the operating room for a related but unplanned procedure during the postoperative period.

3. A patient presents to the doctor's office complaining of fever, cough, and chest pain for 3 days. The physician examines the patient and orders a chest x-ray to determine if the patient has pneumonia. The physician owns the x-ray equipment; the technician takes the x-ray, which is read by the physician. What modifier is appended to the x-ray?
   a. 26
   b. 25
   c. None
   d. 57

4. Modifier 47 is used:
   a. By an anesthesiologist
   b. By a surgeon
   c. By either an anesthesiologist or a surgeon
   d. None of the above

5. Modifier 25 is always appended to:
   a. A diagnosis code
   b. A surgical code
   c. An evaluation and management code
   d. All of the above

6. During a partial colectomy with anastomosis (44140), the surgeon encountered extensive adhesions and an additional loop of small bowel that was stuck in the pelvis. With gentle dissection from afferent and efferent limbs, the adhesion was lysed. Over an hour was spent to lyse the adhesions. What modifier would be appended to CPT code 44140?
   a. 22
   b. 58
   c. 53
   d. 59

7. A patient with chondromalacia of both knees underwent a bilateral arthrodesis (27580) of the knees. What modifier would be appended to the CPT code for the arthrodesis?
   a. 77
   b. 51
   c. 58
   d. 50

8. During a positional nystagmus test, minimum of four positions, with recording (92542), the equipment failed and only two recordings were made. What modifier would be appended to CPT code 92542?
   a. 51
   b. 50
   c. 52
   d. 53

9. Two weeks after an extensive excision of pilonidal cyst (11771), which carries a 90-day global period, the patient returns to the physician's office for E/M services for treatment of her hypertension. What modifier would be appended to the E/M code?
   a. None
   b. 24
   c. 25
   d. 59

10. While on vacation in Texas, Victor tore his Achilles tendon playing tennis. Victor was seen in the emergency room and scheduled for surgery by Dr. Andrews, who repaired the tendon (27652). Victor was instructed to follow up with his orthopedic surgeon when he returned to New York. What modifier would Dr. Andrews append to the CPT code for the Achilles tendon repair?
    a. 54
    b. 55
    c. 56
    d. None

ANSWERS AND RATIONALES

Assign the Appropriate Modifier

1. **Modifier 81** is used to indicate the assistant surgeon was present only for a short time during the procedure.

2. **No modifier** would be reported because the repeat laboratory test due to equipment failure would not be coded.

3. Because the second opinion was requested by the patient's HMO (insurance carrier), **modifier 32 (mandated services)** is appended to the CPT code for the second opinion.

4. Multiple procedures are reported by appending **modifier 51** to the additional procedure(s).

5. When the decision for surgery is made during an E/M encounter, **modifier 57** is appended to the E/M code.

Multiple Choice Answers

1. The correct answer is **a., modifier 79.** The patient was seen during the global period of an unrelated procedure (closed treatment of the Colles' fracture) by the same physician in the office setting; therefore, modifier 79 is appropriate. Answer **b.** is incorrect, as modifier 78 is for an unplanned **return to the operating room** for a *related* procedure. Answer **c.** is incorrect, as modifier 77 is for a repeat procedure by **another physician.** Answer **d.** is incorrect, as modifier 76 is for a **repeat procedure** by the same physician.

2. The correct answer is **b. Modifier 58** is used for a staged or related procedure or service by the same physician during the postoperative period. Answer **a.** is incorrect, as multiple procedures are reported with modifier 51. Answer **c.** is incorrect, as modifier 76 identifies a repeat procedure or service by the same physician. Answer **d.** is incorrect, as modifier 78 identifies an *unplanned* return to the operating/procedure room by the same physician following initial procedure for a related procedure during the postoperative period.

3. The correct answer is **c.** Because the physician owns the equipment and is interpreting the x-ray, the physician will bill for the global service (both the professional and technical components). Therefore, no modifier is necessary. Answer **a.** is incorrect, as

modifier 26 represents the professional component of the service, which must be indicated only when this component is reported separately (when the physician is not providing the technical component). Answer **b.** is incorrect, as modifier 25 is for a significant, separately identifiable E/M service by the same physician on the same day of the procedure or other service and is always appended to an E/M code. Answer **d.** is incorrect, as modifier 57 is used to indicate that an E/M service resulted in the initial decision to perform surgery.

4. The correct answer is **b. Modifier 47** indicates that regional or general anesthesia was provided by the surgeon. Answer **a.** is incorrect, as modifier 47 is never used by an anesthesiologist. Answer **c.** is incorrect, as modifier 47 is utilized only by the surgeon. Answer **d.** is incorrect, as modifier 47 is used by the surgeon.

5. The correct answer is **c. Modifier 25,** as indicated in the CPT modifier description, is always appended to an E/M code. Answer **a.** is incorrect: CPT modifiers are developed for CPT codes and therefore are never appended to diagnosis codes. Answer **b.** is incorrect; when both a surgical procedure and an E/M service are performed on the same day, the E/M service is designated as separate and distinct; therefore, modifier 25 is appended to the E/M code. Answer **d.** is incorrect, as modifier 25 is appended only to an E/M code.

6. The correct answer is **a. Modifier 22** describes increased procedural services. This scenario indicates the surgeon encountered multiple and difficult adhesions during the surgery, which increased the time necessary to complete the procedure by over 1 hour. Answer **b.** is incorrect, as modifier 58 describes a staged or related procedure or service by the same physician during the postoperative period. Answer **c.** is incorrect, as modifier 53 is used to describe a discontinued procedure, and in this scenario, the procedure was not discontinued but required additional work by the physician. Answer **d.** is incorrect, as modifier 59 is used to describe a distinct procedure or service (e.g., different session, procedure, site). This scenario represents one procedure/session that required additional work by the physician to complete the procedure.

7. The correct answer is **d. Modifier 50** represents bilateral procedures. Answer **a.** is incorrect, as modifier 77 is used to describe a repeat procedure by another physician. Answer **b.** is incorrect, as modifier 51 indicates multiple procedures. Because

the procedure is reported as being performed bilaterally (on both knees), with modifier 50 the CPT code is reported only once. Answer **c.** is incorrect, as modifier 58 describes a staged or related procedure or service by the same physician during the postoperative period. In this scenario, the bilateral procedure was performed at one operative session, with staged or related procedures performed when the patient was brought back to the operating room during the postoperative period.

8. The correct answer is **c. Modifier 52** is used to report reduced services. Because the equipment failed before the test could be completed, modifier 52 is appended to indicate the service was provided but not to the full extent of the CPT descriptor. Answer **a.** is incorrect, as modifier 51 represents multiple procedures. Answer **b.** is incorrect, as modifier 50 represents bilateral procedures. Although two positions were recorded, this does not constitute a bilateral procedure. Answer **d.** is incorrect, as modifier 53 is reported when the physician chooses to discontinue a procedure due to circumstances that present a threat to the patient or under extenuating circumstances.

9. The correct answer is **b. Modifier 24** represents an unrelated evaluation and management service by the same physician during a postoperative period. The patient was seen during the postoperative period of the excision of a pilonidal cyst by the same physician for an evaluation of hypertension, which is unrelated to the excision of the cyst. Answer **a.** is incorrect, as it is necessary to append a modifier to indicate the office visit was unrelated to the excision of the cyst. Answer **c.** is incorrect, as modifier 25 is used to describe a separately identifiable E/M service on the *same day* of a procedure or other service, whereas the patient in this scenario returned *2 weeks later* for her unrelated E/M service, during the postoperative period. Answer **d.** is incorrect, as modifier 59 describes a distinct procedural service (e.g., different session, procedure, site). Although the E/M service is a separate service at a different session, the service is provided during the global period and is unrelated to the surgery, which is best described by modifier 24.

10. The correct answer is **a. Modifier 54** represents the surgical care only. Dr. Andrews provided only the surgical service; therefore, he would append modifier 54. Answer **b.** is incorrect, as modifier 55 represents only the postoperative management. This modifier would be used by the patient's orthopedic surgeon in New York, who will provide the follow-up care. Answer **c.** is incorrect, as modifier 56 represents the preoperative management only. Answer **d.** is incorrect, as modifier 54 is appropriate.

CHAPTER 8

Evaluation and Management Codes

Evaluation and Management (E/M) encounters represent the visits provided by a physician or other qualified health-care professional to a patient. There are several different types of E/M services, all of which will require a different amount of work and documentation based on the type of service (e.g., office visit, critical care, preventive visit), place of service (e.g., office, emergency room, nursing home), and the patient's status (e.g., new patient, established patient). These visits are provided at different levels of service. The amount of documentation in the patient's medical records determines the level of service.

Medical Record Documentation

Before we review the history of the documentation guidelines, it is important to know why medical record documentation is important and to understand some of its basic principles. The patient's medical record is a chronological record documenting the care of the patient. This medical record is essential in providing care to the patient, as it provides the physician with needed information regarding not only the patient's state of health but also past treatment and care. This record has several other uses, and for these purposes, it may be utilized and reviewed by individuals other than the patient's physician. Medical records and documentation may be reviewed:

■ By other physicians sharing in or taking over the care of the patient.

■ To appeal a medical claim.
■ For utilization and quality-of-care reviews.
■ For the collection of data for research and education.
■ For the defense of medical malpractice cases.

Regardless of what type of E/M service is provided, some basic principles regarding medical record documentation must be followed. Each record must be complete and legible and should include the following:

1. The patient's name and date of service
2. The reason for the visit, relevant history, physical examination, and any previous diagnostic test results
3. An assessment of the patient including a diagnosis or clinical impression
4. The treatment plan or plan of care for the patient
5. Signature of the provider of service
6. The medical necessity for ordering any diagnostic testing and/or other ancillary services (e.g., physical therapy). If not documented, it should be easily inferred.
7. Any past or present diagnoses; this information should be accessible to the treating or consulting physician.
8. Any appropriate health-risk factors
9. The progress of the patient, changes and response to treatment, and any revision of diagnosis

The documentation in the medical record should also support all CPT, HCPCS, and ICD-9-CM codes reported.

Current Documentation Guidelines

The first Documentation Guidelines (DG) were implemented in 1995 by the Centers for Medicare and Medicaid Services (CMS). In 1997, CMS and the American Medical Association (AMA) introduced new guidelines (see Chapter 1). These new guidelines included physical examinations that are specialty-specific. Many of the physicians expressed discord with these new guidelines. CMS responded by suspending the implementation of the 1997 guidelines pending revision and finalization. Currently, CMS allows you to use either the 1995 or 1997 Documentation Guidelines.

Let's take a look at the differences between the two sets of guidelines.

1995	1997
History: Chief Complaint; History of presenting illness; Review of systems; Past, Family, and Social History Three of three required (see p. 109)	**History:** Chief Complaint; History of presenting illness **OR status of three chronic or inactive conditions;** Review of systems; Past, Family, and Social History Three of three required (see p. 109)
Physical Examination: Body areas and organ systems	**Physical Examination:** Body areas and organ systems as well as elements/bullets under each body area/organ system
Medical Decision Making: Number of diagnosis and treatment options, amount of data reviewed, risk of morbidity and/or mortality Two of three required	Same as 1995

As you can see, the differences between the 1995 and 1997 Documentation Guidelines are with the documentation of the history and physical examination. To get a better understanding of how these differences affect the level of service and which set of guidelines to use, we first look at how the Documentation Guidelines relate to the CPT code or level of service selected.

It is important to note both the E/M Guidelines in the CPT book and the Certified Professional Coder's Exam are based on the 1995 Documentation Guidelines. This review book focuses on and reviews the 1995 Documentation Guidelines.

Determining the Level of Service

The first element we need to determine is **where** the service is taking place. Is the service being provided in a physician's office, a hospital, a nursing home?

Next, we need to determine the **category** of service. What type of service is this? Is this a consultation, a preventive visit, a follow-up office visit?

Then, we need to determine the **status of the patient** (subcategory). Is the patient a new patient or an established patient?

Finally, we need to determine the level of each of the **three key components** of the visit.

Table of contents in the E/M Guidelines section of the CPT book lists all the categories and subcategories of service.

New Patient or Established Patient?

In the physician outpatient setting, a new patient is a patient who hasn't been seen for 3 years by a physician of the same specialty within the same group.

LET'S LOOK AT AN EXAMPLE

Mrs. Jones's newborn baby, James, was seen by Dr. Jacobs in the newborn nursery. Dr. Jacobs examined James, determined the baby was healthy, and discharged him. Dr. Jacobs advised Mrs. Jones to bring James into his office in 10 days for a checkup and vaccinations. Upon presenting to Dr. Jacobs's office, Mrs. Jones completed all the necessary paperwork for the staff to make a new chart, and James was seen by Dr. Jacobs. Is James a new patient or an established patient to Dr. Jacobs's office?

*The Answer Is: **an established patient.*** Dr. Jacobs had already seen James in the newborn nursery; therefore, when he presented to the office, even though it was the first time to the office, it was not the first time Dr. Jacobs saw James.

LET'S LOOK AT ANOTHER EXAMPLE

Dr. Arnold and Dr. Fredricks both work in the same practice, Comprehensive Medical Care. Dr. Arnold's specialty is internal medicine, and Dr. Fredricks is a cardiologist. Mary Anderson went to see Dr. Arnold for a follow-up visit for her hypertension and new complaints of chest pain. Upon examination, Dr. Arnold did not detect any abnormal chest sounds, attributed the chest pain to a mild muscle strain, and reassured Mary. Mary was still concerned, and she made an appointment to see Dr. Fredricks (the cardiologist) for an evaluation. Will Mary be a new or established patient when she sees Dr. Fredricks?

The Answer Is: new. Although both physicians are in the same group, each physician has a different specialty.

Let's take a look at how the level of service is selected. *It is best to follow along by opening your CPT book to the E/M Guidelines section.*

KEY CODING TIP

It is important to identify if the patient is new or established because the documentation requirements are greater for new patients or consultations, which require three of three key components (i.e., history, physical examination, and medical decision), whereas the requirements for established patients are two of three key components.

It is important to note that the *three key components* are the history, physical examination, and medical decision. The remaining four components—counseling, coordination of care, presenting problem, and time—are **contributory components.** Key components must be met or exceeded. Certain E/M categories and subcategories require that all three key components (history, physical, and medical decision) are all documented at the same level; otherwise, the level of service is selected on the basis of the documented lowest component. These E/M categories and subcategories (e.g., new patient visits, initial hospital care, emergency room visits) **can be identified in the CPT book as their descriptors will state, "which *requires these three key components."* (The exception to documentation of the key components, the time exception rule, is discussed later in this chapter.)

Seven components make up a visit:

- History
- Physical Examination
- Medical Decision
- Counseling
- Coordination of Care
- Nature of Presenting Problem
- Time

The Three Key Components
Determining the Level of History (First Key Component)

There are four levels of history: (1) problem-focused, (2) expanded problem-focused, (3) detailed, and (4) comprehensive. As you might imagine, the higher the level of history, the more documentation is required.

Problem-Focused requires a chief complaint, brief history of presenting illness (HPI; one to three elements).

Expanded Problem-Focused requires a chief complaint, brief HPI (one to three elements), and problem-pertinent review of systems (ROS 1).

Detailed requires a chief complaint, extended HPI (4 elements), problem-pertinent ROS extended to include a review of a limited number of additional systems (two to nine ROS), and a pertinent past, family, and social history (PFSH) directly related to the patient's problem (one PFSH).

Comprehensive requires a chief complaint, extended HPI (4 elements), a ROS that is directly related to the problem(s) identified in the HPI plus review of all additional body systems (at least 10), and a complete PFSH (all 3).

Each level of history will include all or some of the following elements: chief complaint (CC), HPI, ROS, PFSH.

CC: This is the reason for the visit. Documentation should include the physician-recommended return, symptom, problem, condition, diagnosis, or any other concern that prompted the encounter (e.g., patient returns for follow-up of hypertension and diabetes, patient presents with complaints of pain and swelling of knee). Each visit should include documentation of a CC, as it provides medical necessity for the visit.

HPI (History of Present Illness) **ELEMENTS**	ROS (Review of Symptoms) **RECOGNIZED SYSTEMS**	
Location	Constitutional	Integumentary
Quality	Eyes	Neurologic
Severity	Ears, nose, mouth, throat	Psychiatric
Duration	Cardiovascular	Endocrine
Timing	Respiratory	Hematologic/lymphatic
Context	Gastrointestinal	Allergic/immunologic
Modifying factors	Genitourinary	
Associated signs and symptoms	Musculoskeletal	

ROS:
The patient's positive responses and pertinent negatives for the system(s) relating to the problem should be documented. For the remaining systems reviewed, a notation indicating all other systems are negative is permissible.

PFSH:
Past history: Patient's past experiences with illnesses, operations, injuries, and treatments
Family history: Review of medical events in patient's family, including diseases which may be hereditary or place the patient at risk
Social history: An age appropriate review of past and current activities

HPI: A chronological description of the development of the patient's illness from the beginning to the present. This includes a list of elements (descriptive adjectives), location, quality, severity, timing, context, modifying factors, and associated signs and symptoms, all of which are related to the presenting problem(s).

ROS: An inventory of body systems obtained through a **series of questions** seeking to identify signs and/or symptoms that the patient may be experiencing or has experienced. Although the ROS includes 14 body areas, it is important to note the ROS is *not* a physical examination, but as stated previously, a series of questions designed to give the physician more insight into the patient's problems. As per the documentation guidelines, the patient's positive responses and pertinent negatives for the system related to the problem should be documented. For the remaining systems reviewed, a notation indicating all other systems are negative is permissible. Therefore, it is not necessary to list the remaining systems individually if the remaining systems have been identified as negative.

PFSH—The PFSH consists of three areas:

■ Past History: A review of the patient's past experiences with illnesses, operations, injuries, and treatments.

■ Family History: A review of the patient's family history, including diseases that may be hereditary or for which the patient may be at risk.

■ Social History: An age-appropriate review of the patient's past and current activities (e.g., smoking, drinking, employment).

The amount of documentation determines the level of history. First, each of the elements (CC, HPI, ROS, PFSH) are assigned to a particular level based on how many requirements are met for that level.

For example: A patient presenting with an insect bite might require a brief history, whereas a patient presenting with severe stomach pain for several days would require a more detailed history. The level of history you select cannot be higher than the lowest level assigned to any of the elements of the history. Let's look at these steps more closely.

	New Patient Visit	99201	99202	99203	99204	99205
	Consultations					
	MUST DOCUMENT ALL 3 KEY COMPONENTS					
History	Chief complaint	Required	Required	Required	Required	Required
	HPI	1–3 elements	1–3 elements	≥ 4 elements		
	ROS		1 system	2–9 systems	≥ 10 systems	
	Past history			1 of the PFSH areas	All 3 of the PFSH areas	
	Family history					
	Social history					

Let's Try One Together

Using the chart presented previously, let's determine the level of history for the following case study of a new patient.

CC: 36-year-old female complaining of Raynaud's syndrome (constriction of the arteries, due to cold or stress).

HPI: Patient complains of Raynaud's over the past couple of years which she describes as coldness in the upper and lower extremities.

Location: upper and lower extremities; quality: coldness; duration: past couple of years.

This statement contains three elements of the HPI. Using the chart, let's circle one to three elements of the HPI.

ROS—Constitutional: denies abnormal weight gain/loss; Cardiovascular: denies chest pain; Respiratory: denies cough and sputum; Gastrointestinal: denies nausea and vomiting; Genitourinary: denies frequency and hematuria; Neurological: denies headaches; Musculoskeletal: denies myalgia and arthritis; Hematological: denies abnormal bleeding and bruising; Skin: denies rashes.

This statement contains nine elements of the ROS. Documenting negative or patient denials of the review of systems is still counted toward the review of systems, as these represent "pertinent negatives." Using the chart, let's circle two to nine systems.

PFSH—Past History: patient states past appendectomy; Family History: no diabetes, carcinoma, coronary artery disease or sudden death; Social History: patient is a social worker, nonsmoker, nondrinker, and no recreational drug use.

This statement covers all three of the history areas. Using the chart, circle all three of the PFSH.

Documentation of the history requires that all three of the elements (HPI, ROS, and PFSH) are documented at the same level *or* that you select the level with the documented lowest element, in this case, the HPI. If we follow the circled HPI up to the level of service (in this case, a new patient), the level of history is 99202 (Level 2, or problem-focused history).

Determining the Level of Physical Examination (Second Key Component)

As with the history, there are four levels of physical examinations: (1) problem-focused, (2) expanded problem-focused, (3) detailed, and (4) comprehensive. *Although the documentation guidelines do not assign a specific amount of documentation required for each body area/organ system, listed in parentheses are the industry standard documentation requirements.*

Problem-Focused: A limited examination of the affected body area or organ system (1).

Expanded Problem-Focused: A limited examination of the affected body area or organ system and other symptomatic or related organ system(s) (2–4).

Detailed: An extended examination of the affected body area(s) and other symptomatic or related organ system(s) (5–7 body areas/organ systems, one in detail).

Comprehensive: A general multisystem examination or a complete examination of a single organ system (8 or more of the 12 *organ systems*).

For examination purposes, the following *body areas* are recognized:

■ Head, including the face
■ Neck
■ Chest, including breasts and axillae
■ Abdomen
■ Genitalia, groin, buttocks

	New Patient Visit	99201	99202	99203	99204	99205
	Consultations					
	MUST DOCUMENT ALL 3 KEY COMPONENTS					
History	Chief complaint	Required	Required	Required	Required	Required
	HPI	1–3 elements	1–3 elements	≥ 4 elements		
	ROS		1 system	2–9 systems	≥ 10 systems	
	Past history			1 of the PFSH areas	All 3 of the PFSH areas	
	Family history					
	Social history					

- Back, including spine
- Each extremity

For examination purposes, the following *organ systems* are recognized:

- Constitutional (e.g., vital signs, general appearance)
- Eyes
- Ears, nose, mouth, and throat
- Cardiovascular
- Respiratory
- Gastrointestinal
- Genitourinary
- Musculoskeletal
- Skin
- Neurological
- Psychiatric
- Hematological/lymphatic/immunological

99201	99202	99203	99204	99205
Problem-Focused	Expanded Problem-Focused	Detailed	Comprehensive	Comprehensive
1 element, body area/ organ system	2–4 elements, body area/ organ system	5–7 elements, body area/organ system— one in detail	8 or more organ systems	8 or more organ systems

Let's Try One Together

Using the chart above, let's determine the level of physical examination for this same Raynaud's patient.

General: Well developed, well nourished, and in no apparent distress.

Blood Pressure: 110/70; Pulse: 78; RR: 12.

Head: normocephalic, atraumatic.

Eyes: Anicteric, EOM (extraocular movements) intact, pink conjunctiva, PERLA (pupils equally reactive to light and accommodation).

Ears/Nose/Throat: Auricles normal, canals with minimal cerumen. Tympanic membrane shows normal light reflex, no erythema. Nasal mucosa without significant erythema, discharge. Oropharynx without exudates or ulcers.

Neck: Supple without JVD (jugular venous distention).

Lungs: Normal breathing pattern, clear to auscultation.

Chest Wall: No focal tenderness, normal, appears without pectus deformity.

Cardiovascular: S1 normal, S2 normal, no murmurs, gallops, rubs.

Abdomen: Bowel sounds positive, soft nontender, no hepatosplenomegaly.

Lymphatic: No abnormal cervical, axillary, inguinal nodes.

Musculoskeletal: Normal gait, strength, and muscle tone.

Extremities: Purple fingers, Raynaud's phenomenon.

Neurological: Motor and sensory exam nonfocal, reflexes normal.

Psychiatric: Alert and oriented ×3, normal memory and affect.

The level of physical examination documented is a "comprehensive," Level 5 physical examination (eight or more body areas/organ systems).

Determining the Level of Medical Decision (Third Key Component)

Three elements are used to determine the level of decision making:

- The number of diagnoses and/or the number of *management options to be considered*. This refers to the presenting problem (e.g., one self-limited or minor problem such as an insect bite, or an undiagnosed new problem with an uncertain prognosis such as a breast lump).

- The amount and/or complexity of data to be ordered. This refers to the diagnostic procedures ordered (e.g., laboratory tests, deep needle biopsy).

- Risk of complications and/or morbidity or mortality. This refers to the *management options selected* (e.g., physical therapy, minor surgery with identified risk factors).

Unlike the history component, which requires all three elements (HPI, ROS, and PFSH) to be documented at the same level (three of three) to qualify for a given type of medical decision making (MDM), *only two of the three elements must be met or exceeded.*

There are four levels of medical decision making: straightforward, low complexity, moderate complexity, and high complexity.

The Documentation Guidelines provide a Table of Risk to help determine the correct level of risk.

TABLE OF RISK

Level of risk	Presenting Problem(s)	Diagnostic Procedure(s) Ordered	Management Options Selected
Minimal	• One self-limited or minor problem, eg, cold, insect bite, tinea corporis	• Laboratory tests requiring venipuncture • Chest x-rays • EKG/EEG • Urinalysis • Ultrasound, eg, echocardiography • KOH prep	• Rest • Gargles • Elastic bandages • Superficial dressings
Low	• Two or more self-limited or minor problems • One stable chronic illness, eg, well controlled hypertension, non-insulin dependent diabetes, cataract, BPH • Acute uncomplicated illness or injury, eg, cystitis, allergic rhinitis, simple sprain	• Physiologic tests not under stress, eg, pulmonary function tests • Non-cardiovacular imaging studies with contrast, eg, barium enema • Superficial needle biopsies • Clinical laboratory tests requiring arterial puncture • Skin biopsies	• Over-the-counter drugs • Minor surgery with no identified risk factors • Physical therapy • Occupational therapy • IV fluids without additives
Moderate	• One or more chronic illnesses with mild exacerbation, progression, or side effects of treatment • Two or more stable chronic illnesses • Undiagnosed new problem with uncertain prognosis, eg, lump in breast • Acute illness with systemic symptoms, eg, pyelonephritis, pneumonitis, colitis • Acute complicated injury, eg, head injury with brief loss of consciousness	• Physiologic tests under stress, eg, cardiac stress test, fetal contraction stress test • Diagnostic endoscopies with no identified risk factors • Deep needle or incisional biopsy • Cardiovascular imaging studies with contrast and no identified risk factors, eg, arteriogram, cardiac catheterization • Obtain fluid from body cavity, eg, lumbar puncture, thoracentesis, culdocentesis	• Minor surgery with identified risk factors • Elective major surgery (open, percutaneous or endoscopic) with no identified risk factors • Presciption drug management • Therapeutic nuclear medicine • IV fluids with additives • Closed treatment of fracture or dislocation without manipulation
High	• One or more chronic illnesses with severe exacerbation, progression, or side effects of treatment • Acute or chronic illnesses or injuries that pose a threat to life or bodily function, eg, multiple trauma, acute MI, pulmonary embolus, severe respiratory distress, progressive severe rheumatoid arthritis, psychiatric illness with potential threat to self or others, peritonitis, acute renal failure • An abrupt change in neurologic status, eg, seizure, TIA, weakness, sensory loss	• Cardiovascular imaging studies with contrast with identified risk factors • Cardiac electrophysiological tests • Diagnostic endoscopies with identified risk factors • Discography	• Elective major surgery (open, percutaneous or endoscopic) with identified risk factors • Emergency major surgery (open, percutaneous or endoscopic) • Parenteral controlled substances • Drug therapy requiring intensive monitoring for toxicity • Decision not to resuscitate or to de-escalate care because of poor prognosis

Number of diagnoses or management options	Amount and/or complexity of data to be reviewed	Risk of complications and/or morbidity or mortality	Type of decision making
Minimal	Minimal or none	Minimal	Straightforward
Limited	Limited	Low	Low complexity
Multiple	Moderate	Moderate	Moderate complexity
Extensive	Extensive	High	High complexity

(Table of Risk from Centers for Medicare and Medicaid Services (CMS) Table of Risk.)

Let's Try One Together

Refer to Table 2, Complexity of Medical Decision Making, located in the CPT book in the E/M Guidelines.

Using the Table of Risk, let's determine the level of medical decision making for the Raynaud's patient.

Diagnostic Testing: EKG, normal sinus rhythm.
Impression: Raynaud's syndrome.

Plan: Will treat with Procardia (prescription medication). Patient to return in 3 months.

The **number of diagnoses and/or management options** (indicated by "Impression") is limited to the Raynaud's syndrome; the **amount and complexity of data** reviewed were minimal (EKG); and the **risk of complications** with regard to management options was moderate (prescription drug management). We can therefore assign these elements to levels as follows:

Number of diagnoses or management options = Limited (low complexity—Level 3)

Amount and/or complexity of data to be reviewed = Minimal (straightforward—Level 2)

Risk of complications and/or morbidity or mortality = Moderate (moderate complexity—Level 4)

Because the level of medical decision making is based on two of the three elements, the level of medical decision is low: Level 3. In this case, because all three of the elements are at different levels, we can select the level in the middle (Level 3).

Putting It All Together

Now that we have identified the level of each of the three key components required to determine the level of service, let's see what level of service the Raynaud's syndrome encounter will be.

The history was documented as expanded problem-focused, Level 2 (99202).

The physical examination was documented as comprehensive, Level 5 (99205).

The medical decision was documented as low complexity, Level 3 (99203).

As we know, key components must be met or exceeded, and because this is a new patient, we are required to have all three of the three key components documented at the same level or we must select the lowest level documented, in this case the history. Therefore, the level of service is Level 2, or 99202.

Remember we said that the documentation requirements are greater for new patients and/or any category or subcategory that requires three of three key components, and established patients require that only two of three key components are met or exceeded. Let's look at how the same documentation of the key components determines the level of service for an *established* patient.

The history was documented as expanded problem-focused, Level 3 (99213). *(Note: Documentation of the history yields a higher level of history for an established patient.)*

The physical examination was documented as comprehensive, Level 5 (99215).

The medical decision was documented as low complexity, Level 3 (99213).

In this scenario, because established patients require that only two of three key components are met or exceeded, this is a Level 3 (99213) encounter, as both the history and medical decision are documented at the same level.

KEY CODING TIP

Some of the E/M examples in the CPC examination give you the documented levels of history, physical examination, and medical decision making. When this information is provided, remember the following:

■ For any category/subcategory requiring three of three key components, either all key components (history, physical, and medical decision) are at the same level or select the level of service based on the documented lowest component.

■ For any category/subcategory requiring two of three key components, we can ignore the documented lowest component and base the level on the two higher documented components, selecting the lower of the two.

Exceptions to the Guidelines

There are two exceptions to these guidelines:

1. The Level 1 (99211) visit for an established patient

2. The time exception for selecting the level of service

Level 1 Established Patient Exception

First let's look at the **Level 1 (99211) established patient visit.** This level is unique, as it is an evaluation that does not require the presence of a physician to provide the service, and typically, 5 minutes is spent performing and supervising these services.

Certain services may be provided by the office staff, such as nursing staff or a medical assistant. In these cases, the services of the nurse or medical assistant are provided "incidental to" the services of the physician. The "incidental-to" rule requires **direct supervision** by the physician: the physician is not required to perform the service but must be in the office suite at the time of the service and immediately available to the patient if need be.

For example: An office visit for a 12-year-old child seen by the nurse for a cursory check of a hematoma 1 day after having blood drawn falls under the incidental-to rule.

More examples of 99211 are located in Appendix C, Clinical Examples of the CPT book.

The Time Exception

There may be some encounters where the three key components are not applicable. For example, in the case of a patient who presents to the office to discuss the results of blood work, an MRI, or a recent biopsy, there is no need to take a history or perform a physical examination.

When counseling and/or coordination of care dominate the encounter (50 percent or more of the total visit time), time may determine the level of service. The time spent must be physician face-to-face time with the patient in the office or outpatient setting or must be floor/unit time in the hospital.

In these cases, the documentation should include the following:

Documentation of Time

- Length of time counseling/coordinating care (e.g., 15 minutes, 25 minutes).

- Total visit time (start time and stop time to be recorded). If the total visit time is the same as the amount of time spent in counseling and/or coordinating care for the patient, it should be stated as such (e.g., 25-minute visit with 25 minutes spent counseling and coordinating care).

- Summary of issues and items discussed.

- Who was present. It is important to note who was present (e.g., husband and wife) because it helps to substantiate the amount of time spent, as now you are answering questions for two people instead of just the patient.

Documentation of Counseling

(Although there are many items bulleted, you need to document only those that are applicable.)

- Discussion of significant medical problems
- Treatment options

- Potential risks and benefits
- Long-term impact and arrangements
- Involvement of family members/caregivers
- Amount of time and discussion to include other providers (only if the patient is present)

LET'S LOOK AT AN EXAMPLE

This is an established patient presenting to the office for results of an MRI and treatment plan.

Office Visit of 10/3/05: Review of MRI films and report dated 9/21/05. MRI of the brain shows mild atrophy and some chronic ischemic changes. Most importantly, the aneurysm is no longer visualized. I reviewed this fact with the patient and his wife. I have also called Dr. Smith to inform him of the result and that as far as I am concerned, anticoagulation is not contraindicated. I have advised the patient to undergo MR angiography in approximately 6 months.

The patient also complains of impaired memory, primarily through his wife. Able to recall unrelated words after distraction, 1/3 on the first trial, 2/3 on the second trial, and 2/3 on the third trial. General fund of knowledge is normal. Able to give correct directions to Dr. office. Able to recall military service number.

The patient is scheduled for more detailed cognitive testing next week, and we will go through with that testing. I don't think we are dealing with much in the way of cognitive impairment.

27-minute visit with *greater than 50% of the visit spent on counseling* regarding the results of MRI, as well as the need for cognitive testing.

How to Code: Many of the E/M codes have a time element listed in their descriptor. Because this is an outpatient established patient, the code range will be 99211–99215. A review of these codes shows CPT code 99214 has a time descriptor of 25 minutes, and CPT code 99215 has a time descriptor of 40 minutes. Because we do not meet the criterion of 40 minutes, we select the next level, in this case 25 minutes, represented by CPT code 99214. Therefore, the correct level of service for this outpatient established patient encounter, based on time, is Level 4 (99214).

E/M Codes—and How to Use Them

Now that we understand how to select the level of service based on the documentation in the patient's medical record, let's review the most common E/M codes.

Office or Other Outpatient Services

New Patient
99201–99205

Established Patient
99211–99215

These services are reported for outpatient office visits. They are classified into five levels of service, which are determined by the Documentation Guidelines.

Hospital Observation Services

These services are used to report E/M services to patients who are not formally admitted to the hospital but are placed in an observation status until they are either admitted to the hospital or well enough to go home. It is important to note that the patient need not be placed in a "designated" observation area in the hospital for these codes to be reported.

Initial Observation Care
99218–99220

These services are classified into three levels of service, which are determined by the Documentation Guidelines. These codes are reported for the initiation of the observation status.

- If the patient is seen in the emergency department and placed in observation status, only the observation status should be reported. The observation status code reported should *include the services* related to the initiation of the observation status that *were provided in the other sites of service* (e.g., emergency room).

- If the patient were to be admitted to the hospital on the same date as the initiation of observation status, you would report only the hospital admission code.

- If the patient were to be admitted to the hospital on a date subsequent to the date of observation initiation, you would report only the observation care on day 1 and the hospital admission code on the subsequent day.

- If the patient were to be admitted and discharged from observation care on the same day, the service would be reported with a code 99234–99236 Observation or Inpatient Care Services (Including Admission and Discharge Services). These codes are represented by three different levels of service, which are determined by the Documentation Guidelines.

- Observation codes may not be reported for patients placed in postoperative recovery, as this is considered part of the surgical package.

Observation Care Discharge
99217

This code is used to report the discharge from observation status *when the patient is discharged on a date other than the admission to observation care.*

Hospital Inpatient Services

Initial Hospital Care
99221–99223

Subsequent Hospital Care
99231–99233

These services are reported for inpatient visits and are classified into three levels of service, which are determined by the Documentation Guidelines. There are separate codes for the initial hospital care (admission) and subsequent hospital care (follow-up visits).

Hospital Discharge Services
99238–99239

There are two levels of hospital discharge services. They both include the final examination of the patient, a discussion of the hospital stay, and instructions for continuing care to include caregivers where applicable, the preparation of discharge records, prescriptions, and referrals forms. Both of these codes are time based. **CPT code 99238** represents discharge day management of 30 minutes or less, and **CPT code 99239** represents discharge day management of more than 30 minutes. These are time-based codes, so time should be documented in the patient's medical record.

Consultations

It is important to note that effective 2010, Medicare no longer recognizes consultation codes. However, the codes are still reimbursed by many insurance carriers and are still listed in the CPT manual for use when appropriate.

Office Consultations
99241–99245

Inpatient Consultations
99251–99255

These services are reported for consultations; they represent two different places of service (inpatient or outpatient). They are classified into five levels of service, which are determined by the Documentation Guidelines. Consults differ from other visits, as they are E/M services that are performed usually by a specialist (consultant) at the request of a physician or other qualified provider for the purpose of providing opinion or advice to the requesting physician or other qualified provider. Additional documentation is required for consultations. *Remember the three-R rule* and include the following documentation:

■ **Request**—The request and the reason for the consultation must be documented in the patient's medical record by both the consultant and the requesting provider.

■ **Render**—The consultant renders and documents appropriate services related to the patient's condition/problem.

■ **Report**—The consultant reports back to the requesting provider, usually in the form of a written report of his or her findings, opinion, and advice.

The consultant may also initiate treatment or diagnostic testing at the time of the consult.

Follow-up visits performed by the consultant at the request of the patient or consultant are reported using the appropriate codes for established patients. (For example, a patient who was diagnosed by the consultant with ulcerative colitis is also followed by the consultant for management of the ulcerative colitis.) If an additional request for an opinion or advice from the consultant regarding a new or the same problem is initiated by another physician or qualified health-care provider, and the request is documented in the patient's medical record, the consultation codes may once again be utilized.

Emergency Department Services
99281–99285

These services are reported for services provided in the emergency department. They are represented by five levels of service, which are determined by the Documentation Guidelines.

Other Emergency Services
99288

Physician direction of emergency medical systems (EMS) emergency care, advanced life support (99288): This code represents the services of a physician who is located in a hospital emergency or critical care department and is in two-way communication with ambulance or rescue personnel outside of the hospital. The physician directs the performance of medical care and or procedures to EMS as the patient is in transit to the hospital.

Critical Care Services
99291–99292

Critical care codes are time-based codes with unique documentation requirements. The guidelines preceding the critical care codes *must be read*. Critical care is defined by CPT as "The direct delivery by a physician(s) of medical care for a critically ill or critically injured person." A critical illness or critical injury is one that acutely impairs one or more vital organ systems such that there is a high probability of impending or life-threatening decline in the patient's condition (e.g., respiratory failure, shock, circulatory failure). It is not mandatory for critical care to be provided in a critical care setting (intensive care unit, respiratory care unit, etc.); critical care may be provided in any setting.

For example: A patient with chest pain does not consider her symptoms severe enough to go to the emergency room. Instead she decides to go to her primary care physician. While waiting her turn to be seen, she goes into cardiac arrest. The physician comes out to the waiting area with a crash cart and medical assistant and provides critical care services to the patient as the receptionist calls for an ambulance. In this scenario, the patient *meets the definition of critically ill* and the *physician provides critical care services.*

So now we know that critical care does not have to be provided in a critical care setting, but what happens if the physician sees a patient in the critical care unit who is recovering or stable? Remember, the patient must meet the definition of being critically ill or critically injured. If the patient does not meet this definition, the services are reported with other appropriate E/M codes (e.g., subsequent hospital visit).

Critical care codes have many services bundled (included) in the code, and as such, the bundled services should not be coded in addition to the critical care codes. Some of the services included are chest x-rays, pulse oximetry, and blood gases (the complete list of bundled codes are located in the critical care guidelines). Any service not included in the code for critical care is separately reportable (e.g., CPR).

Documentation of Time for Critical Care Services

Because critical care codes are time based, the time involved in these services **must** be documented in the patient's record. The time does not need to be continuous; however, for any time spent by the physician providing critical care services, the physician must dedicate his full attention to the patient.

For example: A physician sees a critically ill patient at 9:00 a.m. and provides critical care services until 10:00 a.m. At 1:00 p.m. the nurse calls the physician back to attend to the patient, whose condition is worsening. The physician provides an additional hour of critical care services. In this case, we can add the 1 hour in the morning and the 1 hour in the afternoon and code for 2 hours of critical care services.

Critical care time consists of the following:

- Time at the patient's bedside providing care
- Time spent reviewing test results or imaging studies at the nursing station or on the floor/unit
- Time spent discussing the patient's care with other medical staff at the nursing station or on the floor/unit
- Time spent documenting critical care services in the medical record at the nursing station or on the floor/unit
- Time spent with family members or surrogate decision makers at the nursing station or on the floor/unit obtaining a medical history, reviewing the patient's condition, or discussing the patient's treatment or limitations of treatment, providing the conversations relate directly to the management of the patient and *only* if the patient is unable to participate in such discussion

Time spent outside of the unit or off the floor may not be counted as critical care time (e.g., telephone calls taken at home, in the office, or off the floor/unit).

Codes for documenting critical care time are selected using the following table:

Correct Reporting of Critical Care Services

Total Duration of Critical Care **Less than 30 min (less than 1/2 hr)**	Codes **Appropriate E/M codes**
30–74 min (1/2 hr–1 hr 14 min)	99291 × 1
75–104 min (1 hr 15 min–1 hr 44 min)	99291 × 1 AND 99292 × 1
105–134 min (1 hr 45 min–2 hr 14 min)	99291 × 1 AND 99292 × 2
135–164 min (2 hr 15 min–2 hr 44 min)	99291 × 1 AND 99292 × 3
165–194 min (2 hr 45 min–3 hr 14 min)	99291 × 1 AND 99292 × 4

Any time less than 30 minutes is reported with the appropriate E/M code, as the first 30 minutes is considered part of the E/M service.

Using the table, we code the visit for the previously mentioned patient for whom the physician provided critical care services for nonconsecutive hours, as follows: Because more than 30 minutes of critical care services were provided, we would calculate the total time spent by the physician providing critical care services. In this case, the physician saw the patient for 1 hour in the

morning (9:00 a.m.–10:00 a.m.) and for an additional hour in the afternoon (1:00 p.m.–2:00 p.m.) for a total of 2 hours of critical care services. Using the table, we would report 99291 × 1 (first hour) and 99292 × 2 (two units of CPT code 99292 for each additional half hour).

Nursing Facility Services
Initial Nursing Facility Care
99304–99306
Subsequent Nursing Facility Care
99307–99310

These services are reported for services provided in nursing facilities (e.g., skilled nursing facilities [SNF], long-term care facilities [LTCF], intermediate care facilities [ICF], and psychiatric residential treatment centers). The initial visits may be classified into three levels of service, and the subsequent visits are classified into four levels of service, all of which are determined by the Documentation Guidelines.

Nursing Facility Discharge Services
99315–99316

There are two levels of nursing facility discharge services based on the time involved in the service. Nursing facility discharge services include the final examination of the patient, a discussion of the nursing stay, and instructions for continuing care to include caregivers where applicable, the preparation of discharge records, prescriptions, and referrals forms. Because these codes are time based, time should be documented in the patient's medical record. CPT code 99315 represents discharge day management of 30 minutes or less, and CPT code 99316 represents discharge day management of more than 30 minutes.

Other Nursing Facility Services
99318

This code represents an annual nursing facility assessment of a patient who is usually stable, recovering, or improving.

Domiciliary, Rest Home (e.g., Boarding Home), or Custodial Care Services
New Patient
99324–99328
Established Patient
99334–99337

These E/M services represent services provided in facilities providing room and board and other personal assistance services generally on a long-term basis. They are also used to report E/M services in an assisted living facility. The new patient visits are represented by five levels of service, and the established patient visits are represented by four levels of service, all of which are determined by the Documentation Guidelines.

Domiciliary, Rest Home (e.g., Assisted Living Facility), or Home Care Plan Oversight Services
99339–99340

These time-based codes are used by physicians to report and coordinate the complex and multidisciplinary care modalities of the patient with other medical and nonmedical service providers and family. The patient is not present for these services, and the codes are reported only once a month. CPT code 99339 represents 15–29 minutes, and CPT code 99340 represents 30 minutes or more. Time spent coordinating the care plan for the patient should be documented in the patient's medical record.

Home Services
New Patient
99341–99345

Established Patient
99347–99350

These services are reported for visits provided in the patient's home. They are classified into five levels of service for new patients and four levels of service for established patients, as determined by the Documentation Guidelines.

Prolonged Services
Prolonged Physician Service *With* Direct (Face-to-Face) Patient Contact
99354–99357

Prolonged Physician Service *Without* Direct (Face-to-Face) Patient Contact
99358–99359

Prolonged services represent patient care that is **beyond the usual service** in either the outpatient or inpatient setting. All of the prolonged service codes are add-on codes (indicated by the + symbol in front of the code). Add-on codes are reported in addition to the primary service performed (with other E/M codes at any level) and are never reported alone. Like the critical care codes, prolonged service codes are time-based codes *requiring the time to be documented in the patient's medical record*. The time need not be continuous. As in the case of critical care services, any time less than 30 minutes is reported with the appropriate E/M code.

Examples representing prolonged attendance codes can be found in Appendix C- Clinical Examples of the CPT book. Prolonged Service Codes are calculated with the following table:

Total Duration of Prolonged Services	Code(s)
Less than 30 min (less than 1/2 hr)	Not reported separately
30–74 min (1/2 hr–1 hr 14 min)	99354 × 1
75–104 min (1 hr 15 min–1 hr 44 min)	99354 × 1 AND 99355 × 1
105–134 min (1 hr 45 min–2 hr 14 min)	99354 × 1 AND 99355 × 2
135–164 min (2 hr 15 min–2 hr 44 min)	99354 × 1 AND 99355 × 3
165–194 min (2 hr 45 min–3 hr 14 min)	99354 × 1 AND 99355 × 4

LET'S LOOK AT AN EXAMPLE

A 36-year-old female was stung by a bee on her lip. She presents to her primary care physician's office with swelling of her face and throat along with difficulty breathing. The physician performs and documents a Level 3 E/M service (99213) and administers an epinephrine injection. The patient's condition required intermittent physician evaluations of the patient's breathing and facial swelling. The physician face-to-face time totaled 2 hours after the primary office visit.

How to Code: In this scenario, the intermittent time for the reevaluations by the physician is considered above and beyond the E/M service. The total face-to-face time spent by the physician was 2 hours. As indicated in the prolonged attendance guidelines, the first 30 minutes are not counted as prolonged attendance time; they are considered part of the E/M service. Therefore, we can code for the E/M visit 99213 and the additional time of 2 hours of prolonged service 99354 and 99355 × 2.

Case Management Services

Case management services are subdivided into **anticoagulant management** and **medical team conferences.** Case management services represent the services of a physician or qualified health-care provider responsible for the direct care of the patient, including the coordinating and managing of other health-care services required for the patient.

Anticoagulant Management
99363–99364

Anticoagulant services represent the outpatient management of warfarin therapy. Warfarin is a medication that thins the blood and is used in the treatment and prevention of blood clots and heart attacks. Patients on this medication require routine blood tests to check their INR (International Normalized Ratio).

Anticoagulant services are reported once every 90 days and can be either an initial or subsequent service; each CPT code includes a minimum number of INR tests. These services are represented by two CPT codes, both of which include the review and interpretation of INR testing, patient instruction, dosage adjustment (as needed), and ordering of additional tests. CPT code 99363 represents the initial 90 days of therapy and must include a minimum of eight INR measurements. CPT code 99364 represents each subsequent 90 days of therapy and must include a minimum of three INR measurements.

Medical Team Conferences
99366–99368

There are two types of medical team conferences: those *with* direct face-to-face contact with the patient (99366) and those *without* face-to-face contact with the patient (99367, 99368). To utilize these codes, participation from at least three qualified health-care professionals from different specialties is required, and all of the participants must have performed a face-to-face evaluation of or have treated the patient independently of any team conference within the previous 60 days.

Care Plan Oversight Services

These services represent the time spent by a physician supervising complex or multidisciplinary care modalities requiring ongoing physician involvement in the patient's plan of care. The service includes the following:

- The physician's development and review of care plans
- Subsequent reports of patient status
- Review of related laboratory and other studies
- Communication (including telephone calls) for purposes of assessment or care decisions with health-care professionals, family members, surrogate decision makers, and/or key caregivers involved in the patient's care
- Integration of new information into the medical treatment plan and/or adjustment of medical therapy

The codes are reported for patients under the care of home health agencies (99374–99375), hospice patients (99377–99378), and nursing facilities (99379–99380). Only one physician (the predominant supervisory physician) may report services for a given period of time (once a month). These codes are time-based (15–29 minutes *or* 30 minutes or more), and as such, time spent performing any related service indicated above **must be documented** in the patient's medical record.

Preventive Medicine Services
New Patient
99381–99387
Established Patient
99391–99397

Preventive medicine services are used to report services of healthy individuals with no complaints presenting for their "annual exam" or "routine physical." Preventive visits include an age- and gender-appropriate history, physical examination, counseling/anticipatory guidance/risk factor reduction interventions, and the *ordering* of any age-appropriate laboratory and/or diagnostic tests. These codes are classified according to whether the patient is new or established and are subclassified by the age of the patient.

Once you know if the patient is new or established and the age of the patient, you can then select the appropriate CPT code.

New Patient	Established Patient
99381: under 1 year	99391: under 1 year
99382: 1–4 years	99392: 1–4 years
99383: 5–11 years	99393: 5–11 years
99384: 12–17 years	99394: 12–17 years
99385: 18–39 years	99395: 18–39 years
99386: 40–64 years	99396: 40–64 years
99387: 65 and over	99397: 65 and over

If the physician *performs* an EKG, venipuncture, hearing screen, vaccinations, or other services during a preventive visit, the additional services should be separately reported in addition to the preventive visit code.

With preventive medicine services, the physician is not evaluating or managing (E/M) a problem; however, in certain instances, the physician may evaluate and manage a problem during the course of a preventive visit.

LET'S LOOK AT AN EXAMPLE

One-year-old Eric (established patient) presented to the physician's office for his yearly examination. A comprehensive history was taken, a comprehensive examination was

LET'S LOOK AT AN EXAMPLE—cont'd

performed, anticipatory guidance and counseling was provided, and age-appropriate laboratory and diagnostic tests were performed and/or ordered. During the course of the physical examination, Eric was cranky and pulling at his ears. On examination of his ears, the physician noted erythema of the right tympanic membrane. Eric was diagnosed with otitis media and was given a prescription for Zithromax and a referral to an ears, nose, and throat (ENT) physician.

How to Code: In this scenario, the physician provided two separately identifiable services to the same patient on the same day. CPT allows for the reporting of both the preventive visit and the E/M service at the appropriate level documented on the same day. Both services are reported, and modifier 25 (the modifier for separate E/M service on the same day; this modifier is discussed later in this chapter) is appended to the E/M code. Documentation in the patient's medical record *must support both services*. The diagnosis code of otitis media is linked to the E/M service, and the well-child diagnosis code is linked to the preventive visit. The services provided during this visit are therefore coded as follows:

99392-25, V20.2 (Preventive visit and well-child diagnosis)

99212, 382.9 (Level 2 E/M and otitis media diagnosis)

Counseling for Risk Factor Reduction and Behavior Change Intervention

These codes are classified into three groups: (1) preventive medicine, individual counseling; (2) behavior change interventions, individual counseling; (3) preventive medicine, group counseling.

- Preventive Medicine, Individual Counseling (99401-99404). These codes represent face-to-face services by a physician or other qualified health-care provider **counseling** individual patients **for the purpose of promoting health and preventing illness or injury.** The counseling (e.g., diet and exercise, family problems) varies according to the age of the patient. These codes are time-based, and as such, *time must be documented* in the patient's medical record.

- Behavior Change Interventions, Individual (99406–99409). These codes represent face-to-face services by a physician or other qualified health-care provider counseling individual patients who have *a behavior that is often considered to be an illness* (e.g., tobacco use and addiction, alcohol and/or substance [other than tobacco] abuse). These codes are classified into two categories: smoking and tobacco use cessation and alcohol and/or

substance (other than tobacco) abuse. They are further subclassified by time, and as such, *time must be documented* in the patient's medical record.

- Preventive Medicine, Group Counseling (99411–99412). These codes represent face-to-face services by a physician or other qualified health-care provider counseling **individual patients in a group setting** for the purpose of promoting health and preventing illness or injury. The counseling (e.g., diet and exercise, family problems) varies according to the age of the patient. These codes are time based, and as such, *time must be documented* in the patient's medical record.

Non–Face-to-Face Physician Services

These services are a true reflection of the times we live in; the services are classified into two categories: telephone calls and online medical evaluation.

Telephone Calls
99441–99443

These may be classified into three levels of service. Codes for these services are time-based, and therefore, *time must be documented* in the patient's medical record. These services are provided by a physician to an established patient, parent, or guardian. The telephone call must not be related to an E/M service provided within the previous 7 days nor lead to an E/M service or procedure within the next 24 hours or soonest available appointment. It is recommended to check with the various insurance carriers for their reimbursement policy on telephone calls. Medicare does not reimburse for these services.

Online Medical Evaluation
99444

These services are provided by a physician to an established patient, parent, or guardian. The online service must not be related to an E/M service provided within the previous 7 days. This service is provided via the Internet or a similar electronic communication network. Permanent storage (electronic or hard copy) of the encounter should be kept on file. The service should be provided on a secure HIPAA-compliant network. It is recommended to check with the various insurance carriers for their reimbursement policy for online medical evaluations. Medicare does not reimburse for these services.

Special E/M Services
Basic Life and/or Disability Evaluation Services
99450

Work-Related or Medical Disability Evaluation Services
99455–99456

These codes are used to report evaluations to establish a baseline for life or disability insurance certificates prior to being issued. The codes are classified into two categories: Basic Life and/or Disability Evaluation Services (99450) and Work-Related or Medical Disability Evaluation Services (99455–99456). For work-related or medical disability evaluation services, CPT code **99455** represents an **examination by the treating physician,** and CPT code **99456** represents an **examination performed by someone other than the treating physician.**

Newborn Care Services
99460–99463

Newborn care service codes are used to report services to normal newborns (birth through the first 28 days) in a variety of settings (e.g., hospital, birthing center, home). The codes **(99460–99462)** are classified by the site of service and whether the service is an initial service or a subsequent service. Newborn care service codes are reported once per day. **CPT code 99463** is used to report the admission and discharge at a hospital or birthing center on the same day.

Delivery/Birthing Room Attendance and Resuscitation Services
99464–99465, 99468, 99477

Also listed under Newborn Care Services are codes for **Delivery/Birthing Room Attendance and Resuscitation Services.**

CPT code **99464** represents physician attendance at delivery when requested by the delivering physician. It includes the initial stabilization of the newborn and may be reported in conjunction with other services provided.

CPT code **99465** represents delivery/birthing room resuscitation and may not be reported in addition to attendance at delivery (99464), initial inpatient neonatal critical care (99468), initial hospital care per day for the E/M of a neonate (99477), or initial hospital or birthing care per day for the E/M of a normal newborn (99460).

Inpatient Neonatal Intensive Care Services and Pediatric and Neonatal Critical Care Services

These services are classified into three categories: (1) pediatric critical care patient transport, (2) inpatient neonatal and pediatric critical care, and (3) initial and continuing intensive care services.

Pediatric Critical Care Patient Transport
99466–99467

These codes represent direct face-to-face physical attendance by a physician for interfacility transport of a critically ill or critically injured pediatric patient 24 months of age or less. These codes are time based, and as such, *time must be documented in the patient's medical record.* Time begins when the physician assumes primary responsibility of the pediatric patient and ends when the receiving hospital/facility accepts responsibility for the pediatric patient. Only the time spent in direct face-to-face contact with the patient should be reported. Services less than 30 minutes of face-to-face physician care would not be reported with these codes. Services provided by other members of the transport team should not be reported by the supervising physician.

> **KEY CODING TIP**
> Services for patients being transported to another facility whose care is being directed by two-way communication *(not face-to-face)* are reported with CPT code 99288 Physician direction of emergency medical systems (EMS) emergency care, advanced life support.

Inpatient Neonatal and Pediatric Critical Care
99468–99476

These codes represent critical care services that are provided to neonates and pediatric patients. The same definition of critical care services reviewed under critical care services also apply to the neonate and the pediatric patient (with neonate being defined as 28 days of age or less, and a pediatric patient being defined as 29 days through 24 months of age OR 2–5 years of age). The guidelines preceding the codes (99468–99476) *must be read,* as they list all the services bundled (included) in the inpatient neonatal and pediatric critical care codes. These codes are unique because **they are for "inpatient" critical care for critically ill or critically injured neonates and pediatric patients.**

Critical care services for critically ill or critically injured neonates and pediatric patients of any age provided in the "outpatient" setting (or office) are reported with critical care codes 99291–99292. If critical care services are provided for neonates or pediatric patients in both the outpatient and inpatient settings on the same day, only the appropriate inpatient neonatal or pediatric code would be reported.

Neonatal and pediatric critical care codes are reported once per day, divided according to initial or subsequent visit, and based on the age of the child.

Initial and Continuing Intensive Care Services
99477–99480

These codes represent services to children who are *not* critically ill but nevertheless require intensive observation, frequent interventions, and other intensive services. These services are reported once per day. **CPT code 99477** represents the initial service for the neonate (28 days of age or less), and **CPT codes 99478–99480** represent subsequent visits and are identified by the *weight of the patient.* The patient's weight is categorized as:

■ Very low birth weight (VLBW): present body weight less than 1500 g

■ Low birth weight (LBW): present body weight of 1500–2500 g

■ Normal: 2501–5000 g

E/M Modifiers

The CPT modifiers are a two-position numeric code added to the end of a CPT code that alert the insurance carrier that something is different about the CPT code that is being reported. (For a complete review of modifiers, see Chapter 7.) Let's take a look at the modifiers that are specific to E/M codes and how they are used.

Modifier 24: An unrelated E/M service by the same physician during a postoperative period. This modifier is used when a patient presents during the postoperative period for a service that is unrelated to the surgical procedure performed. Modifier 24 unbundles the E/M service from the global package.

Modifier 25: A significant, separately identifiable E/M service by the same physician on the same day of the procedure or other service. As we saw in the example given earlier in this chapter of the preventive service and the E/M

service provided on the same day to the same patient, modifier 25 alerts the insurance carrier that services that are not normally reported on the same day to the same patient were separate and distinct.

Modifier 32: Mandated services. This modifier is appended to consultations and related services provided at the request of an insurance carrier or as a government, legislative, or regulatory requirement.

Modifier 55: Postoperative management only. In certain cases, the postoperative E/M service is provided by a physician other than the surgeon. In these cases, modifier 55 is appended to the postoperative E/M service. This modifier unbundles the surgical package (preoperative management, surgical procedure, and postoperative management).

Modifier 56: Preoperative management only. In certain cases, the preoperative E/M service is provided by a physician other than the surgeon. In these cases, modifier 56 is appended to the preoperative E/M service. This modifier unbundles the surgical package (preoperative management, surgical procedure, and postoperative management).

Modifier 57: Decision for surgery. Modifier 57 is appended to an E/M code provided on the day before or the day of a surgical procedure with global days greater than 10. For surgical procedures with a global period of 0–10 days, append modifier 25. This modifier also unbundles the E/M service for the consultation or other E/M service where the decision for surgery was made from the global surgical package.

Let's Practice Coding

When taking the exam and while working in your coding career, you will be provided with various E/M scenarios. The best way to determine how to code the E/M services is to highlight key terms. Let's apply our coding knowledge and code the following scenarios.

E/M Scenario 1. At 12:10, an 80-year-old man in full arrest was received in the emergency department by EMS. He was found face down, allegedly struck by a motor vehicle. The patient had multiple lacerations to his head and upper extremities, and his knees were grossly deformed. The full trauma team was in attendance, CPR was provided, and the patient was pronounced dead at 12:50. The patient was identified by his driver's license, and the family was contacted.

One of the key terms to highlight is the **time** (in the case of **time-based services, this is a key piece of documentation**). In this case, we notice the total time spent with this patient is 40 minutes. If provided, the age of the patient should always be highlighted, as some CPT codes are based on the age of the patient. We should also highlight the **place of service**—here, "emergency department." The **condition of the patient** was noted as "full arrest" (critically ill), so we highlight this. Finally, we highlight the "full trauma team," indicating critical care services, and "CPR was provided," as it represents a separately reportable service (CPR is not inclusive with the critical care codes).

In this scenario, the documentation supports 40 minutes of critical care services. When we review the critical care guidelines for inclusive (bundled) services, we notice CPR is not included and therefore should be reported *in addition* to the critical care code.

The appropriate codes for this scenario are:

■ **99291** Critical care, evaluation and management of the critically ill or critically injured patient; first 30–74 minutes

■ **92950** Cardiopulmonary resuscitation (e.g., in cardiac arrest)

Let's Practice Coding—cont'd

E/M Scenario 2. Mom brought 6-month-old Steven (established patient) to the pediatrician's office, complaining of diaper rash. The rash has been present a week, but has been getting worse over the past few days. She tried using cornstarch, which did not help the rash, and Mom was concerned it may have made the rash worse. Review of systems was noted as no fever. Upon examination, the physician noted the skin around the diaper area as an erythematous macular rash. HEENT (head, eyes, ears, nose, and throat) was within normal limits, the lungs were clear to auscultation and percussion, the heart was noted as normal rate and rhythm, and the abdomen was soft and nontender. After documenting the expanded problem-focused history and detailed examination, the physician diagnosed Steven with diaper dermatitis and instructed mom to apply triple paste to the diaper area and to return to the office if the rash became worse, resulting in a straightforward medical decision.

The key terms to highlight are the **age** of the patient, the **place of service,** in this case the "office," and the **levels of the three key components** that make up the office visit **(history, physical, medical decision).** In this case, we have an expanded problem-focused history (Level 3), a detailed physical examination (Level 4), and a medical decision of straightforward complexity (Level 2). We also highlight the **status of the patient**—namely, that this infant is an established patient. When we use the following table to indicate the levels of the three key components, it becomes easy to determine the level of service. Because established patients require two of the three key components, we can select the level of service based on the documentation of the key component in the middle, in this case, the history. **Therefore, this is a Level 3 or 99213 visit.**

CPT EVALUATION AND MANAGEMENT SERVICES OFFICE OR OTHER OUTPATIENT ESTABLISHED PATIENT					
Established patient visit	**99211**	**99212**	**99213**	**99214**	**99215**
KEY COMPONENTS 2 of 3					
History					
Chief complaint	X	X	X	X	X
Problem focused **(Level 2)**		X			
Expanded problem focused **(Level 3)**			X		
Detailed **(Level 4)**				X	
Comprehensive **(Level 5)**					X
Examination					
Problem focused **(Level 2)**		X			
Expanded problem focused **(Level 3)**			X		
Detailed **(Level 4)**				X	
Comprehensive **(Level 5)**					X
Medical decision making					
Straightforward **(Level 2)**		X			
Low complexity **(Level 3)**			X		
Moderate complexity **(Level 4)**				X	
High complexity **(Level 5)**					X
Average time/minutes face to face with patient and/or family	5	10	15	25	40

Let's Practice Coding—cont'd

E/M Scenario 3. Clara Cluny is a 65-year-old female with complaints of urinary frequency. Her sister had the same problem and recommended Clara to the same urologist who had helped her. Clara took her sister's advice and presented to the urologist's office for her initial visit the following week. At the office, the urologist documented a comprehensive history and comprehensive physical examination. Laboratory tests were performed, and Clara was diagnosed with female stress incontinence and hematuria. She was given a prescription for Levsin and instructed to return in 1 month for a cystoscopy, resulting in a medical decision of moderate complexity.

First, we highlight the **age** of the patient. We also highlight "urologist," as this indicates that the patient saw a specialist, and potentially this visit may be a consultation **(type of service).** However, when we look at this encounter more closely, we notice the documentation does not support a consultation. Clara was not sent to the urologist by a physician or a qualified health-care provider, and there was no mention of a report being sent back to the requesting physician. Other key terms to highlight are the **place of service,** in this case the "office"; the word "initial" to indicate Clara is a new patient **(status of patient);** and the **three key components:** "comprehensive history," "comprehensive physical examination," and a "moderate medical decision." Let's use the following new patient table to determine the level of service. We see that the history is Level 4,5; the physical examination is Level 4,5; and medical decision is Level 4. Because new patients require three of three key components, the level of service is determined by the documentation of the lowest of the three key components, in this case, the medical decision. **Therefore, this is a Level 4 99204 visit.**

CPT EVALUATION AND MANAGEMENT SERVICES OFFICE OR OTHER OUTPATIENT NEW PATIENT					
New patient visit	99201	99202	99203	99204	99205
KEY COMPONENTS 3 of 3					
History					
Chief complaint	X	X	X	X	X
Problem focused (**Level 1**)	X				
Expanded problem focused (**Level 2**)		X			
Detailed (**Level 3**)			X		
Comprehensive (**Level 4, 5**)				X	X
Examination					
Problem focused (**Level 1**)	X				
Expanded problem focused (**Level 2**)		X			
Detailed (**Level 3**)			X		
Comprehensive (**Level 4, 5**)				X	X
Medical decision making					
Straightforward (**Level 1, 2**)	X	X			
Low complexity (**Level 3**)			X		
Moderate complexity (**Level 4**)				X	
High complexity (**Level 5**)					X
Average time/minutes face to face with patient and/or family	10	20	30	45	60

Let's Practice Coding—cont'd

E/M Scenario 4. Madison Sampson is 10-month-old established patient who was brought to the pediatrician's office for her routine health exam. Dr. Cortijo performed a comprehensive history and a comprehensive examination. Anticipatory guidance was provided, and vaccinations were ordered.

The key terms to highlight in this encounter are the **age** of the patient, the fact the patient is "established" **(status of patient),** and "routine health exam" **(type of service**—namely, that the reason for the visit was not an illness). The key components "comprehensive history" and "comprehensive examination" are likewise highlighted. Anticipatory guidance and the ordering of age-appropriate services are also highlighted, as these further specify the **type of service**—namely, these are aspects of a preventive visit.

In this scenario, the patient presented for a routine or "preventive visit." All the components of a preventive visit were documented along with the age (10 months) and status of the patient ("established patient"). Therefore, the age-appropriate preventive visit code for an established patient is selected. In this case, for a patient younger than 1 year old, we select CPT code 99391.

Learn More About it

The more you read, the more you know. Increase your knowledge with the following resources:

Recommended Web Sites

CMS Documentation Guidelines / Medicare Learning Network

https://www.cms.gov/MLNEdWebGuide/25_EMDOC.asp

On this site you can download the following source documents:

CMS Evaluation & Management Services Guide

1995 Documentation Guidelines

1997 Documentation Guidelines

STOP-LOOK-HIGHLIGHT

The key to successfully passing the exam and selecting the correct code lies in your knowing how to use your coding book.

To help you navigate through your codebook, and to make sure you have the most important information at your fingertips when you take the exam, highlight key text in the chapter guidelines and subheadings, and insert simple notes and coding tips directly into your codebooks.

When highlighting, use two different color highlighter pens: yellow for standard guidelines and global services, and an alternate color for carve outs and unique notes.

In the E/M Services Guidelines:

■ On page 1 of the E/M Documentation Guidelines under New and Established Patient, highlight the definition of a new patient in the first paragraph, fourth line: "A new patient is one who has not received any professional services from the physician or another physician of the same specialty who belongs to the same group practice, within the past three years."

■ In red ink, write the acronym in parentheses beside the following subheadings:

• Next to Chief Complaint, write *"(CC)."*

• Next to History of Presenting Illness, write *"(HPI)."*

• Next to System Review (Review of Systems), write *"(ROS)."*

• Next to Determine the Complexity of Medical Decision Making, write *"(MDM)."*

■ On page 7 of the E/M Documentation Guidelines under Determine the Extent of the History Obtained, write the following: *"To determine the type of history, all three elements (HPI, ROS, PFSH) must be at the same level, or the type of history is determined by the lowest element."*

■ On page 8 of the E/M Documentation Guidelines under Determine the Extent of Examination Performed, the different types of physical examinations are listed. Write the number of accepted industry-standard body areas/organ systems.

• Next to problem-focused, write *"(1 element/body area)."*

• Next to expanded problem-focused. write *"(2–4 body areas/organ systems)."*

• Next to detailed, write *"(5–7 body area/organ systems, one in detail)."*

• Next to comprehensive, write *"(8 or more body areas/organ systems, or complete examination of a single organ system)."*

■ Under the same subheading, highlight the sentence preceding the list of recognized body areas, and highlight the sentence preceding the list of recognized organ systems.

- On page 9 of the E/M Documentation Guidelines under Determine the Complexity of Medical Decision Making, in the second paragraph, third sentence, highlight the following: "To qualify for a given type of decision making, two of three elements in Table 1 must be met or exceeded."

- On page 9 of the E/M Documentation Guidelines highlight item 3: "When counseling and/or coordination of care dominates (more than 50% of) the physician/patient and/or family encounter (face-to-face time in the office or other outpatient setting or floor/unit time in the hospital or nursing facility), then **time** may be considered the key or controlling factor to qualify for a particular level of E/M services."

- In the blank area on the last page of the Documentation Guidelines, write the following helpful chart, which lists the three key components and their elements:

Components	Elements
History	CC, HPI, ROS, PFSH
Physical examination	Body areas/organ systems
Medical decision	Number of diagnosis or management options, amount and/or complexity of data to be reviewed, risk of complications and/or morbidity or mortality

It is also helpful to copy the new and established patient tables (for determining the level of service) and insert them into (i.e., write them in) your CPT book.
In the E/M Section:
- In the subsection Office or Other Outpatient Services, Established Patient category, in the descriptor of CPT code 99211, the second sentence down, highlight "that may not require the presence of a physician."

- In the subsection Hospital Observation Services, the fourth sentence down, highlight the sentence "It is not necessary that the patient be located in an observation area designed for the hospital."

- In the subsection Hospital Observation Services, under Initial Observation Care, New or Established Patient category, in the guidelines for new or established patients:

  - The second paragraph, sixth sentence down, highlight, "For a patient admitted to the

hospital on a date subsequent to the date of observation status, the hospital admission would be reported with the appropriate Initial Hospital Care code (99221-99223)."

- In your alternate color highlighter, continue to highlight the rest of the paragraph: "For a patient admitted and discharged from observation or inpatient status on the same date, the services should be reported with codes 99234-99236 as appropriate. *Do not report a hospital observation discharge (99217) in conjunction with a hospital admission.*"

- Switching back to your yellow highlighter, in the next paragraph, the seventh line down, highlight "The observation care level of service reported by the supervising physician should include the services related to initial 'observation status' provided in the other sites of service as well as in the observation setting."

- In the subsection Hospital Inpatient Services, Hospital Discharge Services category, highlight the following: "The hospital discharge day management codes are to be used to report the total duration of time spent by a physician for the final discharge day of a patient. The codes include, as appropriate, final examination of the patient, discussion of the hospital stay, even if the time spent by the physician on that date is not continuous, instructions for continuing care to all relevant caregivers, and preparation of discharge records, prescriptions and referral forms."

- In the subsection Consultations, subheading Office or Other Outpatient Consultations, New or Established Patient category:

  - First paragraph, sixth line down, in your alternate color highlighter, highlight the following: "Follow-up visits in the consultant's office or other outpatient facility that are initiated by the physician consultant or patient are reported using the appropriate codes for established patients."

  - Same paragraph, the eleventh line from the beginning of the paragraph, in your yellow or original color highlighter, highlight the following: "If an additional request for an opinion or advice regarding the same or a new problem is received from another physician or other appropriate source and documented in the medical record, the office consultation codes may be used again."

  - At the bottom of the page, write in the following:
    - *Remember the Three "R" Rule*
      - *Request*

• *Render appropriate service*

• *Report back*

■ The subsection ***Critical Care Services*** *must be read.* The key points to highlight in yellow as you read are the following:

• The definition of critical care and critical illness or critical injury (the first 13 sentences in the guidelines).

• In the second paragraph, fourth line down, highlight "Critical care is usually but not always given in a critical care area, such as the coronary care unit, intensive care unit, pediatric intensive care unit, respiratory care unit or the emergency care facility."

• In the fourth paragraph down, highlight in your alternate color highlighter: "Services for a patient who is not critically ill but happens to be in a critical care unit are reported using other appropriate E/M codes."

• In the sixth paragraph, highlight in yellow: "The following services are included in reporting critical care when performed during the critical period by the physician(s) providing critical care:" Following this statement is a list of the services considered to be inclusive.

• The eighth and ninth paragraphs refer to how critical care time may be calculated and what constitutes critical care time. In yellow, highlight both paragraphs.

• In your alternate color highlighter, in the tenth paragraph, highlight "Time spent in activities that occur outside of the unit or off the floor (e.g., telephone calls whether taken at home, in the office, or elsewhere in the hospital) may not be reported as critical care, because the physician is not immediately available to the patient."

• In the critical care timetable chart, under Total Duration of Critical Care, highlight "less than 30 minutes," and under Codes, highlight "appropriate E/M codes."

■ In the subsection Prolonged Services, subheading Prolonged Physician Service With Direct (Face-to-Face) Patient Contact, highlight the following in yellow:

• The first paragraph, which indicates these codes are reported in addition to E/M services at any level.

• The second paragraph, which indicates that the time need not be continuous.

• In the prolonged attendance time chart, under Total Duration of Prolonged Services, highlight

"less than 30 minutes," and under Code(s), highlight "not reported separately."

■ In the subsection Case Management Services, subheading Anticoagulant Management:

• Highlight in yellow the second paragraph: "When reporting these services, the work of anticoagulant management may not be used as a basis for reporting an evaluation and management (E/M) service or care plan oversight time during the reporting period."

• Three lines down from there, in your alternate color highlighter, highlight "If a significantly separately identifiable E/M service is performed, report the appropriate E/M service code using modifier -25."

■ In the subsection Preventive Medicine Services, in the guidelines, highlight the following:

• In the second paragraph, highlight in yellow: "The extent and focus of the services will largely depend on the age of the patient."

• Highlight in your alternate color highlighter the third paragraph, which provides guidance for an E/M service provided at the same time as a preventive visit.

• Highlight the fourth paragraph in your yellow highlighter: "An insignificant or trivial problem/abnormality that is encountered in the process of performing the preventive medicine evaluation and management service and which does not require additional work and the performance of key components of a problem-oriented E/M service should not be reported."

• In the sixth paragraph down, highlight in yellow: "Codes 99381–99397 include counseling/anticipatory guidance/risk factor reduction interventions which are provided at the time of the initial or periodic comprehensive preventive medicine examination."

• In your alternate color highlighter, highlight the last paragraph, which indicates the additional services that are separately reportable with a preventive visit.

■ The subsection ***Inpatient Neonatal Intensive Care Services and Pediatric and Neonatal Critical Care Services*** *must be read.* The key points to highlight as you read are the following:

• Under the subheading Inpatient Neonatal and Pediatric Critical Care, highlight the first line: "The same definitions for critical care services apply for the adult, child, and neonate."

• The fifth paragraph down, highlight the following: "The pediatric and neonatal critical care codes include those procedures listed for the critical care codes (99291, 99292). In addition the following procedures are also included (and are not separately reported) in the pediatric and neonatal critical care service codes (99468–99472, 99475, 99476), the intensive care service codes (99477–99480), and the pediatric critical care patient transport codes (99466, 99467). Following this paragraph is a list of those services which are considered inclusive."

- After the list of inclusive codes, in your alternate color highlighter, highlight "Any services performed which are not listed above may be reported separately."

■ In the subsection Inpatient Neonatal Intensive Care Services and Pediatric and Neonatal Critical Care Services, subheading Initial and Continuing Intensive Care Services, the fourth sentence down, highlight "Codes 99478–99480 are used to report subsequent services provided by a physician directing the continuing intensive care of the low birth weight (LBW 1500–2500 grams) present body weight infant, very low birth weight (VLBW less than 1500 g) present body weight infant, or normal (2501–5000 g) present body weight newborn who does not meet the definition of critically ill but continues to require intensive observation, frequent interventions, and other intensive care services."

E/M Vocabulary Words

At the end of the E/M section, also write the following vocabulary words:

Chief Complaint: A concise statement, usually in the patient's own words, describing the reason for the visit (e.g., symptom, complaint, condition).

Concurrent Care: Occurs when similar services are rendered to the same patient by more than one physician on the same day.

Consultation: A service provided by a physician at the request of another physician or appropriate source to evaluate and make recommendations on specific medical conditions or problems.

Inpatient: A patient who receives services after being admitted to a hospital or nursing facility.

Outpatient: A patient who receives services in a physician's office, ambulatory facility, or at a hospital or clinic but who is not admitted overnight.

Transfer of Care: Occurs when a physician who is currently treating a patient for medical problems turns over care of the patient to another physician who in turn agrees to accept responsibility for the patient and has not provided consult services to the patient from the initial encounter.

E/M Acronyms and Abbreviations

At the end of the E/M section also write in the following acronyms and abbreviations:

CC–**C**hief **C**omplaint
CPO–**C**are **P**lan **O**versight
DG–**D**ocumentation **G**uidelines
E/M–**E**valuation and **M**anagement
ENT–**E**ars, **N**ose, and **T**hroat
HEENT–**H**ead, **E**yes, **E**ars, **N**ose, **T**hroat
HPI–**H**istory of **P**resenting **I**llness
INR–**I**nternational **N**ormalized **R**atio
LBW–**L**ow **B**irth **W**eight
MDM–**M**edical **D**ecision **M**aking
PERLA–**P**upils **E**qually **R**eactive to **L**ight and **A**ccommodation
ROS–**R**eview of **S**ystems
VLBW–**V**ery **L**ow **B**irth **W**eight

TAKE THE CODING CHALLENGE

To accurately code, you must be able to locate, read, and comprehend the section guidelines and guidelines that pertain to each subsection, subheading, and category codes. **If you can read, you can code.** Challenge yourself to see if you can find where the following guidelines in the E/M section are located.

Guideline Questions

1. The location of guidelines alerting the coder to code any vaccine/toxoid products; immunization administrations; ancillary studies involving laboratory, radiology, other procedures, or screening tests (e.g., vision, hearing, developmental) identified with a CPT code from 99381–99387 or 99391–99397:

_____.

2. The location of guidelines alerting the coder that a patient does not have to be located in an observation area designated by the hospital to report these codes:

_____.

3. The definition of very low birth weight can be found in these guidelines:

_____.

4. The location of guidelines alerting the coder that follow-up visits in the consultant's office or other outpatient facility that are initiated by the physician consultant or patient are reported using the appropriate codes for established patient office visits:

_____.

5. The location of guidelines alerting the coder that the services are intended to describe the outpatient case management of warfarin therapy:

_____.

Multiple Choice

1. A 34-year-old established female patient presents with a complaint of a sore throat. Patient states she has had the sore throat for 2 days and describes the severity as mild. She has no fever, no earache, no nausea or vomiting. After documenting the expanded problem-focused history, the physician performed a problem-focused examination and rapid strep test on the patient, which was positive. The low-complexity medical decision was documented with the patient receiving a prescription for antibiotic medication and an appointment to follow up in 10 days. Select the correct level of service.
   a. 99395
   b. 99213
   c. 99212
   d. 99203

2. Lily Zelefsky, a new patient to Dr. Franklin, presented in the office for an evaluation of her unexplained recent weight gain and dizziness. The detailed history was documented. The comprehensive physical examination revealed HEENT was within normal limits; heart and lungs were within normal limits; abdomen was noted as positive bowel sounds and soft and nontender; alert and oriented × 3; no focal defects; no clubbing, cyanosis, or edema was noted. Dr. Franklin ordered a complete blood workup, referred Lily to a nutritionist for her weight gain, and prescribed meclizine for the dizziness, resulting in a moderate decision. Select the correct level of service.
   a. 99243
   b. 99213
   c. 99253
   d. 99203

3. When reporting time for critical care services, time that can be counted as critical care time includes:
   a. Any time spent engaged in work directly relating to the individual's patient care, either at the patient's bedside or elsewhere on the floor or unit
   b. Only time spent engaged in work directly relating to the individual's patient care, performed at the patient's bedside
   c. Any time spent engaged in work directly relating to the individual's patient care, either at the patient's bedside or elsewhere on the floor or unit, as well as time spent in telephone calls taken at home or in the office directly relating to the individual's patient care
   d. Time spent performing additional procedures that are not bundled into critical care services

4. A patient who is admitted and discharged from hospital observation status on the same day is reported with:
   a. The appropriate level of initial observation status code and the appropriate level of hospital discharge code
   b. Only one code should be reported, the initial observation care code
   c. Only one code should be reported, the observation care discharge
   d. The appropriate level of observation or inpatient care services, including admission and discharge services on the same day

5. Documentation of a preventive visit consists of:
   a. An age- and gender-appropriate history, physical examination, and counseling/anticipatory guidance/risk factor reduction interventions
   b. An age- and gender-appropriate history, physical examination, and counseling/anticipatory guidance/risk factor reduction interventions, and the E/M of any significant abnormalities noted during the physical examination
   c. An age- and gender-appropriate history, physical examination, and counseling/anticipatory guidance/risk factor reduction interventions, and the ordering of age-appropriate laboratory/diagnostic procedures
   d. An age- and gender-appropriate history, physical examination, and counseling/anticipatory guidance/risk factor reduction interventions, and any age-appropriate vaccinations and vaccine administration

6. A neurological consultation in the emergency department was requested for a 28-year-old male who was brought in by ambulance after having a seizure while driving home from work. A comprehensive history obtained from the patient's mom included her son's occupation as a computer gaming programmer, and he has been experiencing visual disturbances the past few weeks. The neurologist completed a comprehensive single organ system (neurological) physical examination and ordered a CT and MRI of the brain to help determine the cause of the seizure. The medical decision was of moderate complexity. Select the correct level of service.
   a. 99254
   b. 99244
   c. 99284
   d. 99204

7. John, a 64-year-old, was sent to a urologist at the request of his primary care physician for an evaluation of hematuria (blood in urine). The urologist performed and documented a detailed history and physical examination. John was scheduled to come back in a week for a cystoscopy. Risks and benefits of the procedure were discussed at length, and the medical decision was of moderate complexity. Select only the office service.
   a. 99243
   b. 99243, 52000
   c. 99243–57
   d. 99243–57, 52000

8. While skiing, Melissa fell and hit her head. She did not lose consciousness; however, immediately after the fall, a bump on her head appeared and she developed a minor headache. After being evaluated in the emergency department, she was placed in observation status for 10 hours to assess the outcome of the fall. After the emergency department physician determined her condition no longer required monitoring, she was discharged to go home on the same day. Documentation included a comprehensive history and physical examination, and the medical decision was of low complexity. Select the correct level of service.
   a. 99218
   b. 99234
   c. 99284
   d. 99217

9. Tara is a 30-year-old new patient who presented to the gynecologist's office for a routine checkup. After documenting a comprehensive history and physical, Dr. Kennity counseled Tara on contraceptive management and ordered routine blood workup. Select the correct level of service.
   a. 99395
   b. 99215
   c. 99205
   d. 99385

10. Prolonged attendance codes are reported:
    a. In addition to an E/M code at any level
    b. When the service provided is beyond the usual service in either the inpatient or outpatient setting
    c. On the basis of the documented time, even if the time spent is not continuous
    d. All of the above

ANSWERS AND RATIONALES

Answers to Guideline Questions

1. CPT codes 99381–99387 or 99391–99397 represent preventive medicine services. The guidelines that alert the coder that additional services may be reported in addition to the preventive visit codes are located in the E/M section, subsection Preventive Medicine Services, in the last paragraph of guidelines.

2. They key term in this question is "observation." The appropriate guidelines refer to the utilization of hospital observation services and are located in the E/M section, subsection Hospital Observation Services, the fourth sentence in the guidelines.

3. Infants and neonates of very low birth weight who are not critically ill may require intensive services; therefore, the definition of very low birth weight can be found in the guidelines for Initial and Continuing Intensive Care Services.

4. The key terms in this question are "consultant" and "outpatient." The appropriate guidelines refer to subsequent visits provided by a consultant in the outpatient setting and are located in the E/M section, subsection Consultation, subheading Office or Other Outpatient Consultations, category New or Established.

5. The key terms in this question are "outpatient," "case management," and "warfarin," all of which refer to the case management of patients who are on warfarin therapy. The appropriate guidelines are located in the E/M section, subsection Case Management Services, subheading Anticoagulant Management.

Multiple Choice Answers

1. The correct answer is **b.** The level of history is expanded problem-focused (Level 3), the physical examination is problem-focused (Level 2), and the medical decision is low (Level 3). For established patients, two of three key components must be met or exceeded. In this case, both the history and medical decision are at the same level, resulting in CPT code 99213. Answer **a.** is incorrect, because although 99395 is an established patient code for a 34-year-old patient, it is a *preventive* visit code, whereas in this encounter the patient was evaluated for a sore throat. Answer **c.** is incorrect, because although this is a code for an established patient who has been evaluated and managed for an illness, it is at the wrong level (Level 2). For established patients, two of three key components must be met or exceeded; in this case only the physical examination was at Level 2. Answer **d.** is incorrect, because although this code represents E/M of an illness, it is for a new patient, and the patient in this scenario is established.

2. The correct answer is **d.** Lily is a new patient seen in the outpatient setting. The documentation included a detailed history (Level 3), a comprehensive physical examination (Level 5), and a moderate medical decision (Level 4). For *new* patients, three of three key components must be met or exceeded, and therefore in this case, the key component documented at the lowest level, Level 3 (99203), determines the level of service. Answers **a.** and **c.** are incorrect, as they both represent *consultation* codes—with 99243 representing an outpatient consultation and 99253 representing an inpatient consultation. In this scenario, advice or opinion from Dr. Franklin by another physician or qualified health-care professional was not requested or documented. Answer **b.** is incorrect, as it represents an established patient.

3. The correct answer is **a.** The critical care service guidelines specifically list what is and what is not considered critical care. Certain services that are not provided at the patient's bedside but are provided on the floor or unit may be counted as critical care time (e.g., time spent at the nursing station on the floor reviewing test results). Answer **b.** is incorrect, as it does not include time spent on the floor or unit engaged in work directly related to the patient's care. Answer **c.** is incorrect, as the critical care service guidelines are very clear: time spent in activities that occur outside of the unit or off the floor may not be counted as critical care time. Answer **d.** is incorrect, as any services performed that are not listed as inclusive (bundled) into critical care services are separately reported.

4. The correct answer is **d.** Patients admitted and discharged from observation status on the same date are reported with the appropriate level code from observation or inpatient care services (including admission and discharge services) on the same date. Answer **a.** is incorrect, as it includes a hospital discharge code, which would be reported only if the patient were admitted to the hospital. Answer **b.** is incorrect. Reporting only the hospital observation codes does not capture the discharge services provided. Answer **c.** is incorrect, as it does not capture the services provided while the patient was in the observation status.

5. The correct answer is **c.** Information on the components of a preventive visit is located in the Preventive Medicine Services guidelines; it is important to note that preventive visit includes the "ordering" of the age-appropriate vaccines. Answer **a.** is incorrect, as it does not include the ordering of age-appropriate laboratory/diagnostic procedures. Answer **b.** is incorrect, as any significant abnormalities encountered, documented, and evaluated at the time of a preventive medicine service would be reported with the appropriate problem-oriented E/M service code and *not* be considered part of a preventive visit. Answer **d.** is incorrect, as any vaccinations and vaccine administration services provided during a preventive medicine service are separately reported.

6. Answer **b.** is correct. This is a consultation, as the advice of a neurologist was requested. It is an *outpatient* consultation, as the patient was seen in the emergency department of the hospital; the three key components were documented as comprehensive history (Level 5), comprehensive physical (Level 5), and medical decision of moderate complexity (Level 4). Consultations require that three of three key components be met or exceeded; therefore, this is a Level 4 (99244) consultation. Answer **a.** is incorrect, as CPT code 99254 represents an "inpatient" consultation. Answer **c.** is incorrect, as CPT code 99284 represents an emergency department visit. Although the patient was seen in the emergency department, the emergency department physician called in the neurologist for his advice and opinion, making this an outpatient (the emergency department is considered an outpatient area of the hospital) consultation. Answer **d.** is incorrect, as CPT code 99204 represents a new patient office visit.

7. The correct answer is **a.** We are asked to code only for the office service, in this case an outpatient consultation (patient was seen in the urologist's office at the request of the primary care physician). The three key components were documented as detailed history (Level 3), detailed physical examination (Level 3), and a medical decision of moderate complexity (Level 4). Consultations require that three of three key components be met or exceeded; therefore, this is a Level 3 (99243) outpatient consultation. Answer **b.** is incorrect, as it

includes the cystoscopy, which we were not asked to code. Answer **c.** is incorrect, as modifier 57 Decision for surgery is reported only when the E/M was provided the day before or the day of the surgery. In this scenario, the patient is returning a week later for the cystoscopy. Answer **d.** is incorrect, as it includes the modifier, which is not applicable, and the cystoscopy, which we were not asked to code.

8. The correct answer is **b.** The patient was admitted and discharged from observation status on the same day; therefore, the appropriate level of observation status admission and discharge on the same day would be reported. The key components were documented as a comprehensive history, a comprehensive physical examination, and a low medical decision. Observation status admission and discharge on the same day requires that three of three key components be met or exceeded, resulting in CPT code 99234. Answer **a.** is incorrect, as it only represents the observation status and not the services provided for the discharge. Answer **c.** is incorrect, as it represents an emergency department visit. When observation status is initiated in the course of an encounter in another site of service (e.g., emergency department), all E/M services provided are considered part of the initial observation care when provided on the same day. Answer **d.** is incorrect, as it represents the observation discharge and does not include the services for the observation care.

9. The correct answer is **d.** Gynecologists provide a single organ system preventive examination. The comprehensive nature of preventive medicine service codes reflects an age- and gender-appropriate history/examination and is not synonymous with the comprehensive examination required in E/M codes. Age-appropriate counseling was provided, and the appropriate diagnostic tests were ordered. Answer **a.** is incorrect, as it represents an established patient preventive visit. Answer **b.** is incorrect, as it represents an established patient E/M problem-oriented encounter. Answer **c.** is incorrect, as it represents a new patient E/M *problem-oriented* encounter.

10. Answer **d.** is correct. This information is located in the prolonged attendance code guidelines.

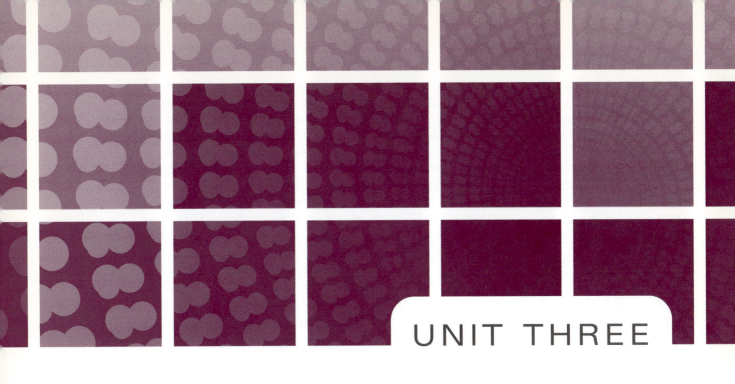

Specialty Coding

CHAPTER 9

Anesthesia

Anesthesiology is the field of medicine that specializes in sedating patients during surgery through the administration of anesthesia medication. The anesthesiologist is responsible for monitoring the patient's vital signs and life functions during the procedure to ensure that the patient remains stable. Anesthesiologists can also provide long-term treatment and management of pain through the use of medication.

There are two organizations responsible for the development of anesthesia codes and guidelines: the American Medical Association (AMA) and the American Society of Anesthesiologists (ASA). Although the guidelines of both organizations are similar, the ASA Relative Value Guide (RVG) contains some codes for anesthesia services that may not be found in the CPT book.

Anesthesia services are coded differently than other services in the CPT book. In fact, the anesthesia section of the CPT book is even formatted differently than the other sections of the CPT book. The anesthesia section is organized on the basis of anatomic site and then on the type of procedure, whereas the other sections are organized according to anatomic site, procedure, condition, description, or approach.

Unlike the other CPT codes, anesthesia codes are based on units of time (i.e., the time during which anesthesia was administered). Additionally, *one* anesthesia code may represent the anesthesia services used in *two or more* procedures; in other words, there is no specific one-to-one relationship between the anesthesia codes and the procedure codes. This differs from the other CPT codes, which represent only the service that they describe.

What Is Anesthesia and Who Administers It?

Anesthesia is the partial or complete loss of sensation achieved by the administration of an anesthetic agent (medicine for the relief of pain), usually by injection or inhalation. Anesthesia can be administered by the following different types of providers:

- **Anesthesiologist:** A physician who specializes in anesthetic administration, pain relief, and the care of patients before, during, and after surgery.
- **Anesthetist:** A specially trained registered nurse who administers anesthetics.
- **Certified Registered Nurse Anesthetist (CRNA):** A registered, advance-practice nurse who has acquired additional education and training and has passed a national certification examination to administer anesthesia and provide anesthesia-related care.
- **Other Physicians: According to CPT, regional or general anesthesia may be provided by the surgeon.**

What Are the Different Types of Anesthesia?

The type of anesthesia provided is determined on the basis of the type of surgery being performed as well as on the medical condition of the patient. There are several different types of anesthesia. Some are named according to their site (e.g., lumbar), some are named by category (e.g., frost for cryoanesthesia), and some have more familiar terms, such as the following:

- **General Anesthesia.** General anesthesia causes a patient to be unconscious, requiring assisted ventilation (help with breathing) during surgery. The anesthetic can be inhaled through a mask or tube (inhalation), can be administered through an intravenous line, or administered rectally. General anesthesia may be administered for surgeries as complex as cardiac bypass and for less complicated surgeries such as a thyroid needle biopsy.

If you or someone you know received anesthesia for a surgical procedure and complained afterward of a sore or raspy throat, a "general anesthesia" was most likely administered. During the administration of general anesthesia, a breathing tube may be placed into the windpipe to maintain proper breathing. Once the surgery is completed, the breathing tube is removed, which may leave the patient with the sore or raspy throat.

- **Spinal Anesthesia.** This type of anesthesia is usually used for procedures on the lower half of the body (e.g., lower abdominal, pelvic, rectal, or lower extremity). With spinal anesthesia, the anesthetic is injected into the area around the spinal cord to block pain sensation during surgery.
- **Epidural.** This is very similar to a spinal anesthetic and may also be used for surgery on the lower limbs. However, with an epidural, the anesthetic agent is administered through a catheter placed into the epidural space (the space outside the dura, the membrane that covers the spinal cord and nerve roots in the spine and runs the length of the spine). Epidurals are commonly used as an anesthetic during labor.
- **Regional.** This type of anesthesia numbs only the portion of the body on which the operation will be performed. It is achieved by an injection of local anesthetic into the area of nerves that provide feeling to that part of the body. There are many different types of regional anesthesia, such as trigger-point injections and nerve blocks. Spinal anesthesia and epidurals are also considered regional anesthesia.
- **Local Anesthesia.** Local anesthesia is the numbing of a small area limited to the site where the anesthetic is injected or applied topically by spray, cream, ointment, gel, or powder. Although regional and local anesthesia appear to be similar, it is important to note the difference. Regional anesthesia provides numbness to larger areas because the nerve blocks are involved, whereas local anesthesia is limited to the area where the anesthetic is applied.
- **Moderate (Conscious) Sedation.** This type of anesthesia provides a decreased level of consciousness that does not put the patient to sleep. Patients can respond to verbal commands, and no interventions are required to maintain a patent airway.
- **Tumescent Anesthesia.** This is a method of obtaining anesthesia for large areas using very dilute concentrations of local anesthetic. This allows for treatment of large areas with less bleeding (e.g., for liposuction).
- **Field Block.** This is conduction anesthesia in which small nerves are not anesthetized individually, as in nerve block anesthesia, but instead are blocked en

masse by local anesthetic solution injected to form a barrier proximal to the operative site.

■ **Patient-Controlled Analgesia (PCA).** PCA is a system that allows the patient to self-administer pain medication through the use of a patient-controlled analgesic pump. The system allows the patient to administer an analgesic drug such as morphine whenever the pain returns. The system is preset so that an excessive amount of medication cannot be administered.

Although not a type of anesthesia, another service provided by anesthesiologists is a *blood patch.* A blood patch is an injection of a small amount of the patient's own blood at the site of the spinal tap. The blood acts to patch the hole in the outer membrane of the spinal cord (dura) that was created by the procedure.

How the Anesthesia Section is Organized

The CPT codes in the anesthesia section (with the exception of the last four subsections) are divided first by anatomic site and then by the specific type of procedure. *More than one CPT procedure code may be represented by one anesthesia code.*

For example: Look up the CPT code 01400, Anesthesia for open or surgical arthroscopic procedures on knee joint; not otherwise specified. This one anesthesia CPT code can be used for CPT codes 29866–29868, all of which relate to arthroscopic surgical procedures of the knee.

Because there are approximately 4000 surgical, medical, and radiological procedures that are represented by approximately 260 anesthesia codes, utilization of a crosswalk is recommended. The crosswalk will crosswalk the anesthesia services to CPT codes, and vice versa. The ASA publishes *A Guide for Surgery/Anesthesia CPT Codes.*

The last four subsections are not organized by anatomic site. They are:

■ Radiological Procedures: 01916–01936

■ Burn Excisions or Débridement: 01951–01953

■ Obstetric: 01958–01969

■ Other Procedures: 01990–01999

Anesthesia CPT codes include the preoperative, intraoperative, and postoperative care. This includes all **usual** preoperative and postoperative visits to the patient and routine intraoperative care such as administration of fluids and/or blood and monitoring services. It is important to note that although postoperative care usually includes pain management, some pain management may be reported separately, such as a spinal injection for significant pain.

If the anesthesiologist provides care that is **unusual** or beyond that which is included in the service, it may be reported in addition to the basic anesthesia service. Examples of this type of care include unusual forms of monitoring such as Swan-Ganz, intra-arterial, and central venous.

Coding for Moderate (Conscious) Sedation

The CPT codes for moderate (conscious) sedation are located in the Medicine Section of the CPT book. These codes are selected on the basis of the time element and the age of the patient and are used when the physician providing the service also provides the moderate (conscious) sedation. There are many CPT codes that **include** moderate (conscious) sedation as part of the procedure or service. For these services that include moderate (conscious) sedation, you would **NOT** report the moderate (conscious) sedation code with the service code. Codes that include the moderate (conscious) sedation are easily identified, as they have the bull's-eye (•) symbol before the CPT number. Also, Appendix G of the CPT book includes a full list of CPT codes that include moderate (conscious) sedation.

For example: A colonoscopy is an excellent example of a surgical code that would be performed with moderate (conscious) sedation. In the CPT book, look up CPT code 44388, Colonoscopy through stoma; diagnostic, with or without collection of specimen(s) by brushing or washing (separate procedure). You will notice this CPT code has a bull's-eye (⊙). This indicates that the moderate (conscious) sedation is included in the service for the colonoscopy. Therefore, if a colonoscopy was performed and moderate (conscious) sedation was provided, only the CPT code for the colonoscopy should be reported.

Calculating the Anesthesia Payment

Anesthesia services are billed differently than other services. There is a standard formula, which for the most part is nationally accepted:

$$\text{Base Units (B)} + \text{Time Units (T)} +$$
$$\text{Modifying Units (M)} \times \text{Conversion Factor (CF)}$$
$$\text{OR}$$
$$(B + T + M) \times \text{Conversion Factor}$$

Base Unit. The ASA Relative Value Guide (RVG) assigns a base value/base unit to each CPT code based on the complexity of the anesthesia service. The terms *base value* and *base unit* are the same (Table 9–1).

Time. This part of the calculation is based on the time (total number of minutes) during which the anesthesia was administered. Time begins when the anesthesiologist begins to prepare the patient for the induction of anesthesia in the operating room (or in an equivalent area) and ends when the anesthesiologist is no longer in personal attendance; that is when the patient may be safely placed under postoperative supervision. Time must be documented in the patient's chart.

Insurance carriers may independently determine the amount of time in a unit; usually, 15 minutes equals one unit.

Time is another area where anesthesia is unique, as anesthesia is recorded in military time.

Civilians use a 12-hour clock system whereby the same time notation comes up twice in a day. The use of a.m. or p.m. distinguishes the difference between the two times. Arranging to meet a friend at 6:30 and failing to use an a.m. or p.m. designation could result in confusion about which time to meet.

Military time is divided into hours starting at midnight as 0000. Using midnight as a starting point, hours increase by 100. For example, 1:00 a.m. in civilian time is 0100 in military time. Noon becomes 1200 hours and is the beginning point of noticeable change from civilian time. For example, 1:00 p.m. in civilian time becomes 1300 hours in military time. The use of military time provides accuracy and eliminates confusion when recording anesthesia time. For example, you would see anesthesia time written as 13:02–15:48 (military time). In civilian time, this would translate to 1:02 p.m.–3:48 p.m.

Modifying Unit. Modifying units indicate any additional conditions or circumstances that may make the administration of the anesthesia service more complex. There are two basic modifying characteristics: (1) qualifying circumstances and (2) physical status modifiers.

■ *Qualifying Circumstances.* In some cases, anesthesia services may be provided in situations that make the administration of the anesthesia more difficult. These circumstances include extraordinary condition of the patient, unusual risk factors, or significant operative conditions. These CPT codes are shown in Table 9–2. The CPT codes representing qualifying circumstances: Are located in your CPT book under Anesthesia Guidelines and also in the Medicine Section under Qualifying Circumstances for Anesthesia, listed numerically. (Note: All of the qualifying circumstances codes listed in the CPT book are also listed in Table 9–2.)

■ Provide additional information about the administration of the anesthesia service.

■ Are used in addition to the anesthesia CPT code (the + sign indicates these codes are add-on codes).

■ Begin with "99" and are considered adjunct codes; this means they can never be reported alone.

■ May be reported along with other, additional qualifying circumstances. In other words, if necessary, more than one qualifying circumstance may be reported.

■ *Physical Status Modifiers.* These modifiers (shown in Table 9–3) are used to indicate the patient's condition at the time anesthesia was administered. Additionally, the codes for these physical status modifiers:

■ Are located in your CPT book under "Anesthesia Guidelines." (Note: All of the physical status

▌ TABLE 9–1 Examples of Base Units (B)

CPT Code	CPT Description	Base Unit Value
01360	Anesthesia for all open procedures on lower one-third of femur	5 + TM
01380	Anesthesia for all closed procedures on knee joint	3 + TM
01382	Anesthesia for diagnostic arthroscopic procedures of knee joint	3 + TM
01402	Anesthesia for open or surgical arthroscopic procedures on knee joint; total knee arthroplasty	7 + TM
00600	Anesthesia for procedures on cervical spine and cord; not otherwise specified	10 + TM

▌ TABLE 9–2 Qualifying Circumstances

CPT Code	CPT Description	Relative Value
+ 99100	Anesthesia for patient of extreme age, younger than 1 year and older than 70	1
+ 99116	Anesthesia complicated by utilization of total body hypothermia	5
+ 99135	Anesthesia complicated by utilization of controlled hypotension	5
+ 99140	Anesthesia complicated by emergency conditions (specify)	2

TABLE 9–3 Physical Status Modifiers

Physical Status Modifier	CPT Description	Relative Value
P1	A normal, healthy patient	0
P2	A patient with mild systemic disease	0
P3	A patient with severe systemic disease	1
P4	A patient with severe systemic disease that is a constant threat to life	2
P5	A moribund patient who is not expected to survive without an operation	3
P6	A declared brain-dead patient whose organs are being removed for donor purposes	0

TABLE 9–4 Conversion Factors (CF)

Locality	Anesthesia Conversion Factor
Atlanta, Georgia	20.86
Idaho	18.93
Manhattan, New York	22.03

Code 01382 Anesthesia for diagnostic arthroscopic procedures of knee joint *has a base value of 3* (see Table 9–1). The time is determined by taking 60 minutes and dividing it by the 15-minute time increment. In this case, the **time equals 4** units. Modifier P3 describes a patient with severe systemic disease and has a **value of 1** (see Table 9–3). The total of 8 is then multiplied by the conversion factor for Manhattan, which is $22.03 (see Table 9–4). The total reimbursement is $176.24:

Base Value = 3 + Time = 4 + Modifiers = 1 = Total 8
8 × 22.03 (CF) = Total Reimbursement $176.24

If the same service was provided in Idaho, the total of 8 would be multiplied by the conversion factor of $18.93 for a total reimbursement of $151.44.

modifier codes listed in the CPT book are also listed in Table 9–3.)

■ Serve to identify the level of complexity of the anesthesia service provided to the patient.

■ Begin with a letter P, have a number from 1 to 6, and are appended to the end of the CPT code. The ascending numbers correspond to the increasing degree of severity of poor health, with the exception of P6, which refers to a declared brain-dead organ donor.

■ Should be supported by documentation in the patient's chart.

■ Are not assigned by the coder but determined by the anesthesiologist.

Also keep in mind:

■ P1, P2, and P6 all have a base value of "0" because the condition(s) they represent do not affect the service provided.

Conversion Factor (CF). This is the dollar value assigned for each unit and is based on the geographical location where the service takes place (Table 9–4). Because it is more expensive to provide a service in Manhattan, New York, than it is in Atlanta, Georgia, the conversion factor for Manhattan is higher than for Atlanta.

Putting It All Together

Mary Jones is a 58-year-old with severe hypertension. She lives in New York and undergoes a 60-minute anesthesia period for a diagnostic arthroscopy of the knee.

Let's Do The Next One Together

Using the tables above, calculate the reimbursement for Mr. Morrison's procedure:

Mr. Morrison is a 72-year-old male living in Atlanta. Georgia. He has maintained good health, but due to problems with his knee, he will undergo a 2-hour knee arthroplasty to replace severely damaged cartilage of the knee.

KEY CODING TIP
When reading from an operative report or a progress note, highlight key words that you will need to calculate the reimbursement or to code for the service. This will allow you to focus only on the information you need.

Let's look at the scenario. Certain facts are important to accurately code for the anesthesia service. We need to know the **age of the patient,** so let's highlight *72-year-old.* We also need to know **where the service took place**, so let's highlight *Atlanta, Georgia.* It is important to note the **status of the patient** along with **any unusual circumstances,** so let's highlight the fact that he *maintained good health.*

continued

Let's Do The Next One Together—cont'd

We also need to know the **total time** for the procedure, so let's highlight *2-hour*. Finally, we need to know **what procedure** was performed; in this case, it is anesthesia services for an arthroplasty, so let's highlight *knee arthroplasty*. Your paragraph should look like this:

*Mr. Morrison is a 72-year-old male living in Atlanta, Georgia. He has **maintained good health,** but due to problems with his knee, he will undergo a 2-hour knee arthroplasty to replace severely damaged cartilage of the knee.*

Now we have all the information we need to calculate the reimbursement for this service. Let's fill in the blanks.

By looking at Table 9–1, we know that the base unit value (B) for an arthroplasty (CPT code 01402) is **7**. We can calculate the time by dividing 120 minutes (2 hours) by 15 (remember, 15 minutes is equal to one unit); this gives us a total of **8** units for our time (T). After reading the scenario, we can determine that this is a normal, healthy patient; physical status modifier of P1 would have been appended by the anesthesiologist. This modifier has a zero value. However, because of the age of the patient (72 years), we do have a qualifying circumstance (anesthesia for patient of extreme age, younger than 1 year and older than 70 years): by looking at Table 9–2, we see that this modifier carries a value of **1**.

Base = __7__ + Time = __8__ + Modifiers = __1__ = Total __16__
Total __16__ × CF __20.86__ =
Total Reimbursement: __$333.76__

LET'S TRY ANOTHER

Marcus Wilson is a 51-year-old resident of Idaho who underwent a cervical decompression for his neck pain. Aside from suffering from mild psoriasis, he is in good health. The 3-hour procedure was performed and completed without incident.

Let's look at this scenario and highlight the important facts to properly code for the anesthesia service. We need to know the **age of the patient,** so let's highlight *51-year-old*. We also need to know **where the service took place,** so let's highlight *Idaho*. It is important to note the **status of the patient** along with **any unusual circumstances,** so let's highlight *mild psoriasis* (which in this case is a mild systemic disease). We also need to know the **total time** for the

procedure, so let's highlight *3-hour*. Finally, we need to know **what procedure** was performed; in this case, it is anesthesia service for a cervical decompression to relieve the neck pain. Your paragraph should look like this:

Marcus Wilson is a 51-year-old resident of Idaho who underwent a cervical decompression for his neck pain. Aside from suffering from mild psoriasis, he is in good health. The 3-hour procedure was performed and completed without incident.

Now we have everything we need to calculate the reimbursement for this service. Let's fill in the blanks utilizing the tables presented earlier.

By looking at Table 9–1, we know that the base unit value (B) for a cervical decompression (CPT code 00600) is **10**. We can calculate the time by dividing 180 minutes (3 hours) by 15 (remember, 15 minutes is equal to one unit); this gives us a total of **12** units for our time (T). After reading the scenario, we can determine that the patient has a mild systemic disease; therefore, the physician appended the P2 (see Table 9–3) physical status modifier (this modifier has a value of 0). Additionally, because of the age of the patient (51 years), we do not have any qualifying circumstance based on age or any other type of qualifying circumstance.

Base = __10__ + Time = __12__ + Modifiers =
__0__ = Total __22__
Total __22__ × CF __18.93__ =
Total Reimbursement: __$416.46__

Multiple Procedures

Now you have the concept. But what happens when multiple surgical procedures are performed during the same anesthetic administration? In some cases, a patient may have multiple surgeries performed at the same operative session. When this happens, the services of the anesthesiologist are reported with only the anesthesia code with the highest base unit.

For example: For a patient undergoing a clavicle biopsy (base unit value = 3) and a radical mastectomy (base unit value = 5), only the base unit value of 5 is reported.

Concurrent Care

CRNAs can work independently or under the direction of an anesthesiologist. Many insurance carriers cover anesthesia services when the anesthesiologist is physically and personally involved in the care of the patient simultaneously with the CRNA. This is called *concurrent care.*

In order to bill concurrent care, the anesthesiologist must be present at the induction and emergence from anesthesia and be able to be immediately available in case of an emergency. Additionally, the anesthesiologist must:

1. Perform the preanesthesia evaluation and examination.
2. Prescribe the anesthesia.
3. Participate personally in the induction of and emergence from the anesthesia procedure.
4. Ensure that any part of the anesthesia plan not personally performed by the anesthesiologist is performed by a qualified individual.
5. Monitor the course of anesthesia administration at frequent intervals.
6. Remain physically present to provide diagnosis and treatment in an emergency situation.
7. Provide postanesthesia care.

Modifiers

Anesthesiologists use both CPT and HCPCS modifiers. Let's take a look at HCPCS modifiers first.

HCPCS Modifiers

These modifiers describe who performed the service, alert the carrier regarding concurrent care cases, and identify monitored anesthesia care (MAC).

AA: Anesthesia services performed personally by anesthesiologist.

AD: Medical supervision by a physician: more than four concurrent anesthesia procedures.

G8: MAC for deep, complex, complicated, or markedly invasive surgical procedures.

G9: MAC for patient who has history of severe cardiopulmonary condition.

QK: Medical direction of two, three, or four concurrent anesthesia procedures involving qualified individuals.

QS: MAC services.

QX: CRNA service; with medical direction by a physician.

QY: Medical direction of one CRNA by an anesthesiologist.

QZ: CRNA service; without medical direction by a physician.

CPT Modifiers

CPT modifiers are two-digit numeric numbers that are always appended to the end of a CPT code. CPT modifiers provide additional information about the service without changing the description of the CPT code. A complete listing of all the CPT modifiers is located in Appendix A of the CPT book.

Modifiers 22 and 23 are modifiers most commonly used by anesthesiologists.

Modifier 22—Increased Procedural Service

When the work required to provide a service is substantially greater than typically required, it may be identified by adding modifier 22 to the usual procedure code. Documentation must support the substantial additional work and the reason for the additional work (e.g., increased intensity, time, technical difficulty of procedure, severity of patient's condition, physical and mental effort required).

Modifier 23—Unusual Anesthesia

Occasionally, a procedure that usually requires either no anesthesia or local anesthesia, because of unusual circumstances, must be done under general anesthesia. This circumstance may be reported by adding modifier 23 to the procedure code of the basic service.

For example: A patient presents with a laceration on the hand, which requires sutures. The suture repair would usually be performed with a local anesthetic. However, if a hyperactive child presented for the suture repair, the physician may recommend general anesthesia to assure the child would remain still during the procedure.

The following anesthesia modifiers are _not_ used by anesthesiologists:

Modifier 47—Anesthesia by Surgeon. Regional or general anesthesia provided by the surgeon may be reported by adding modifier 47 to the basic service. (This does not include local anesthesia.) **Note:** Modifier 47 would not be used as a modifier for the anesthesia procedures.
Modifier 47:

- Is used when the physician personally performs regional or general anesthesia for a surgical procedure he or she is also performing (i.e., is not an anesthesiologist).
- Would be appended to the surgical code.
- Is not applicable to anesthesia codes.
- Is not reported for moderate conscious sedation.

Modifier 51—Multiple Procedures. This **modifier is not applicable to anesthesia codes.** Rather, Modifier 51 is used when reporting the procedures themselves (in which case, the modifier is appended to the additional procedures), *not* the anesthesia used in the procedures. (See Chapter 7 for more details on the use of this modifier.) Remember that when coding for anesthesia services for multiple procedures, only the procedure with the highest base value is reported. **Therefore, modifier 51 would not be used for anesthesia codes.**

Let's Practice Coding

Now that you have a good understanding of anesthesia services and have prepared your CPT book, you are ready to code.

Locating Anesthesia Codes. To locate a CPT code for an anesthesia service in the CPT book, go to the index, look up the word *Anesthesia,* and then, beneath Anesthesia, look for either the anatomic site or the procedure (as subentries of *Anesthesia*). Let's try one.

Let's look up the anesthesia code for corneal transplant of the eye.
By Anatomical Site: We first go to the CPT index and look up *Anesthesia,* and then the subentry *Eye.* When we find *Eye,* we see that we can select *Cornea,* which brings us to CPT code 00144.

    Anesthesia
        Eye.................00140-00148
            Cornea.....................00144

When we look up 00144 in the Anesthesia section of the CPT book, the code descriptor reads:

00144—Anesthesia for procedures on eye; corneal transplant

By Procedure: In some cases, you could also locate the anesthesia code by looking up Anesthesia in the CPT index and then by type of procedure—in this case, "corneal transplant." Let's do that as an exercise. Look up *Anesthesia* in the CPT index, and then look up the subentry *Corneal transplant.* Notice it will also take you to CPT code 00144.

    Anesthesia
        Corneal Transplant.................00144

Now look up the anesthesia code for a biopsy of the liver.
By Anatomical Site: Look up *Anesthesia* in the CPT index and then the subentry *Liver.*
    Anesthesia
        Liver......................00702, 00796

Notice you have two CPT codes to select from: 00702, 00796.

Now look up both codes in the Anesthesia section and compare them with the codes you found in the index. We see that the code descriptors read:

00702–Anesthesia for procedures on upper anterior abdominal wall; percutaneous liver biopsy
00796–Anesthesia for intraperitoneal procedures in upper abdomen including laparoscopy; liver transplant (recipient)

The correct choice is CPT code 00702, as it describes the liver biopsy.

By Procedure: Look up *Anesthesia* in the CPT index, then the subentry *Biopsy,* and then its subentry *Liver.*
    Anesthesia
        Biopsy.................00100
            Liver...................00702

So now you know two ways to look up anesthesia CPT codes.

Learn More About It

The more you read, the more you know. Increase your knowledge with the following resources:

Recommended Web Sites
American Society of Anesthesiologists
http://www.asahq.org
American Medical Association
http://www.ama-assn.org
Centers for Medicare and Medicaid Services— Anesthesia Center
http://www.cms.hhs.gov/center/anesth.asp

Recommended Books
Current Year Version of Relative Value Guide
Author: American Society of Anesthesiologists
SKU–30509-3SI
Publisher: American Society of Anesthesiologists
520 N. Northwest Highway, Park Ridge, Ill. 60068-2573
(847) 825-5586
Current Year Version CROSSWALK Book: A Guide for Surgery/Anesthesia CPT Codes
Author: American Society of Anesthesiologists
SKU–PM10CW
Publisher: American Society of Anesthesiologists

520 N. Northwest Highway, Park Ridge, Ill. 60068-2573
(847) 825-5586

STOP-LOOK-HIGHLIGHT

The key to successfully passing the exam and selecting the correct code lies in your knowing how to use your coding book.

To help you navigate through your codebook, and to make sure you have the most important information at your fingertips when you take the exam, highlight key text in the chapter guidelines and subheadings, and insert simple notes and coding tips directly into your codebooks.

When highlighting, use two different color highlighter pens: yellow for standard guidelines and global services and an alternate color for carve-outs and unique notes.

In the Anesthesia Guidelines:

In the middle of the second paragraph, in yellow, highlighst "These services include the usual preoperative and postoperative visits, the anesthesia care during the procedure, the administration of fluids and/or blood and the usual monitoring services (e.g., ECG, temperature, blood pressure, oximetry, capnography, and mass spectrometry)." **This is the definition of what is inclusive in anesthesia services.** With your alternate color highlighter, go on to highlight "Unusual forms of monitoring (e.g., intra-arterial, central venous, and Swan-Ganz) are not included." **This defines what is not inclusive.**

In the fourth paragraph, in yellow, highlight *"To report moderate (conscious) sedation provided by a physician also performing the service for which conscious sedation is being provided, see codes 99143-99145."* And also, in red pen, write *"These codes are located in the Medicine section."* This note will be **a reminder that the CPT codes for moderate (conscious) sedation are located in the Medicine section and not the Anesthesia section.**

■ Under Time Reporting, in yellow, highlight the second sentence: "Anesthesia time begins when the anesthesiologist begins to prepare the patient for the induction of anesthesia in the operating room (or in an equivalent area) and ends when the anesthesiologist is no longer in personal attendance, that is, when the patient may be safely placed under postoperative supervision." **This defines anesthesia time.**

■ Under Qualifying Circumstances, highlight in yellow, "More than one qualifying circumstance may be selected." In red pen, add *"Qualifying circumstances can also be found in the Medicine section."*

● On the Anesthesia Guidelines page, in red pen, write the following:
   Anesthesia Modifiers Commonly Used
   • *22 Unusual Procedural Services*
   • *23 Unusual Anesthesia*
   Anesthesia Modifiers Not Used
   • *47 Anesthesia by Surgeon*
   • *51 Multiple Procedures*

● *01999 is the CPT code for Unlisted Anesthesia Service*

● *Formula for calculating anesthesia payments is Base (B) + Time (T) + Modifying Factors (M) = Total Units × Conversion Factor (CF)*

● *When multiple surgical procedures are performed during the same session, only the anesthesia code with the highest base unit is reported*

Under Moderate (Conscious) Sedation Guidelines located in the Medicine section of the CPT book (99143-99150):

■ In the first paragraph, highlight in yellow, "Moderate (conscious) sedation is a drug-induced depression of consciousness during which patients respond purposefully to verbal commands, either alone or accompanied by light tactile stimulation. No interventions are required to maintain a patient airway, and spontaneous ventilation is adequate. Cardiovascular function is usually maintained."

■ In the third paragraph, highlight in your alternate color highlighter, "When providing moderate sedation, the following services are included and NOT reported separately." **Everything bulleted below this statement is included in the CPT code for moderate (conscious) sedation.**

■ In red ink underneath the title Moderate (Conscious) Sedation, write, *"These codes are used when the physician providing the service is also providing the moderate (conscious) sedation."*

In Appendix A, Modifiers:

■ In the description of modifier 47, highlight "Note: Modifier 47 would not be used as a modifier for the anesthesia procedures."

■ With a red pen, underneath modifier 51, write, *"Multiple procedures would not be considered applicable to anesthesia services. Therefore this modifier would not be used by anesthesiologists."*

Anesthesia Vocabulary Words

In your CPT book on the blank Note page for Anesthesia, write the following anesthesia vocabulary words:

Anesthesia: Anesthesia is the partial or complete loss of sensation, which is achieved by the administration of an anesthetic agent (medicine for the relief of pain), usually by injection or inhalation.

Blood patch: This is **not** a type of anesthesia but a procedure used by anesthesiologists. The blood patch consists of an injection at the spinal tap site of a small amount of the patient's own blood. This acts to close a cerebrospinal fluid leak.

Endotracheal: Administration of gaseous drugs through an endotracheal tube (ET) or mask to achieve general anesthesia.

Epidural: An injection of an anesthetic agent through a catheter placed into the epidural space. Also known as peridural, epidural, epidural block, spinal, intraspinal, and subarachnoid.

General anesthesia: Induces a controlled state of unconsciousness. The drugs producing this state can be administered by inhalation, intravenously, intramuscularly, or rectally.

Local anesthesia: The numbing of a small area limited to the site where the anesthetic is injected or applied topically by spray, cream, ointment, gel, or powder.

Moderate (conscious) sedation: Provides a decreased level of consciousness that does not put the patient to sleep. Patients can respond to verbal commands, and no interventions are required to maintain a patent airway.

Patient-controlled anesthesia: A system that allows the patient to be in control of his or her pain medication by a patient-controlled analgesic pump. The system allows the patient to administer an analgesic drug such as morphine to control pain whenever he or she is hurting. The system is preset so an excessive amount of medication cannot be administered.

Regional anesthesia: Anesthesia that is used to block painful sensations in a region of the body and is produced by a field block or nerve block. Also known as conduction anesthesia or block anesthesia.

Tumescent anesthesia: A method for obtaining anesthesia for large areas using very dilute concentrations of local anesthetic. This allows for treatment of large areas with less bleeding (e.g., for liposuction).

Anesthesia Acronyms and Abbreviations

In your CPT book on the blank Note page for Anesthesia, write the following acronyms and abbreviations:

ASA: **A**merican **S**ociety of **A**nesthesiologists

CRNA: **C**ertified **R**egistered **N**urse **A**nesthetist

ET: **E**ndotracheal **T**ube

MAC: **M**onitored **A**nesthesia **C**are

PCA: **P**atient-**C**ontrolled **A**nesthesia

RVG: **R**elative **V**alue **G**uide

TAKE THE CODING CHALLENGE

Assign the Appropriate Anesthesia Code

1. Cesarean delivery only

   _____

2. Lumbar puncture

   _____

3. Heart transplant

   _____

4. Upper gastrointestinal endoscopy

   _____

5. Radical hysterectomy

   _____

Multiple Choice

1. Mr. Jones has a severe systemic disease and undergoes anesthesia for a total hip replacement (base value 10) and diagnostic arthroscopy of the knee (base value 3). The base value for both procedures is determined by:
   a. Adding both base values together
   b. Subtracting the lower base value from the higher base value
   c. The procedure with the highest base value will determine the base value
   d. Each procedure keeps its own base value

2. Time for anesthesia services begins when:
   a. The surgeon begins the surgery
   b. The anesthesia is administered by the anesthesiologist
   c. The anesthesiologist begins to prepare the patient for the induction of anesthesia
   d. None of the above

3. A 48-year-old patient with severe systemic disease presents for surgery in the lower abdomen for repair of a ventral hernia. The code for anesthesia services for this patient would be:
   a. 00832-P3
   b. 00830-P3
   c. 00834-P2
   d. 00832-P2

4. CRNA is the acronym for:
   a. Central Registered Nurse Assistant
   b. Certified Registered Nurse Anesthetist
   c. Concurrent Registered Nurse Anesthetist
   d. Concurrent Regional Nurse Assistant

5. Needle biopsy pleura (32400) is performed on a 75-year-old patient. The code(s) for anesthesia services for this patient would be:
   a. 00520
   b. 00522
   c. 00522, 99100
   d. 00520, 99100

6. The following modifiers are not applicable for anesthesia services:
   a. 47 and 51
   b. 22 and 23
   c. 22 and 47
   d. 23 and 51

7. What type of sedation provides a deep level of consciousness that does not put the patient to sleep and allows the patient to respond to verbal commands?
   a. General
   b. Patient-controlled
   c. Moderate or conscious
   d. Tumescent

8. Which of the following is inclusive when reporting anesthesia services?
   a. The usual preoperative and postoperative visits and the anesthesia care during the procedure
   b. The administration of fluids and/or blood
   c. The usual monitoring services (e.g., ECG, temperature, blood pressure, oximetry, capnography, and mass spectrometry)
   d. All of the above

9. Moderate (conscious) sedation codes are:
   a. Adjunct codes to the anesthesia service
   b. Only used by CRNAs
   c. Age-specific
   d. Located at the end of the anesthesia section

10. What type of anesthesia modifier indicates the patient's status at the time anesthesia was administered?
    a. HCPCS
    b. Qualifying circumstance
    c. Physical status
    d. 22

CODING CHALLENGE ANSWERS AND RATIONALES

Assign the Appropriate Anesthesia Code

1. The correct answer is 01961 Anesthesia for cesarean delivery only. You can look this up in the CPT index under **Anesthesia,** then **Cesarean delivery.** You will be presented with two code selections, 01961 and 01963. When you look both CPT codes up in the Anesthesia section, you can compare the two code descriptors.
   01961 Anesthesia for *cesarean delivery only*
   01963 Anesthesia for *cesarean hysterectomy without any labor analgesia/anesthesia care*
   When you read the descriptors of the two codes, you will notice CPT code 01963 is for a cesarean hysterectomy without any labor analgesia/anesthesia care. Because we are coding for a cesarean delivery only, CPT code 01961 would be the correct code.

2. The correct answer is 00635 Anesthesia for procedures in lumbar region; diagnostic or therapeutic lumbar puncture. You can look this up in the CPT index under **Anesthesia** and then **Lumbar Puncture.** You will be presented with only one option, 00635. The complete descriptor for CPT code 00635 includes the description of a diagnostic or therapeutic lumbar puncture, which is the correct code.

3. The correct answer is 00580 Anesthesia for heart transplant or heart/lung transplant. You can look this up in the CPT index under **Anesthesia,** then **Heart,** then **Transplant.** You will be presented with only one option: 00580. The complete descriptor for CPT code 00580 includes the description of a heart transplant, which is the correct code.

4. The correct answer is 00740 Anesthesia for upper gastrointestinal endoscopic procedures, endoscope introduced proximal to duodenum. You can look this up in the CPT index under **Anesthesia,** then **Gastrointestinal Endoscopy.** You will be presented with only one option: 00740. The complete descriptor for CPT code 00740 includes the description for upper gastrointestinal endoscopic procedures, which is the correct code.

5. The correct answer is 00846 Anesthesia for intraperitoneal procedures in lower abdomen including laparoscopy; radical hysterectomy. You can look this up in the CPT index under **Anesthesia,** then **Hysterectomy,** and then **Radical.** You will be presented with only one option: 00846. The complete descriptor for CPT code 00846 includes the description for a radical hysterectomy, which is the correct code.

Multiple Choice Answers

1. The correct answer is **c.** The procedure with the highest base value will determine the base value. According to the ASA, when multiple surgical procedures are performed during a single anesthetic administration, only the anesthesia code with the highest base unit value is reported.

2. The correct answer is **c.** The anesthesiologist begins to prepare the patient for the induction of anesthesia. According to the ASA, "Anesthesia time begins when the anesthesiologist begins to prepare the patient for the induction of anesthesia in the operating room (or in an equivalent area) and ends when the anesthesiologist is no longer in personal attendance, that is, when the patient may be safely placed under postoperative supervision." This information is also located in the CPT book in the Anesthesia Guidelines under Time Reporting.

3. The correct answer is **a.** By looking at the four choices, we can immediately eliminate answers **c.** and **d.** as both answers include the P2 modifier, which is for patients with "**mild** systemic disease," and our patient has "**severe** systemic disease." Answer **b.** is incorrect, as CPT code 00830 is *Anesthesia for hernia repairs in lower abdomen; **not otherwise specified.*** CPT code 00832 is *Anesthesia for hernia repairs in lower abdomen; **ventral** and incisional **hernias*** and includes the correct modifier, P3, for the severe systemic disease, making answer **a.** the correct choice.

4. The correct answer is **b.**

5. The correct answer is **c.** By looking at the four choices, we can immediately eliminate answers **a.** and **b.** as neither includes the qualifying circumstance add-on code 99100 for patients of extreme age, younger than 1 year and older than 70. Answer **d.** has an incorrect CPT code, 00520 *Anesthesia for closed chest procedures; (including bronchoscopy) not otherwise specified.* CPT code 00522 *Anesthesia for closed chest procedures; **needle biopsy of pleura*** accurately describes the procedure and includes the qualifying circumstance (99100) to describe the extreme age of the patient, which makes c the correct choice.

6. The correct answer is **a.** Modifier 47 is used when the anesthesia is provided by the surgeon, and modifier 51 is for multiple procedures. When multiple procedures are provided during a single anesthetic administration, only the anesthesia code with the highest base value is reported. Modifier

22 may be used by anesthesiologists, as it describes an increased procedural service, and modifier 23 may also be used, as it describes unusual anesthesia. Because answers **b., c.,** and **d.** all include modifier(s) that can be used, the correct choice is **a.**

7. The correct answer is **c.**, moderate or conscious sedation. Answer **a.** is incorrect, as general anesthesia causes the patient to become unconscious. Answer **b.** is incorrect, as patient-controlled anesthesia is a system that allows patients to be in control of their pain medication by using a controlled analgesic pump. Answer **d.** is incorrect: tumescent anesthesia is a method that uses dilute concentrations of local anesthetic.

8. The correct answer is **d.** The Anesthesia Guidelines in the CPT book list all of the services described in answers **a., b.,** and **c.** as being inclusive when reporting anesthesia services.

9. The correct answer is **c.** Answer **a.** is incorrect, as the CPT codes for moderate conscious sedation (99143-99150) are not adjunct codes to anesthesia services. Answer **b.** is incorrect, as they are not specific to only CRNAs. Answer **d.** is incorrect, as moderate conscious sedation codes are located in the Medicine section of the CPT book and not the Anesthesia section.

10. The correct answer is **c.** Answer **a.** is incorrect, as the HCPCS modifiers describe who performed the services, identify concurrent cases, and describe who monitored anesthesia care. Answer **b.** is incorrect, as qualifying circumstances describe difficult circumstances under which anesthesia was provided. Answer **d.** is incorrect, as modifier 22 describes an increased procedural service.

CHAPTER 10

Surgery

Anatomical knowledge of the various body areas/ organ systems is the key to correct coding from the different surgery subsections. In this chapter, we cover some of the common services from each of the body areas/organ systems located in the Surgery section. Most of the subsections are organized according to anatomical site and are then further divided according to the type of procedure. Because the Surgery section is the largest section of the CPT book, let's first review the organization of the Surgery section of the CPT manual.

How the Surgery Section of the CPT Book Is Organized

The Surgery section includes both **diagnostic procedures,** such as endoscopies and biopsies, and **therapeutic procedures,** such as removals and repairs.

The Surgery section is further divided into subsections based on body area/organ system (e.g., Integumentary, Musculoskeletal). The subsections are then organized by the type of procedure (removal, repair, and so on).

Notes, which provide coding guidance, appear at the beginning of each Surgery subsection, after the headings, or they may appear immediately after subheadings. These notes provide coding guidance relating to the type of procedure and are extremely helpful, as many surgical procedures can be performed differently.

For example: Breast biopsy may be performed by core needle (19100) or open incisional (19101). In both cases, a breast biopsy is performed; however, the different CPT codes describe how the breast biopsy is performed.

Let's Review the Surgery Guidelines

The guidelines are located in the beginning of the Surgery section. It is important to understand these guidelines, as they apply to all the codes in the Surgery section.

The Surgical Package

A single physician fee is billed/paid for all necessary services before, during, and after surgery. The CPT codes for surgical procedures therefore usually include a number of different services, including:

- Preoperative (before) services
- Intraoperative (during) services
- Postoperative (after; also known as the global period) services

  CPT lists the services included in the surgical package as:

- Local infiltration, metacarpal/metatarsal/digital block or topical anesthesia
- Subsequent to the decision for surgery, one related evaluation and management (E/M) encounter on the date immediately prior to or on the date of the procedure (including history and physical)
- Immediate postoperative care, including dictating operative notes, talking with the family and other physicians
- Writing orders
- Evaluating the patient in the postanesthesia recovery
- Typical postoperative follow-up care

It is equally important to remember the following services are *not* included in the surgical package:

- General anesthesia.
- Complications, exacerbations, recurrence, or any other diseases or injuries during the postoperative period are separately reportable.

Surgical procedures are categorized as either a major surgical procedure or a minor surgical procedure. Each of these procedures includes a postoperative or global period (the time following the surgical procedure). **Major surgical procedures** have a 90-day global period. The global period begins the day following the surgery and includes a 1-day preoperative period. General anesthesia services are *not* bundled and are reported separately by the anesthesiologist.

Minor surgical procedures have either a 0- or a 10-day global period, and the visit the day of a minor surgical procedure is typically included in the reimbursement for the procedure and includes the preoperative evaluation to address the problem, explaining any risks and benefits of the procedure and obtaining the patient's consent. The postoperative period includes the day of the surgery and/or the 10 days following the minor surgical procedure depending on the global days assigned to the minor surgical procedure.

For *minor* surgical procedures, the preoperative and postoperative services are usually reported separately.

Example of a major procedure: A patient presents to a general surgeon upon request of his primary care physician for evaluation of a potential hernia. The general surgeon examines the patient and determines the patient has an inguinal hernia in need of repair. The surgery is scheduled for 3 weeks from the date of the office visit.

When the patient presents for the hernia repair, the general surgeon will provide a brief history and physical on the patient (preoperative), perform the hernia repair (intraoperative), and see the patient at follow-up a week after the surgery to assure the patient is healing properly (postoperative). The surgeon will be paid one fee for all three components of the surgical package.

It is important to note that postoperative visit includes the typical postoperative follow-up care. Any complications, exacerbations, recurrence, or the presence of other diseases or injuries requiring additional services should be separately reported.

Special Report

A special report should be sent with surgical procedures that are billed with an unlisted surgical CPT code (see "Unlisted Service or Procedure" in the Surgery Guidelines), for surgical procedures with modifier 22 appended, for any Category III code (temporary codes for emerging technology), and for any service that is rarely provided or unusual. A special report should include the following:

■ A definition or description of the nature, extent, and need for the procedure

■ The time, effort, and any special equipment necessary to provide the service

Separate Procedure

In CPT, the term "separate procedure" is used to designate certain procedures that are integral to a larger service/procedure (bundled). These codes are easily identified in CPT, as the words "separate procedure" are included in their CPT descriptor.

These CPT codes designated as separate procedures identify certain procedures that (1) may be billed by

themselves when that is the only service provided, or (as occurs more often) (2) would not be billed because they are performed as part of a larger service or procedure (bundled).

For example: CPT code 45378 Colonoscopy, flexible, proximal to splenic flexure; diagnostic, with or without collection of specimen(s) by brushing or washing, with or without colon decompression (separate procedure) may be performed by itself as a diagnostic colonoscopy. However, when it is performed along with CPT code 45380 Colonoscopy, flexible, proximal to splenic flexure; with biopsy, single or multiple, the diagnostic colonoscopy (45378) would not be separately reported, as it is an integral part of the colonoscopy with biopsy (45380)—that is, it is bundled into the colonoscopy with biopsy.

The Multiple Surgery Rule[1]

The multiple surgery rule applies when a physician performs multiple surgical procedures on the same patient during the same operative session. When these procedures are not integral to a larger procedure, they are separately payable and should be listed individually. In these cases, Medicare and many of the insurance carriers will reimburse as follows:

■ 100% of the fee schedule amount is allowed for the procedure with the highest unit value.

■ 50% of the fee schedule amount is allowed for the second through the fifth procedures.

■ Each procedure thereafter requires that documentation be submitted with a copy of the operative report.

However—

Add-on codes, listed in Appendix D, and modifier 51 exempt codes, listed in Appendix E of the CPT book, are exempt from the multiple surgery rule and are allowed at 100% of the fee schedule allowance.

KEY CODING TIP

When reporting multiple surgeries, it is important to always code the highest paying procedure first.

The Multiple Endoscopy Rule[2]

This rule is similar to the multiple surgery rule, as it reduces the reimbursement amount for multiple endoscopies;

---

[1]Although the multiple surgery rule is not discussed in the CPT Guidelines, it is the purpose of modifier 51 to identify multiple surgical procedures. The multiple surgery rule may be considered a billing rule, as it is important from a reimbursement perspective that the CPT codes are listed according to the highest paying procedure.

[2] Like the multiple surgery rule, the multiple endoscopy rule is not discussed in the CPT Guidelines but may be considered a billing rule. The reimbursement with the multiple endoscopy rule, however, is greatly different from that with the multiple surgery rule.

however, the reimbursement reduction is calculated differently than the multiple surgery reduction. When multiple endoscopies are performed, Medicare and many insurance carriers will pay the full amount of the higher valued endoscopy and then a *percentage* of the next highest endoscopy based on the relative value units (RVUs) of each CPT code.

For example, if the following endoscopies were performed:

■ 45378 Diagnostic colonoscopy (separate procedure)

■ 45380 Colonoscopy with biopsy

■ 45385 Colonoscopy with polyp removal

the provider would code for the colonoscopy with biopsy (45380) and the colonoscopy with polyp removal (45385). As explained earlier, he or she would not code for the diagnostic colonoscopy (45378), as it is considered an integral part of the colonoscopy with biopsy, or bundled.

The provider will be reimbursed the full value for the higher value endoscopy, in this case the colonoscopy with polyp removal, which has an RVU of 13.85 **plus** the difference between the next highest endoscopy, the colonoscopy with biopsy with an RVU of 12.28, and the base endoscopy, diagnostic colonoscopy with an RVU of 10.23, or 2.05 RVUs, for a total payment of 15.90 RVUs (13.85 + 2.05 = 15.90).

Materials Supplied by Physician

In many cases, supplies and materials that are over and above those which are usually included with the procedure may be reported separately with CPT code 99070 Supplies and materials (except spectacles), provided by the physician over and above those usually included with the office visit or other services rendered (list drugs, trays, supplies, or materials provided) OR with the specific HCPCS code.

The surgery guidelines also include the following:

■ A complete list of "subsection information." This is an index of the surgical procedure CPT codes by body area/organ system.

■ A complete listing of unlisted surgical procedures by body area/organ system. These unlisted codes are also located in the CPT index and can be found throughout the Surgery section. Unlisted CPT codes are reported when a service or procedure cannot be identified by a Category I or Category III CPT code.

The Surgery Codes—and How to Use Them

Because this is a review book, we cover some of the common services from each of the body areas/organs systems located in the Surgery section. As mentioned at the beginning of this chapter, anatomical knowledge of the various body areas/organ systems is the key to correct coding from the different Surgery subsections.

As we go through each subsection, you will notice that most of the subsections are organized according to anatomical site and are then further divided according to the type of procedure. Before looking at each subsection individually, let's review some of the common categories.

Débridement: Surgical removal of foreign material and dead tissue from a wound.

Destruction: The ablation of tissue by any method (e.g., electrosurgery, cryosurgery, laser).

Endoscopy: Visual examination of the interior of a hollow body organ by use of an endoscope.

Excision: Removal by cutting.

Incision: A surgical cut made in the body to perform surgery.

Incision and drainage: A procedure performed on an abscess whereby a cut is made into the lining of the abscess allowing the pus to escape either by a drainage tube or by leaving the cavity open to the skin.

Laparoscopy: Surgical technique in which operations in the abdomen are performed through small incisions.

Manipulation: The realignment of a fractured bone or joint.

Repair: To remedy, replace, or heal as in a wound or lost part.

A more extensive list of vocabulary words is given later in this chapter.

Integumentary (Skin)
10040–19499

Let's take a look at some of the more common procedures coded from the Integumentary subsection of the Surgery section.

Excision of Lesions

A lesion is any abnormal tissue damaged by disease or trauma (e.g., growth, sore). The lesion codes are divided on the basis of whether they are malignant or benign, the location of the lesion, size of the lesion, and number of lesions. The excision codes include the local anesthesia and simple closure. CPT defines excision as "full thickness (through the dermis) removal of a lesion, including margins, and includes simple (non-layered) closure when performed."

The size of a lesion is determined by measuring the lesion diameter plus the most narrow margins required for complete excision in centimeters (Fig. 10-1). This will equal the total excised diameter. Therefore, the physician will excise not only the lesion but also margins around the lesion to assure the lesion is completely removed.

For example: A lesion that measures 0.9 cm (excised diameter) will also have the margins excised, in this case 0.3 cm (margin) and 0.3 cm (margin). To determine the total diameter, you add the excised diameter and the margins: 0.9 cm + 0.6 cm (margins) = 1.5 cm (total excised diameter).

Lesions may also be removed by other methods, such as paring or cutting (peeling or scraping away the lesion), biopsy (the removal of a sample of tissue for diagnosis), or shaving (only the suspect area is removed by a cut parallel to the surface surrounding the skin by scalpel), and in the case of skin tags, removal may be by scissoring or any sharp method, ligature strangulation, electrosurgical destruction, or a combination of methods.

LET'S LOOK AT AN EXAMPLE

Melissa Schmidt presented for an excision of a benign lesion on the right side of her face; the lesion measured 2.0 cm. The operative report indicated the margins measured 0.2 cm and 0.2 cm. The excised diameter of the lesion is 2.0 cm + 0.4 cm (0.2 cm + 0.2 cm) = 2.4 cm. In this case, the correct CPT code would be 11443 Excision, other benign lesion including margins, except skin tag (unless listed elsewhere), face, ears, eyelids, nose, lips, mucous membrane; excised diameter 2.1–3.0 cm.

How to Code: We would code the encounter using the Key Coding Tip and highlighting the key points of information: the **type of removal** noted is excision; the **type of lesion** is benign; the **site of the lesion** is the face; and the **size of the lesion** (i.e., the total excised diameter) is 2.4 cm.

KEY CODING TIP

To properly code surgical removal of lesions, carefully read the documentation to determine the following:

1. The type of lesion removal (excision, shaving, and so on)
2. The site of the lesion
3. The size of the lesion (the **total** excised diameter)
4. The number of lesions
5. The type of lesions (malignant or benign)

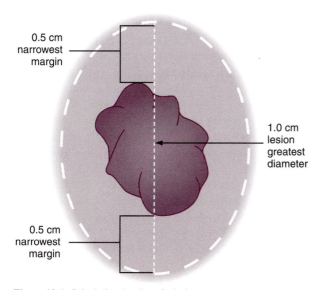

0.5 cm narrowest margin

1.0 cm lesion greatest diameter

0.5 cm narrowest margin

Figure 10-1. Calculating the size of a lesion.

Repair Codes

The repair codes are **divided by** the **site** of the repair, the **complexity** of the repair, and the **length** of the repair. The CPT subsection notes listed under the Repair (Closure) heading are a must-read, as they provide instructions on how to properly report repair codes, and they give definitions of the **three different types of repair** (i.e., levels of complexity): **simple, intermediate, and complex.**

Wound closure by sutures, staples, or tissue adhesives such as Dermabond (cyanoacrylate, a tissue skin adhesive) used singly, in combination with each other, or in combination with adhesive strips, qualify as a repair closure. However, the use of **adhesive strips on their own does not qualify as a repair closure,** and in cases where adhesive strips is the sole method of closure, the appropriate E/M code should be reported.

Let's review the different types of repairs.

Simple Repair: Used for superficial wounds (e.g., epidermis, dermis, subcutaneous tissues without involvement of deeper structures) requiring a one-layer closure. Includes local anesthesia and chemical electrocauterization of wounds not closed.

Intermediate Repair: Used for wounds that require layer closure or single-layer closure of heavily contaminated wounds.

Complex Repair: Used for wounds requiring more than a layer closure (e.g., traumatic lacerations or avulsions).

The repair codes in CPT group together various anatomical sites in one code descriptor.

For example: CPT code 12001 Simple repair of superficial wounds of scalp, neck, axillae, external genitalia, trunk and/or extremities (including hands and feet); 2.5 cm or less.

It is important to note when **multiple wounds** are repaired, you would **add together** the **lengths of wounds of the same level of complexity** that are located on the **same anatomical sites that are grouped together.**

For example: A 4-cm simple repair of the trunk and a 2-cm simple repair of the arm would be added together, as they are both simple repairs (same complexity), and their respective anatomical sites are grouped together in the CPT descriptor. In this case, you would report CPT code 12002 Simple repair of superficial wounds of scalp, neck, axillae, external genitalia, **trunk** and/or **extremities** (including hands and feet); **2.6 cm to 7.5 cm.**

When multiple wounds are repaired, you would list the most complex repair as the primary procedure and the additional less complicated repair would be listed as secondary with modifier 51 appended.

Additionally, débridement, exploration, and ligation may or may not be included in the repair code depending on the extent of the service provided. Simple débridement, simple exploration, and simple ligation are all included in the wound repair.

Débridement would be considered as a separate procedure only when the wound is grossly contaminated and requires extensive débridement or when débridement is performed without an immediate primary closure.

KEY CODING TIP

To select the correct repair code, carefully read the documentation to determine the following:

1. The site of the repair
2. The complexity of the repair
3. The length of the repair
4. Whether multiple wounds are of the same complexity and from anatomical sites that are grouped together

---

LET'S LOOK AT AN EXAMPLE

While running through a department store, 10-year-old Jamie tripped and fell through the plate glass window, sustaining lacerations on his face, ears, and legs. In the emergency room, the physician documented a 2.1-cm simple repair of the face, 1.1-cm simple repair of the ear, and a 3.2-cm intermediate repair of the right leg, and 1.1-cm simple repair of the left leg.

How to Code: Note that we add together the repair of the face and ear, as they are both the same complexity

and because their anatomical sites may be grouped together, and we therefore arrive at a total wound length of 3.2 cm. The simple repair of the left leg would be assigned a separate code, as would the intermediate repair of the right leg. Finally, we would list the intermediate repair first as the most complex repair. Putting this all together, we would code the encounter as follows:

12032 Repair, intermediate, wounds of scalp, axillae, trunk and/or extremities (excluding hands and feet); 2.6 cm to 7.5 cm

12013 Simple repair of superficial wounds of face, ears, eyelids, nose, lips and/or mucous membranes; 2.6 cm to 5.0 cm

12001 Simple repair of superficial wounds of scalp, neck, axillae, external genitalia, trunk and/or extremities (including hands and feet); 2.5 cm or less

Musculoskeletal System
20005–29999

When coding from the Musculoskeletal subsection, it is important to have a good foundation in both anatomy and medical terminology. The first page of the Musculoskeletal subsection provides you with definitions of the different types of treatment for fracture care. Because fracture care is a common orthopedic procedure, let's take a closer look at fractures.

Fractures. First let's consider the different **types of fractures.** A fracture can be a **closed** fracture (the wound is not open, the bone does not protrude from the skin), **open** fracture (either the bone can be visualized through an open wound or the bone protrudes from the skin), or **dislocation** (the bone is displaced from its joint).

Now let's look at the different **types of treatments.** **Closed treatment** is when the fracture site is not surgically opened. With closed fracture care, the fracture may be treated with or without manipulation (realignment of the bones). **Open treatment** is when the fracture site is surgically opened, and internal fixation may be used. **Percutaneous skeletal fixation** is when the fracture treatment is neither open nor closed, but fixation (hardware, e.g., pins, screws) is placed across the fracture site.

There are **two types of fixation devices: external fixation** devices (placing pins or screws through the bone and secured together outside the skin with clamps and rods) and **internal fixation** devices (pins or screws are placed through or within the fracture; this is known as *open reduction with internal fixation [ORIF]*).

All of these services include the application of the first cast or traction device.

It should be kept in mind that, as is mentioned in the CPT book, "the type of fracture (e.g., open, compound, closed) does not have any coding correlation with the type of treatment (e.g., closed, open, or percutaneous) provided." Instead, the CPT codes for fracture care and joint injuries are categorized by the type of treatment (e.g., manipulation, fixation, or immobilization) provided. These treatment types are applicable to either open or closed fractures or joint injuries (reference the Musculoskeletal System subsection Coding Guidelines). Therefore, an open fracture may receive a closed treatment, and a closed fracture may receive an open treatment.

For example: A closed fracture (one in which the wound is not open and the bone does not protrude from the skin) may be treated by surgically opening and exposing the fracture to view and treating the fracture with internal fixation (open treatment).

Fracture Types

Fracture Type	Definition
Open fracture/ Compound fracture	The bone can be visualized through an open wound or protrudes through the skin
Closed fracture	A simple, uncomplicated fracture The bone does not protrude through the skin, and there are no open wounds
Dislocation/Luxation	The displacement or misalignment of a bone from its joint
Subluxation	The partial displacement of a bone from its joint

Fracture Treatments

Fracture Treatment	Definition
Closed treatment	The fracture site is not surgically opened The bone is immobilized by cast or strapping The bones are realigned by manipulation or reduction The bone is realigned by skeletal traction
Open treatment	The fracture is surgically opened
Percutaneous skeletal fixation	External fixation: pins or screws are placed through the bone and are secured outside of the skin Internal fixation: pins or screws are placed through or within the fracture

LET'S LOOK AT AN EXAMPLE

Paul Frank's fractured wrist required open treatment of a carpal scaphoid fracture with internal fixation.

How to Code: We would first identify the location of the fracture as carpal scaphoid and the treatment as open with fixation for CPT code 25628 Open treatment of carpal scaphoid (navicular) fracture, includes internal fixation, when performed.

Arthrocentesis, Aspiration, or Injection of Major Joint or Bursa. Arthrocentesis is a common procedure by which a sterile needle is used to drain fluid from a joint. The codes are divided according to the size of the joint injected: small (e.g., a finger or toe), intermediate (e.g., an elbow or ankle), and major (e.g., a shoulder or knee). The local anesthetic is included in the code for the aspiration.

It is important to note that in some cases, a drug (e.g., cortisone) may be injected into the joint to relieve inflammation, and in some cases, the injection is carried out under ultrasonic guidance. In these cases, the ultrasound and drug injected would be reported separately.

LET'S LOOK AT AN EXAMPLE

The patient was placed in supine position with a rolled blanket underneath the left knee to gently flex the joint. The skin overlying the area to be injected was cleaned in a sterile fashion using Betadine. Under ultrasonic guidance, the left knee was injected with 2% lidocaine and 2 mL of Hyalgan. The patient tolerated the procedure well.

How to Code: In this case, we would report one code for the injection into the left knee. The ultrasonic guidance is reported with a second code, and a third code is selected for the drug injected (Hyalgan). The anesthetic (lidocaine) is inclusive with the procedure and is not separately reportable. The LT modifier would be appended to the injection code to properly identify the site of injection. We would therefore select the following codes:

20610-LT Arthrocentesis, aspiration and/or injection; major joint or bursa (e.g., shoulder, hip, knee joint, subacromial bursa)

76942 Ultrasonic guidance for needle placement (e.g., biopsy, aspiration, injection, localization device), imaging supervision and interpretation

J7321 Hyaluronan or derivative, Hyalgan or Supartz, for intra-articular injection, per dose

Application of Casts and Strapping. These CPT codes are to be utilized when the cast application or strapping is a replacement procedure performed during or after follow-up care or when provided as an initial service performed without a restorative treatment.

It is important to remember the physician who applies the initial cast, strapping, or splint and who assumes the follow-up fracture care should not use the code for the application of a cast, strapping, or splint, as this is included in the fracture care codes.

LET'S LOOK AT AN EXAMPLE

Josephine was caught in a rain storm and as a result her right short-arm cast became wet and flexible. She was seen in the office where her physician replaced the right short-arm cast.

How to Code: In this case, it would be appropriate to code the replacement cast, as replacement casts are not included in the fracture care codes. The RT modifier is appended to indicate the service was provided on the right arm. Therefore, we would code as 29075-RT Application, cast; elbow to finger (short arm).

Endoscopy/Arthroscopy. Arthroscopy is a minimally invasive operation by which the surgeon can examine the joint with a scope and can make repairs through a small incision.

Arthroscopy codes are located at the end of the Musculoskeletal subsection, and it is important to note the *diagnostic arthroscopy is always included in the surgical arthroscopy* and therefore should not be reported separately.

Once again, anatomy is key when coding arthroscopic procedures. For example, the knee has three compartments: medial, lateral, and patellofemoral. If both a meniscectomy and a synovectomy are performed on the same knee but in different compartments, they are separately reported.

Respiratory
30000–32999

The Respiratory subsection is organized according to anatomical site (from the nose to the lungs), and the endoscopy codes are located within each anatomical site.

To properly code respiratory procedures, it is important to know the different types of examinations and the different types of approaches by which a surgical procedure can be performed.

There are **two types of examinations:** an **indirect examination,** which refers to the examination being performed by use of a tongue depressor and a mirror to view the larynx, vocal cords, and so on, and a **direct examination,** where the view is **by endoscopy** (use of a scope).

For example: In CPT code 31510 Laryngoscopy, **indirect;** with biopsy, the laryngoscopy is performed by indirect method, and in CPT code 31535 Laryngoscopy, **direct,** operative, with biopsy, the biopsy is performed by direct method.

There are also **two different types of approaches** to surgical procedures for the respiratory system: an **external** approach, which is **through the skin,** and an **internal** approach, which is **through the respiratory system.**

For example: In CPT code 30300 Removal foreign body, intranasal, the foreign body is removed through the nose (respiratory system); however, in CPT code 30320 Removal foreign body, intranasal; by lateral rhinotomy, the foreign body is removed by a full-thickness skin incision from the nostril along the nasal rim and continuing superiorly.

KEY CODING TIP

When coding endoscopies, you should keep in mind the following:

1. Code to the fullest extent of the procedure (e.g., begins at the mouth and ends at the bronchial tube).
2. Code the correct approach (through the skin or through the respiratory system).
3. The diagnostic endoscopy is always included in the surgical endoscopy.
4. Bilateral procedures are often coded. Remember to use the RT and LT modifiers as applicable.
5. In cases of multiple endoscopies, sequence the primary procedure first.

LET'S LOOK AT AN EXAMPLE

Mr. Smith presented to the pulmonologist for a diagnostic bronchoscopy. Upon diagnostic examination, a foreign body was removed and a biopsy was taken during the same operative session.

How to Code: In this case, because a surgical endoscopy was also performed, we would not code for the diagnostic bronchoscopy, as it is included in the surgical procedure (considered an integral part of the bronchoscopy). We can, however, code for multiple endoscopies, the bronchoscopy with foreign body removal, and bronchoscopy with bronchial biopsy. We would select the following codes:

31635 Bronchoscopy, rigid or flexible, with or without fluoroscopic guidance; with removal of foreign body
31625 Bronchoscopy, rigid or flexible, with or without fluoroscopic guidance; with bronchial or endobronchial biopsy(s), single or multiple sites

LET'S LOOK AT ANOTHER EXAMPLE

Mr. Smith had a nasal polyp removed from his left nostril, and two polyps were removed from his right nostril.

How to Code: In this case, we can code the procedure twice and append the appropriate modifiers to show the service was provided in both nostrils, as the CPT code descriptor for the nasal polyp removal is a unilateral code. We would not code 30110 twice for the right side for the two polyps, as the CPT codes include multiple polyps. We would therefore code the procedure as follows:

30110 LT Excision, nasal polyp(s), simple
30110 RT-51 Excision, nasal polyp(s), simple

Cardiovascular
33010–37799

Most notable about the Cardiovascular subsection is that cardiovascular services can be reported from three sections of the CPT book. The Surgery section is used to report the cardiovascular surgical procedures, the Medicine section is used to report nonsurgical cardiovascular procedures, and the Radiology section is used to report radiological imaging services and diagnostic services.

For example:

33500 Repair of coronary arteriovenous or arteriocardiac chamber fistula; with cardiopulmonary bypass: **Surgical Procedure located in the Cardiovascular Surgery subsection.**

93000 Electrocardiogram, routine ECG with at least 12 leads; with interpretation and report: **Nonsurgical Cardiovascular Procedure located in the Medicine section.**

75557 Cardiac magnetic resonance imaging for morphology and function without contrast material: **Diagnostic Cardiovascular Procedure located in the Radiology section.**

Types of Cardiovascular Procedures. An **interventional** cardiovascular procedure is an invasive cardiac procedure that is reported with a code from the Cardiovascular Surgery subsection and a code from the Radiology section for the radiological supervision and guidance. **Invasive** procedures are those that break the skin, with the most invasive being open heart surgery, whereas one example of a minimally invasive procedure is minimally invasive direct coronary artery bypass (MIDCAB). **Noninvasive** procedures are those in which the skin is not broken, such as an exercise stress test.

The codes in the Cardiovascular subsection are organized according to anatomical site and then divided according to the procedure performed. For example, the codes under **Heart and Pericardium** (anatomical site) are organized on the basis of the type of procedure (e.g., patient-activated event recorder, shunting), and the codes under **Arteries and Veins** (anatomical site) include embolectomy/thrombectomy and transluminal angioplasty (procedures).

Pacemakers. One of the common cardiovascular procedures is the implantation of a **pacemaker** (a small device placed in the chest to help control arrhythmias [abnormal heart rhythms]) or pacing cardioverter-defibrillator (a small, battery-powered electrical impulse generator placed in the patient's chest to detect and correct cardiac arrhythmias by delivering a jolt of electricity). Both devices include a pulse generator (battery and electronic device) and electrodes (leads).

There are **two types** of pacemakers and pacing cardioverter-defibrillators: **single chamber,** which has a single electrode and is placed in the right atrium **or** right ventricle, and **dual chamber,** which has two electrodes; one is placed in the right atrium, **and** the other electrode is placed in the right ventricle.

KEY CODING TIP
Before selecting the CPT code for pacemakers or pacing cardioverter-defibrillators, determine the following:
1. The type of device utilized (single chamber or dual chamber)
2. The type of placement (initial, repair, upgrade, or replacement)
3. Where the lead is placed (atrium, ventricle, or both)
4. Extent of procedure performed (replacement of an electrode or the entire system)
5. Surgical approach used for placement (epicardial [opening the chest] or transvenous [through a vein])
6. If the placement is temporary or permanent
7. If fluoroscopy was used

Let's Try One Together
Mrs. Jones was diagnosed with sick sinus syndrome (a condition that makes the heart beat too slowly). Under fluoroscopic guidance, her physician performed a subcutaneous insertion of a permanent pacemaker pulse generator with transvenous placement of electrodes in both the right atrium and the right ventricle.

continued

Let's Try One Together—cont'd

We would code the procedure using the Key Coding Tip and highlighting the key pieces of information. We first note the service is provided under fluoroscopic guidance (which can be separately coded), the pacemaker was placed via a subcutaneous insertion, the type of pacemaker was identified as **permanent,** the placement of the electrodes was transvenous **(the surgical approach used for placement),** and in this case, the electrodes were placed in both the right atrium and the right ventricle **(where the lead is placed).** This provides us with the information we need to locate the correct code. In the CPT Index, we would look up Pacemaker, Heart, followed by Insertion. This will give us a code range of 33206–33208. When we look up the code range in the Cardiovascular subsection, we can identify the correct code by the placement (transvenous) and the location (right atrium and right ventricle).

Mrs. Jones was diagnosed with sick sinus syndrome (a condition that makes the heart beat too slowly). Under fluoroscopic guidance her physician performed a subcutaneous insertion of a permanent pacemaker pulse generator with transvenous placement of electrodes in both the right atrium and the right ventricle.

We therefore are able to correctly code this encounter as:

33208 **Insertion** or replacement of **permanent pacemaker** with transvenous electrode(s); **atrial and ventricular**

And because the procedure was performed under fluoroscopic guidance, a radiology code must also be assigned:

71090 Insertion **pacemaker, fluoroscopy** and radiography, radiological supervision and interpretation

The Digestive System
40490–49999

The Digestive System subsection is organized by anatomical site and further divided by procedure type. The codes within the digestive system begin at the mouth and end with the anus. They are further divided by anatomical site and procedure.

Endoscopic Procedures. As with the respiratory system, there are many endoscopy codes related to gastrointestinal procedures. Again, the endoscopies can be performed as a diagnostic procedure or as a surgical procedure. If a surgical endoscopy is performed (e.g., endoscopy with biopsy), the diagnostic procedure is always included with the surgical procedure and therefore should not be reported separately.

There are multiple endoscopy categories within the Digestive System subsection. The two most common are upper gastrointestinal (GI) endoscopy, which is performed on the upper GI tract (esophagus, diaphragm, stomach, gallbladder, bile duct, liver, and duodenum), and the lower GI tract endoscopy (most of the intestines and the anus).

When coding for endoscopies, you should remember to code to the fullest extent of the procedure performed.

For example: A proctosigmoidoscopy includes an examination of the rectum and sigmoid colon.

A sigmoidoscopy includes an examination of the entire rectum and sigmoid colon and might include a portion of the descending colon.

A colonoscopy includes an examination of the entire colon (rectum to cecum) and may include the terminal ileum.

Additionally, multiple endoscopies may be performed at the same session.

LET'S LOOK AT AN EXAMPLE

During Mr. Walker's diagnostic colonoscopy, Dr. Simmons removed three polyps by bipolar cautery and one by snare technique.

How to Code: We would not code for the diagnostic colonoscopy, as it is included in the surgical procedure (removal of polyps). We would, however, code multiple endoscopies: one for the polyp removal by bipolar cautery and one for the removal by snare technique. Although three polyps were removed by bipolar cautery, we would report the code only once, as the CPT code descriptor includes the removal of both single and multiple polyps. CPT code 45385 would be sequenced first, as it is the more complex procedure, as identified by its RVU or reimbursement amount.

45385 Colonoscopy, flexible, proximal to splenic flexure; with removal of tumor(s), polyp(s), or other lesion(s) by snare technique

45384 Colonoscopy, flexible, proximal to splenic flexure; with removal of tumor(s), polyp(s), or other lesion(s) by hot biopsy forceps or bipolar cautery

Repair of Hernias. Another common code within the gastrointestinal subsection is the repair of hernias. A hernia is an abnormal bulging or protrusion of tissue or an organ through an abnormal opening usually in the abdomen or groin area.

Hernias may be initial or recurrent, strangulated (the blood supply is cut off), incarcerated (hernia of the bowel that cannot return to its normal place), or reducible (an uncomplicated hernia that can be put back to its original site either spontaneously or after manipulation).

KEY CODING TIP

Before selecting the CPT code for a hernia repair, determine the following:

1. The site of the hernia (inguinal, lumbar, or femoral).
2. Whether the hernia is initial or recurrent.
3. The age of the patient (the CPT codes are based on the age of the patient).
4. The clinical presentation of the hernia (reducible, incarcerated, strangulated).
5. If a mesh was used (this is an add-on code to the hernia débridement and repair codes 11004–11006, 49560–49566).

LET'S LOOK AT AN EXAMPLE

Three-year-old Michael presented for an incarcerated umbilical hernia repair.

In this case, we have information on the age of the patient (3 years old), the clinical presentation of the hernia (incarcerated), and the location of the hernia (umbilical). We do not have information on whether the hernia is initial or recurrent. Therefore, the correct CPT code would be:

49582 Repair **umbilical hernia, younger than age 5 years; incarcerated** or strangulated

This particular hernia code does not differentiate between initial or recurrent.

The Urinary System
50010–53899

The Urinary subsection is organized according to anatomical site and further divided by procedure type (incision, excision, and so on). Anatomical knowledge of the urinary system is essential for accurate coding. Let's review some urinary terminology:

Bladder: A solid, muscular, and elastic-type organ that collects and holds urine excreted by the kidneys.

Kidneys: Paired organs responsible for urine production.

Urethra: A singular tubular structure used to expel urine from the bladder.

Ureter: One of a pair of thick-walled tubes that carries urine from the kidney to the urinary bladder.

Because the spelling is very similar for urethra (urethral) and ureter (ureteral), care must be taken to carefully read the documentation for the correct term.

Urinary Calculi Removal. The removal of urinary calculi (stones) is a common procedure that can be performed using a variety of methods (e.g., open incision, endoscopic). In a nephrolithotomy, the calculus is removed through an open incision into the kidney (50060). Nephrolithotomy may also be performed as a secondary surgical operation for calculus (50065), as a complication by congenital kidney abnormality (50070), or for a removal of a large staghorn calculus (a stone that fills the calyces [a cuplike extension of the renal pelvis] and renal pelvis) (50075).

In a percutaneous nephrostolithotomy (PCNL) or pyelostolithotomy, the kidney stones are removed by a small incision into the patient's back via insertion of an endoscope over a guide wire to crush or extract the calculi. There are two CPT codes to describe this procedure, and they are based on the size of the calculi.

50080 Percutaneous nephrostolithotomy or pyelostolithotomy, with or without dilation, endoscopy, lithotripsy, stenting, or basket extraction; **up to 2 cm**

50081 Percutaneous nephrostolithotomy or pyelostolithotomy, with or without dilation, endoscopy, lithotripsy, stenting, or basket extraction; **over 2 cm**

Extracorporeal shock wave lithotripsy (ESWL) is a procedure that uses shock waves directly to the kidney stone to break a large stone into smaller ones that will pass through the urinary system.

LET'S LOOK AT AN EXAMPLE

Under radiological guidance, the physician identified two kidney stones, one in each kidney. The patient was placed on the lithotripsy table and was administered general anesthetic. Shock waves were directed through a water cushion placed against the patient's body at the location of each kidney. The pulverization process was viewed via video x-ray by the physician, who then determined the stone fragments were small enough to harmlessly pass through the patient's urinary system over the next few days.

How to Code: In this case, we would highlight the radiological guidance, the two kidney stones, one in each kidney, and the lithotripsy (procedure performed). The CPT code for the service performed is 50590 Lithotripsy, extracorporeal shock wave. The radiological guidance is included in the procedure and is not separately reportable.

continued

LET'S LOOK AT AN EXAMPLE—cont'd

Finally, because the service was performed bilaterally, we would append modifier 50 (bilateral procedure) to the CPT code. To accurately report the service provided, we would therefore code it as 50590-50.

Male Genital System
54000–55899

The Male Genital System subsection is organized according to anatomical site and further divided by procedure (incision, destruction, excision, and so on). Most of the CPT codes are listed under the subheading *penis* in the *repair* category.

As men age, they may develop many conditions related to the prostate, such as infections, inflammation, benign prostatic hyperplasia (BPH: enlargement of the prostate), or prostate cancer.

An enlarged prostate interferes with the flow of urine from the bladder, causing difficult and/or frequent urination. As such, many of the procedure codes used to treat **BPH** are located in both the Urinary section and the Male Genital System section.

Prostate cancer may involve surgery, in which case the treatment will vary based on the extent of the disease. The surgical procedures for the treatment of prostate cancer are located in the Male Genital System subsection under the subheading "Prostate," categories "excision, laparoscopy, other procedures," and include:

- Radical prostatectomy: Removal of the entire prostate gland, the seminal vesicles, and some surrounding tissue (CPT code 55810).
- Laparoscopic radical prostatectomy: Minimally invasive procedure (CPT code 55866).
- Cryoablation: Freezing of the prostate (CPT code 55873).

LET'S LOOK AT AN EXAMPLE

The patient was brought into the operating room, and the lower abdomen was prepped and draped in the standard fashion. An incision was made in the skin between the base of the scrotum and the anus. A curved instrument was advanced up through the urethra to the prostate. Through the perineal incision, the physician manipulated the instrument and dissected the tissues to expose the prostate. The curved instrument was then replaced with a straight instrument, and the entire prostate gland was removed along with the seminal vesicles and the vas deferens. The bladder outlet was revised, and the bleeding was controlled by ligation. A catheter was placed in the bladder, and the dissected tissues and the incision were closed by layer suturing.

How to Code: The key words to highlight are **the approach** (perineal incision), **the procedure** (removal of the prostate), and the **extent of the procedure** (along with the seminal vesicles and the vas deferens). Based on these key pieces of information, we would select as the correct CPT code 55810 Prostatectomy, perineal radical.

Female Genital System
56405–58999

This subsection is organized by anatomical site and further divided by procedure type (e.g., incision, destruction, repair).

Included in this subsection are many minor procedures that can be performed in a physician's office, such as a colposcopy (examination of the tissues of the vagina and cervix via endoscope) and insertion of an intrauterine device (IUD).

A number of services are also performed laparoscopically or with the use of a hysteroscope. As reviewed with previous procedures performed, the diagnostic laparoscopy or hysteroscopy is always included in the surgical laparoscopy or hysteroscopy and therefore would not be separately reported.

Many of the services in this subsection are performed as part of a major procedure; therefore, it is important to read the code descriptors and notes carefully to determine if a procedure is bundled or considered to be inclusive of a major procedure. For example, a pelvic examination under anesthesia (57410) may be performed to provide information that will be helpful with a surgical procedure performed at the same time. When this occurs, the pelvic examination under anesthesia is considered bundled or inclusive to the surgery and is not separately reported.

Vulvectomy (the surgical removal of part or all of the vulva) codes (56620–56640) are organized by the type of procedure (e.g., simple, radical) and the extent of the procedure (partial, complete).

The definitions for simple, radical, partial, and complete are located under the subheading Vulva, Perineum, and Introitus.

Simple procedure: Removal of skin and superficial subcutaneous tissue.

Radical procedure: Removal of skin and deep subcutaneous tissues.

Partial procedure: Removal of less than 80% of the vulvar area.

Complete procedure: Removal of greater than 80% of the vulvar area.

Hysterectomy (removal of the uterus) procedures (58150–58294) are organized by approach (abdominal, vaginal) and extent (removal of tubes, ovaries). Carefully read the code descriptors to determine what is included in the code.

LET'S LOOK AT AN EXAMPLE

A total abdominal hysterectomy, bilateral salpingo-oophorectomy, and a pelvic examination under anesthesia would all be reported with one CPT code: 58150 Total abdominal hysterectomy (corpus and cervix), with or without removal of tube(s), with or without removal of ovary(s).

How to Code: The CPT code descriptor includes the removal of the fallopian tubes and ovaries; therefore, the salpingo-oophorectomy would not be separately reported. The examination under anesthesia is bundled into the major procedure and also would not be separately reported. It is important to note the code descriptor includes the language "with or without tube(s) with or without removal of ovary(s)," indicating this code is a bilateral procedure code and modifier 50 is not applicable.

Maternity Care and Delivery
59000–59899

The codes in this subsection describe procedures related to pregnancy and obstetric care. Obstetric care is divided according to the three stages of pregnancy—antepartum care (before childbirth), delivery services, and postpartum care (after birth)—and is represented by separate codes for each stage or with codes for the global package (antepartum care, delivery, and postpartum care).

The notes within this subsection must be read, as they provide clear coding guidance as to the services included in the CPT code for each stage of pregnancy.

Antepartum Care. The antepartum care includes the initial and subsequent history; physical examinations; recording of weight, blood pressures, fetal heart tones; routine chemical urinalysis; and monthly visits to 28 weeks of gestation, biweekly visits to 36 weeks of gestation, and weekly visits until the time of delivery. It is equally important to note that **any other visits or services during the antepartum period are not included.**

For example: If a pregnant woman sees her obstetrician during the antepartum period for evaluation of a sore throat and is treated for pharyngitis, the physician may report a separate E/M visit during the antepartum period, as the main reason for the visit is the sore throat

and not the pregnancy, which would be considered as incidental.

The codes for antepartum care include multiple visits: for example, CPT codes 59425 Antepartum care only; 4 to 6 visits and 59426 Antepartum care only; 7 or more visits. **E/M codes would be used to report the first three antepartum visits.**

Delivery Services. The delivery services include the hospital admission, the history and physical examination, management of uncomplicated labor, and a vaginal or cesarean delivery. **Any complications of labor and delivery or medical problems are separately reportable.**

Postpartum Care. Postpartum care begins after delivery and includes any uncomplicated inpatient and outpatient postpartum visits. **Any unrelated medical problems or complications relating to the pregnancy may be separately reported.**

The division of the obstetric package allows for different physicians to report separate portions of the obstetric service. For example, one physician might provide all of the antepartum and postpartum care, and another may provide the delivery service. Or, during the course of a pregnancy, a patient might change physicians, allowing each physician to report the extent of his or her services for antepartum care provided.

LET'S LOOK AT AN EXAMPLE

At the time of Elaine Fields's cesarean delivery, Dr. Smith, who provided all of Elaine's antepartum care and who will continue to follow Elaine during the postpartum period, performed a fallopian tube ligation at Elaine's request.

How to Code: In this scenario, we can see that Dr. Smith provided the entire obstetric package, and the baby was delivered by cesarean section. Additionally, Elaine elected to have her tubes ligated at the time of delivery. In this case, we would report CPT code 59510 Routine obstetric care including antepartum care, cesarean delivery, and postpartum care for the entire obstetric package and CPT code 58611 Ligation or transection of fallopian tube(s) *when done at the time of cesarean delivery* or intra-abdominal surgery.

The Nervous System
61000–64999

The codes within the Nervous System subsection are organized according to anatomical site (Skull, Meninges, and Brain; Spine and Spinal Cord; Extracranial Nerves; Peripheral Nerves; and Autonomic

Nervous System) and are further divided by the type of procedure performed.

Pain management services are coded from this subsection. Pain management can be provided by surgery, other procedures (injections), or medication. The types of injections that provide pain relief for the patient are:

Nerve block: Injection of an anesthetic (nerve block) into somatic and sympathetic nerves for diagnostic purposes, pain relief. Somatic nerves control voluntary body movements through the action of skeletal muscles and the reception of external stimuli (e.g., sight, hearing, touch). Sympathetic nerves are automatic (not consciously controlled) and are responsible for mobilizing the body's energy and resources (fight-or-flight response) during stress.

Nerve blocks are commonly used in the management of postoperative pain. For example, a patient who underwent a total knee replacement may receive a femoral nerve block (64450) for management of postoperative pain.

Facet joint injection: Many pain management injections are given in the "facet joint." Facet joints are joints located between the vertebral and are present on both sides of the spine (there are two facet joints at each level of the vertebral column), providing flexibility to the spine (e.g., allowing you to bend at the waist). Each facet joint is supplied by two nerves. An injection into the facet joint is called a *facet joint nerve block.*

Transforaminal epidural injection: An epidural injection is given to provide relief from certain types of low back and neck pain. The transforaminal approach is a very selective injection around a specific nerve root.

KEY CODING TIP

Before selecting the CPT code for pain management, determine the following:

- The type of injection (nerve block, facet injection, epidural)
- If a nerve block, which nerves are involved (somatic, sympathetic, facet joint nerve)
- If a facet injection, whether it is done at a single or multiple level
- Whether the injection is performed unilaterally or bilaterally
- If a spinal injection, whether the injection is performed at multiple spinal regions (e.g., cervical, thoracic, or lumbar)
- The type of medication injected

LET'S LOOK AT AN EXAMPLE OF A TRANSFORAMINAL EPIDURAL INJECTION

The patient was placed prone on the fluoroscopy table. The patient's back was prepped and draped in the usual sterile fashion. Subcutaneous lidocaine was instilled into the superficial soft tissues of the patient's back for local anesthesia. Under fluoroscopic guidance, a 25-g, 3.5-in spinal needle was advanced just inferior and lateral to the L5 pedicle. Then 1.0 of nonparticular radiocontrast was slowly instilled through the needle. It demonstrated filling of the nerve root sleeve with extension of the contrast along the adjacent epidural space. A mixture of 1 mL lidocaine and 40 mg Kenalog was instilled slowly through the needle. The needle was removed, and the same procedure was performed for the right L5 nerve root. The patient reported significant pain relief. The patient's skin was cleansed, and the adhesive bandage was placed over the puncture site. There were no complications during or immediately after the procedure.

How to Code: In this case, **the lumbar area is involved,** and the procedure was **performed bilaterally** at the L5 spinal level under fluoroscopic guidance. The **type of medication** injected was 40 mg of Kenalog, and the lidocaine is not separately reported, as it is considered inclusive to the procedure. Because the service was provided bilaterally (the same procedure was performed for the right L5 nerve root), we will append modifier 50 to the CPT code for the injections. In this case the fluoroscopy is not separately reported as it is an inherent part of the CPT code descriptor for the injection. Therefore, we would report the following codes:

64483-*50* Injection(s), anesthetic agent and/or steroid, transforaminal epidural, with imaging guidance (fluoroscopy or CT); lumbar or sacral, single level

Next, we would select from the HCPCS codes to report the drug injected—namely, from the J codes (Drugs Administered Other than Oral Method):

J3301 ×*8* Injection, triamcinolone acetonide, not otherwise specified, 10 mg

Note that the HCPCS code is reported with 8 units to identify the 80 mg of Kenalog administered (40 mg on each side).

Eye and Ocular Adnexa
65091–68899

This subsection is organized according to anatomical site and further divided by the type of procedure (e.g., retinal repair). As with many of the previous subsections, anatomical knowledge is a key element to correct code selection. (See the anatomical diagram in Chapter 2.)

Of interest in this subsection are the prophylaxis (the prevention of disease) codes, as they are reported for repetitive services. The prophylaxis code descriptors (67141, 67145, 67208–67220, 67227, 67228, 67229) include treatments that are provided at one or more sessions that occur at different encounters within a defined treatment period.

For example: With CPT code 67141 Prophylaxis of retinal detachment (e.g., retinal break, lattice degeneration) without drainage, **1 or more sessions;** cryotherapy, diathermy, you would only report this code once to include all the treatments provided during the defined treatment period.

Care should be taken to read not only the CPT code descriptor but any additional notes listed in parentheses under the CPT code descriptor, as these may provide additional coding guidance.

For example:

65175 Removal of ocular implant

(For orbital implant [implant outside the muscle cone] insertion, use 67550; removal, use 67560.)

Cataract (clouding of the lens of the eye) removal codes are some of the more common codes in this subsection. There are three types of methods used to remove the lens and cataracts:

Phacoemulsification: The lens is broken into fragments inside the capsule by ultrasound and removed by aspiration.

Extracapsular cataract extraction (ECCE): The lens of the eye is removed, and the elastic capsule that covers the lens is left partially intact to allow implantation of an intraocular lens (IOL).

Intracapsular cataract extraction (ICCE): The complete lens of the eye within its capsule is removed, and the patient's vision is corrected by contact lens or extremely thick glasses.

LET'S LOOK AT AN EXAMPLE

June Newton, a 67-year-old, presented to the ophthalmologist with complaints of increasing difficulty with glare when driving in the nighttime. On review of systems, there were no complaints of eye pain, flashes, or floaters. On completion of a comprehensive ophthalmological examination, June was diagnosed with a cataract and surgery was recommended. The surgery consisted of removal of the cataract piecemeal using an irrigation and aspiration technique from the right eye with insertion of an intraocular lens. There were no complications during or immediately after the procedure, and the patient tolerated the procedure well.

How to Code: The key words to highlight in this encounter when coding for the surgical procedure are the removal of the cataract from the right eye by irrigation and aspiration with no complications.

At first glance, there are two CPT codes that appear to be suitable:

66982 Extracapsular cataract removal with insertion of intraocular lens prosthesis (one stage procedure), manual or mechanical technique (e.g., irrigation and aspiration or phacoemulsification), **complex,** requiring devices or techniques not generally used in routine cataract surgery (e.g., iris expansion device, suture support for intraocular lens, or primary posterior capsulorrhexis) or performed on patients in the amblyogenic developmental stage

66984 Extracapsular cataract removal with insertion of intraocular lens prosthesis (1 stage procedure), manual or mechanical technique (e.g., irrigation and aspiration or phacoemulsification)

Although both codes appear to be similar, CPT code 66982 is for complex procedures such as utilization of unusual surgical techniques or surgeries performed on pediatric or complex adult patients who may have weakened or absent lens support structures.

Because June's surgery was not complex, the correct CPT code would be 66984. In addition, we would append the RT modifier to indicate that the procedure was performed on the right eye. Therefore, we would report the procedure with the following code: 66984-RT.

Common Surgical Prefixes and Suffixes

Common Surgical Prefixes

Prefix	Meaning	Example
A(n)-	Absence, without	Anuria (lack of urine output)
Ambi-	Around, all sides	Ambidextrous (using both hands)
Ante-	Before, in front of	Anterior (front of body)
Brady-	Slow	Bradycardia (slow heart rhythm)
Dys-	Difficult, painful	Dysuria (painful urination)
Hyper-	Above, beyond	Hypernatremia (excess sodium)
Hypo-	Low, decrease	Hyponatremia (low sodium)

continued

Common Surgical Prefixes—cont'd

Prefix	Meaning	Example
Infra-	Beneath	Infrarenal (below the kidneys)
Intra-	Within, into	Intramuscular (into the muscle)
Mal-	Bad, abnormal	Malformation (abnormally formed)
Mega-	Great, large	Megacolon (enlarged colon)
Poly-	Much, many	Polydipsia (excessive thirst)
Pseudo-	False	Pseudocyst (accumulation of fluid resembling a true cyst)
Supra-	Above, upon	Supraorbital (above the orbit)
Tachy-	Rapid	Tachycardia (rapid heart beat)
Trans-	Across, through	Transdermal (through the skin)

Common Surgical Suffixes

Suffix	Meaning	Example
-Ectomy	Surgical removal	Splenectomy (removal of spleen)
-Itis	Inflammation	Colitis (inflammation of the colon)
-Oma	Tumor	Fibroma (fibrous tumor)
-Osis	Condition	Fibrosis (formation of fibrous tissue)
-Plasia	Growth	Dysplasia (abnormal tissue growth)
-Plasty	Surgical repair	Angioplasty (repair of blood vessels)
-Plegia	Paralysis	Paraplegia (paralysis of lower body)
-Poiesis	Production	Hematopiesis (production of blood cells)
-Rrhea	Fluid discharge	Rhinorrhea (runny nose)
-Scope	Observe	Endoscope (tool for observing the interior of the body)
-Stomy	Opening	Colostomy (opening into the colon through the abdominal wall)
-Taxis	Movement	Ataxia (lack of coordination)
-Tomy	Incision	Thoracotomy (surgical opening of the chest wall)
-Trophy	Growth	Hypertrophy (overgrowth)

Let's Practice Coding

Now that we have reviewed the surgery guidelines and the various subsections of the Surgery section, let's practice our skills and code some operative reports.

First let's review some coding basics.

When coding an operative report, it is best to have a highlighter at hand to highlight key portions of the report. This will help to determine what procedures were performed, whether any procedures are bundled, and whether any modifiers are applicable.

Operative reports read like a newspaper article. You have your **headline** and your **story**.

Your headline is a good place to start to gather information about the surgery performed. It provides you with information as to:

■ Who participated in the procedure. Was it one physician, or was there an assistant at surgery or a co-surgeon? If so, who are your coding for? This is important information to know *before* you start to read the report so you can properly identify the work of the physician you are coding for.

■ Why the procedure was performed and the nature/type of the operation. It is here where you will find clinical information about the patient and the type of procedure that is to be performed. You would *never* select your CPT code from the heading, which indicates the nature of the operation, as in some cases the operation performed as dictated in the body of the operative report will differ from the nature of the operation stated within the heading section of the report.

Following your headline is the **story**. This is the body of the operative report, which is divided into three sections: the opening, the procedure(s) performed, and the closing.

The opening generally provides information as to how the patient was prepared, positioned, and anesthetized for the surgery.

The physician will then dictate the procedure(s) performed. Here you will find all the details of the surgical procedures that were performed, what part of the surgery was performed by each surgeon (if multiple surgeons participated), and whether any complications or additional work was performed by the surgeon(s). It is within this section that you will highlight key words about the procedure. You will want to identify and highlight the anatomical structures involved, the type of procedure, the approach, the extent of the procedure, and size or number if applicable (e.g., lesions).

The closing will provide information as to how the patient tolerated the procedure and the condition of the patient as he or she was brought into the recovery room.

LET'S LOOK AT AN EXAMPLE

Operative Report
Operation Date: 1/5/2010
Surgeon: Dr. Ben Casey
Preoperative Diagnosis: Right breast ductal carcinoma in situ
Postoperative Diagnosis: Same
Nature of Operation: Needle localization, right breast lumpectomy
Anesthesia: General with laryngeal mask
Operative Indications: This is a 59-year-old female patient who was recently diagnosed with a lesion in the right breast. It was a 6-mm lesion. Biopsy was positive for ductal carcinoma in situ. The patient could not undergo MRI, and plan was made for lumpectomy. Risks, benefits, and alternatives were discussed in detail. Breast conservation surgery versus mastectomy was discussed with the patient, and plan was made for lumpectomy with radiation.
Operative procedure: The patient was brought to the operating room and laid in supine position and was given general anesthesia with laryngeal mask. Previously, on the day of the surgery, the patient had undergone needle localization on the area of the clip. The right breast was prepped and draped in the usual sterile technique.
Circumareolar incision was taken down through the skin and subcutaneous tissue. Dissection was done. The needle was delivered into the wound. Then, using a Bovie, lumpectomy was performed around the needle. X-ray of the specimen showed that the clip in the specimen was present. Additional margins were taken. The lumpectomy was oriented for pathology. Hemostasis was achieved.
Closure was done with 3-0 Vicryl and 4-0 Biosyn. Dressing was done. The patient was extubated and brought to the recovery room in stable condition.

How to Code: First we highlight who performed the surgery. In this case, it was only one physician, Dr. Ben Casey. Next we would highlight "previously, on the day of the surgery, the patient had undergone needle localization on the area of the clip." This lets us know we should not code for the needle localization, which was listed in the heading of the operative report under nature of the operation, as this was not performed by the surgeon at the time of the surgery but was performed prior to the surgery by another physician. (This is an example of why you would never code from the heading of the operative report.) We can identify the procedure performed as a lumpectomy, which is reported with CPT code 19301 Mastectomy, partial (e.g., lumpectomy, tylectomy, quadrantectomy, segmentectomy). Finally we would append modifier RT to indicate this was performed on the right breast (19301-RT).

LET'S LOOK AT ANOTHER EXAMPLE:

Operative Report
Operation date: 12/15/2009
Surgeon: Dr. Marcus Welby
Preoperative Diagnosis: Skin nevus, trunk
Postoperative Diagnosis: Same
Nature of Operation: Complex closure after removal of skin nevus, trunk
Anesthesia: General
Operative Indications: This is a 61-year-old patient who has a history of breast cancer. She presented for excision of a nevus of the skin, trunk.
Operative Procedure: The patient was prepped and draped in the usual sterile fashion after induction of general anesthesia. An elliptical incision was made surrounding the nevus. This was taken out with sharp dissection. The resulting wound was then closed in layers using 3-0 Maxon sutures and then 4-0 Biosyn in subcuticular fashion. Steri-Strips were applied. The patient tolerated the procedure well.

How to Code: First we highlight who performed the surgery. In this case, it was only one physician, Dr. Welby. Next we would highlight the incision surrounding the nevus and that it was taken out with sharp dissection. Additionally we would highlight the wound was closed in layers.
  As we go to select the code for the excision of the skin nevus (a benign overgrowth of skin pigment which forms cells), we can apply the Key Coding Tip for excisions. In this case, the type of lesion is benign (skin nevus), the site was not identified in the body of the operative report but was indicated in the nature of the operation and the operative indications as "trunk." The size of the excised skin nevus was not documented; therefore, we can only select the CPT code that lists the lowest size. There was only one lesion removed by sharp dissection (excision). The documentation supports CPT code 11400 Excision, benign lesion including margins, except skin tag (unless listed elsewhere), trunk, arms or legs; excised diameter 0.5 cm or less.
  The wound was closed in layers; this is not bundled with the excision code (only simple, non-layered closure is included); therefore, we can also code for the closure as 12031 Repair, intermediate, wounds of scalp, axillae, trunk and/or extremities (excluding hands and feet); 2.5 cm or less, once again selecting the CPT code that describes the smallest size, as the operative report did not document the size of the wound.

Learn More About It

The more you read, the more you know. Increase your knowledge with the following resources.

Recommended Web Sites

There are many Web sites that show videos of surgical procedures and organ systems. You can Google surgical videos to find your favorite sites or Google specific surgical procedures and organ systems. Some common surgical procedures are also shown in 3D. Some sites are:

Knee replacement: http://www.youtube.com/watch?v= dqtOQ2WnYBM&feature=fvw

Tracheotomy: http://www.youtube.com/watch?v= d_5eKkwnIRs&feature=related

Mitral valve surgery: http://www.youtube.com/watch?v= EnJQh_W3r3A&feature=pyv&ad=5358990562&kw= heart%20surgery

The respiratory system: http://www.youtube.com/watch?v= bwXvqSqAgKc&feature=related

STOP-LOOK-HIGHLIGHT

The key to successfully passing the exam and selecting the correct code lies in knowing how to use your coding book.

To help you navigate through your codebook, and to make sure you have the most important information at your fingertips when you take the exam, highlight key text in the chapter guidelines and subheadings, and insert simple notes and coding tips directly into your codebooks.

When highlighting, use two different color highlighter pens: yellow for standard guidelines and global services and an alternate color for carve-outs and unique notes.

On the Surgery Guidelines Page:

■ On the first page of guidelines under the CPT Surgical Package Definition, write in red ink: *"Includes the Preoperative, Intraoperative and Postoperative."*

■ At the bottom of the CPT Surgical Package Definition, write in red ink: *"General anesthesia is not included."*

■ Under Materials Supplied by Physician, write in red ink: *"When applicable, report with appropriate HCPCS code."*

■ On the last page of the surgery guidelines under Special Report, write in red ink: *"Special reports should be sent with any unlisted CPT code, Category III codes, or when modifier 22 is appended."*

■ At the bottom of the last page of the surgery guidelines, it is helpful to write: *"CPT code 99024 Postoperative follow-up visit, normally included in the surgical package."* This is a quick reference to the CPT code for services provided during the

postoperative period. This CPT code is not reimbursable, as the service is part of the surgical package. Many providers utilize this code to track their postoperative encounters.

■ On the first page of the surgery guidelines under the CPT Surgical Package Definition, on the fifth line in the first paragraph, highlight in yellow: "In defining specific services 'included' in a given CPT surgical code, the following services are always included in addition to the operation per se."

■ On the first page of the surgery guidelines under Follow-Up Care for Therapeutic Surgical Procedures, highlight the third line down in yellow: "Complications, exacerbations, recurrence, or the presence of other diseases or injuries requiring additional services should be separately reported."

■ On the first page of the surgery guidelines under Materials Supplied by Physician, highlight in yellow the fourth line down: "List drugs, trays, supplies, and materials provided. Identify as 99070 or specific supply code."

■ On the first page of the surgery guidelines under Separate Procedure, highlight in yellow the entire paragraph. Continuing on the second page in your alternate color highlighter, highlight the remainder of the paragraph describing separate procedures.

■ On the last page of the surgical guidelines under Special Report, highlight in yellow the third line down: "pertinent information should include an adequate definition or description of the nature, extent, and need for the procedure, and the time, effort, and equipment necessary to provide the service. Additional items which may be included are:"

In the Integumentary Subsection:

■ Right above the beginning of the subsection, write in red ink: *"Measurement in the CPT is by the metric system."*

■ Under the notes for Excision-Benign Lesions, write in red ink:

Key Coding Tips for Lesions
■ *The type of lesion removal (excision, shaving)*
■ *The site of the lesion*
■ *The size of the lesion*
■ *The number of lesions*
■ *If the lesions were malignant or benign*

■ Under the notes for Excision-Benign Lesions, write in red ink: *"Excision codes include local anesthesia and simple closure."*

■ Under the notes for Repair (Closure), write in red ink:

Key Coding Tips for Repairs

- *The site of the repair*
- *The complexity of the repair*
- *The length of the repair*
- *Whether multiple wounds are from the same complexity and from anatomical sites that are grouped together*

■ Under Excision-Benign Lesions, highlight in yellow on the third line down: "includes local anesthesia." In the second paragraph, highlight "includes simple (non-layered) closure when performed" and "Code selection is determined by measuring the greatest clinical diameter of the apparent lesion plus that margin required for complete excision (lesion diameter plus the most narrow margins required equals the excised diameter)." In the third paragraph, the third line down, highlight using your **alternate color highlighter:** "Repair by intermediate or complex closure should be reported separately."

■ Repeat the same highlighting for Excision—Malignant Lesions.

■ Under Repair (Closure), highlight in yellow: "Use the codes in this section to designate wound closure utilizing sutures, staples, or tissue adhesives (e.g., 2-cyanoacrylate), either singly or in combination with each other, or in combination with adhesive strips." In your **alternate color highlighter,** continue to highlight: "Wound closure utilizing adhesive strips as the sole repair material should be coded using the appropriate E/M code."

■ Under Repair (Closure), highlight in yellow the words "Simple repair, Intermediate repair and Complex repair." This section will provide you with coding guidance as to what is and isn't included with each repair type.

■ Under Repair (Closure), highlight in yellow under the types of repair, "Instructions for listing services at time of wound repair." The four numbered steps that follow will provide you with detailed information on how to report repair codes.

In the Musculoskeletal Subsection:

■ On the first page of the Musculoskeletal subsection at the bottom of the page, write in red ink: *"ORIF = open reduction with internal fixation."*

■ After CPT code 20610 Arthrocentesis major joint or bursa write in red ink: *"Injected drugs are reported separately, local anesthetic is included."*

■ Above Arthroscopy of the Knee (above CPT code 29866), write in red ink: *"The knee has 3 compartments: medial, lateral, patellofemoral."*

■ On the first page of the subsection, highlight in yellow the heading "Definitions" and also the key words "Closed Treatment, Open Treatment, and Percutaneous Skeletal Fixation, and Manipulation." This will provide you with the definitions of the different types of fracture treatments.

■ On the same page, highlight in yellow the paragraph under the definition of Percutaneous Skeletal Fixation. "The type of fracture (e.g., open, compound, closed) does not have any coding correlation with the type of treatment (e.g., closed, open, or percutaneous) provided."

■ Under Application of Casts and Strapping Subheading, highlight in yellow in the first paragraph: "The listed procedures apply when the cast application or strapping is a replacement procedure used during or after the period of follow-up care, or when the cast application or strapping is an initial service performed without a restorative treatment or procedure(s) to stabilize or protect a fracture, injury, or dislocation and/or to afford comfort to a patient."

■ Under the same subheading, in the next paragraph, with **your alternate color highlighter,** highlight: "A physician who applies the initial cast, strap or splint and also assumes all of the subsequent fracture, dislocation or injury care cannot use the application of casts and strapping codes as an initial service, because the first cast application is included in the treatment of fracture and/or dislocation codes."

■ Under the subheading Endoscopy/Arthroscopy, highlight in yellow the first sentence: "Surgical endoscopy/arthroscopy always includes a diagnostic endoscopy/arthroscopy."

In the Respiratory Subsection:

■ On the blank Note page, before the Respiratory subsection or at the end of the Respiratory subsection, write in the following:

- *Respiratory types of exams, indirect by tongue depressor and mirror, direct by endoscope.*
- *Approaches, external approach—through the skin and internal approach through the respiratory system.*
- *The Endoscopy Rules*
  - *The fullest extent of the procedure (e.g., begins at the mouth and ends at the bronchial tube) is coded.*
  - *The approach (through the skin or through the respiratory system) is coded.*
  - *The diagnostic endoscopy is always included in the surgical endoscopy.*

- *Bilateral procedures are often coded. Remember to use the RT and LT modifiers.*
- *In cases of multiple endoscopies, sequence the primary procedure first.*

In the Cardiovascular Subsection:

- At the top of the first page, write: *"Uses codes from the Cardiovascular, Medicine, and Radiology sections."*
- At the bottom of the first page, write the following definitions:

  "Invasive procedure—breaks the skin. Noninvasive—does not break the skin."

- In the category of Pacemaker or Pacing Cardioverter-Defibrillator, where space is available, write:

  Key Coding Tip

  - *The type of device utilized (single chamber or dual chamber)*
  - *The type of placement (initial, repair, upgrade, or replacement)*
  - *Where the lead is placed (atrium, ventricle, or both)*
  - *Extent of procedure performed (replacement of an electrode or the entire system)*
  - *The surgical approach used for placement: epicardial (opening the chest) or transvenous (through a vein)*
  - *If the placement is temporary or permanent*
  - *If fluoroscopy was used*

- Under the heading Pacemaker or Pacing Cardioverter-Defibrillator, highlight in yellow the first sentence: "A pacemaker system includes a pulse generator containing electronics, a battery, and one or more electrodes (leads)."
- Under the same heading, in the second paragraph, highlight in yellow: "A single-chamber pacemaker system includes a pulse generator and one electrode inserted in either the atrium or ventricle. A dual-chamber pacemaker system includes a pulse generator and one electrode inserted in the right atrium and one electrode inserted in the right ventricle."
- Under the same heading, in the third paragraph, highlight in yellow the same passages for a pacing cardioverter-defibrillator system.
- Under the same heading, in the paragraph before last, highlight in yellow the following: "When the 'battery' of a pacemaker or a pacing cardioverter-defibrillator is changed, it is actually the pulse generator that is changed. Replacement of a pulse generator should be reported with a code for removal of the pulse generator and another code for insertion of a pulse generator."

In the Digestive System Subsection:

- In the category Repair (Hernioplasty, Herniorrhaphy, Herniotomy) at the bottom of the page, write:

  Key Coding Tip

  - *The site of the hernia (inguinal, lumbar, or femoral)*
  - *Is the hernia initial or recurrent*
  - *The age of the patient*
  - *The clinical presentation of the hernia (reducible, incarcerated, strangulated)*
  - *If a mesh was used (this is an add-on code to the hernia débridement and repair codes 11004–11006, 49560–49566)*

- In the Endoscopy heading above CPT code 45300, highlight in yellow the definitions of the key terms proctosigmoidoscopy, sigmoidoscopy, and colonoscopy.
- In the same area, *under the definitions, highlight the first paragraph: "For an incomplete colonoscopy, with full preparation for a colonoscopy, use a colonoscopy code with the modifier 52 and provide documentation."*
- *In the same area, under definitions, highlight the second paragraph: "Surgical endoscopy always includes the diagnostic endoscopy."*
- *In the category Repair (Hernioplasty, Herniorrhaphy, Herniotomy), highlight in yellow the first three paragraphs in their entirety. Paragraph 1: "The hernia repair codes in this section are categorized primarily by the type of hernia (inguinal, femoral, incisional, etc)." Paragraph 2: "Some types of hernias are further categorized as 'initial' or 'recurrent' based on whether or not the hernia has required previous repair(s)." Paragraph 3: "Additional variables accounted for by some of the codes include patient age and clinical presentation (reducible versus incarcerated or strangulated)."*

In the Subsection Male Genital System:

- *Under the subheading Prostate, under the category Excision, highlight in yellow: "(For transurethral removal of prostate, see 52601–52604)" and "(For transurethral destruction of prostate, see 53850–53852)."*

In the Urinary System Subsection:

- On the top of the first page in this subsection, write: *"The codes are first divided anatomically, and many procedures are performed via endoscope."*
- On the same page, at the top, write: *"KUB = Kidney(s), Ureter(s), and Bladder."*

In the Female Genital System Subsection:

■ In the Corpus Uteri subheading under Hysterectomy Procedures, write in red ink: *"Carefully read the operative report to determine the approach and removal."*

■ In the Vulva, Perineum, and Introitus subheading, highlight the definitions of a simple, radical, partial, and complete procedure.

In the Maternity Care and Delivery Subsection:

■ Write the following in red ink: *"Fetal gestation averages 40 weeks, or 266 days," "VBAC is Vaginal Birth After Cesarean Delivery,"* and *"VBACS is Vaginal Birth After Cesarean Section."*

■ After the fourth paragraph, write in red ink: *"Postpartum care is up to 6 weeks after delivery."*

■ *Highlight the following in the second paragraph: "Antepartum care includes the initial and subsequent history; physical examinations; recording of weight, blood pressures, fetal heart tones; routine chemical urinalysis; and monthly visits up to 28 weeks' gestation, biweekly visits to 36 weeks' gestation, and weekly visits until delivery." In your alternate color highlighter, continue to highlight the last sentence: "Any other visits or services within this time period should be coded separately."*

■ *In yellow, highlight the following in the third paragraph: "Delivery services include admission to the hospital, the admission history and physical examination, management of uncomplicated labor, vaginal delivery (with or without episiotomy, with or without forceps), or cesarean delivery." In your alternate color highlighter, highlight: "Medical problems complicating labor and delivery management may require additional resources and should be identified by utilizing the codes in the medicine and evaluation and management services section in addition to codes for maternity care."*

■ *In yellow, highlight the fourth paragraph, which defines postpartum care in its entirety: "Postpartum care includes hospital and office visits following vaginal or cesarean section delivery."*

■ *Right above CPT code 59425 Antepartum care only 4–6 visits, highlight in yellow: "(For 1–3 antepartum care visits, see appropriate E/M code(s))."*

In the Nervous System Subsection:

■ At the end of the Nervous System subsection, on the last page or on the blank Note page, write:

Key Coding Tip for Nerve Blocks

■ *What nerves were involved (somatic, sympathetic, facet joint nerve)?*

■ *If a facet injection, was it at a single or multiple level?*

■ *Was the injection performed unilaterally or bilaterally?*

■ *If spinal injection, was the injection performed at multiple spinal regions (e.g., cervical, thoracic, or lumbar)?*

■ *What type of medication was injected?*

In the Subsection Eye and Ocular Adnexa

■ Above CPT code 97141, highlight in yellow the first paragraph under Prophylaxis: "Codes 67141, 67145, 67208–67220, 67227, 67228, 67229 include treatment at one or more sessions that may occur at different encounters. These codes should be reported once during a defined treatment period."

Surgery Subsection Vocabulary Words

In your CPT book on an available blank Note page or a page you designated for vocabulary words, write in the following surgical vocabulary words:

Surgical Terms

Débridement: Surgical removal of foreign material and dead tissue from a wound.

Destruction: The ablation of tissue by any method (e.g., electrosurgery, cryosurgery, laser, and so on).

Endoscopy: Visual examination of the interior of a hollow body organ by use of an endoscope.

Excision: Removal by cutting.

Incision: A surgical cut made in the body to perform surgery.

Incision and drainage: A procedure performed on an abscess whereby a cut is made into the lining of the abscess, allowing the pus to escape either by a drainage tube or by leaving the cavity open to the skin.

Laparoscopy: Surgical technique in which operations in the abdomen are performed through small incisions.

Manipulation: The realignment of a fractured bone or joint.

Repair: To remedy, replace, or heal as in a wound or lost part.

Integumentary System (Skin)

Cyanoacrylate: A tissue skin adhesive.

Dermis: The deep vascular inner layer of the skin. The dermis contains nerve endings, sweat glands, oil glands, hair follicles, and blood vessels.

Epidermis: The outer layer of the skin. The epidermis provides a protective physical and biological barrier to the environment and prevents loss of water.

Lesion: An abnormal tissue damaged by disease or trauma (e.g., growth, sore).

Subcutaneous Tissue: The deepest layer of the skin located beneath the dermis. It includes fat cells, connective tissues, blood vessels, and nerves.

Musculoskeletal System

Arthrocentesis: A common procedure by which a sterile needle is used to drain fluid from a joint.

Arthroscopy: A minimally invasive operation by which a surgeon can examine the joint with a scope and make repairs through a small incision.

External fixation: The application of pins or screws through the bones and secured together outside the skin with clamps and rods.

Internal fixation: The application of pins or screws placed through or within a fracture.

Manipulation: The application of manually applied force to restore a fracture or dislocation to its normal anatomical alignment.

Meniscectomy: Surgical removal of the meniscus of the knee.

Synovectomy: Surgical excision of part or all of the synovial membrane (joint lining) of a joint.

Respiratory System

Bronchus: A passage of airway in the respiratory system that directs air into the lungs.

Bronchoscopy: Examination of the trachea and the bronchi through a rigid or flexible tube (bronchoscope).

Direct examination: An examination by view of endoscope.

Indirect examination: An examination performed by use of tongue depressor and a mirror.

Cardiovascular System

Arrhythmia: Abnormal rhythm of the heart

Invasive procedures: Procedures that break the skin.

Noninvasive procedures: Procedures that do not break the skin.

Digestive System

Endoscopic retrograde cholangiopancreatography: An examination and x-ray of the pancreatic duct, hepatic duct, common bile duct, duodenal papilla, and gallbladder via endoscope.

Esophagogastroduodenoscopy: An examination of the upper part of the gastrointestinal tract up to the duodenum via endoscope.

Femoral hernia: A common type of groin hernia caused by a protrusion of an internal organ through a weakness in the containing wall.

Hiatal hernia: A protrusion of part of the stomach through the diaphragm.

Incarcerated hernia: Hernia that cannot return to its normal place.

Incisional hernia: A hernia that occurs at the site of a previous surgical incision.

Inguinal hernia: The most common type of hernia in males. This occurs when a part of the small intestine pushes through an opening in the abdominal muscle.

Reducible hernia: An uncomplicated hernia that can be put back to its original site either spontaneously or after manipulation.

Strangulated hernia: A hernia in which the affected organs lost their blood supply due to compression or constriction.

Ventral hernia: A hernia that occurs in the abdominal wall and not the groin area.

Urinary System

Benign prostatic hyperplasia: Enlargement of the prostate.

Bladder: A solid, muscular, and elastic-type organ that collects and holds urine excreted by the kidneys.

Kidney: Paired organs responsible for urine production.

Nephrolithotomy: Removal of stones from the kidney.

Ureter: One of a pair of thick-walled tubes that carries urine from the kidney to the urinary bladder.

Urethra: A singular tubular structure used to expel urine from the bladder.

Maternity Care and Delivery

Antepartum: The prenatal period before childbirth.

Postpartum: The period after delivery of a baby, usually the 6 weeks after birth.

Nervous System

Facet joint: Facet joints connect each vertebra with the vertebra directly above and below it and are designed to allow the vertebral bodies to rotate.

Nerve block: A procedure whereby an anesthetic agent is injected directly near a nerve to block pain.

Eye and Ocular Adnexa Subsection

Cataract: A disease that clouds the natural lens of the eye.

Prophylaxis: A measure taken for the prevention of disease or a condition.

Surgery Subsection Acronyms and Abbreviations

In your CPT book on an available blank Note page or a page you designated for vocabulary words, write in the following acronyms and abbreviations.

BPH–**B**enign **P**rostatic **H**yperplasia

CABG–**C**oronary **A**rtery **B**ypass **G**raft

ECCE–**E**xtra**c**apsular **C**ataract **E**xtraction

EGD–**E**sopha**g**ogastro**d**uodenoscopy

ENT–**E**ars, **N**ose, and **T**hroat

ERCP–**E**ndoscopic **R**etrograde **C**holangio**p**ancreatography

ESWL–**E**xtracorporeal **S**hock **W**ave **L**ithotripsy

ICCE–**I**ntra**c**apsular **C**ataract **E**xtraction

IOL–**I**ntra**o**cular **L**ens

MIDCAB–**M**inimally **I**nvasive **D**irect **C**oronary **A**rtery **B**ypass

OBGYN–**Ob**stetrics and **Gyn**ecology

ORIF–**O**pen **R**eduction with **I**nternal **F**ixation

PCD–**P**acer **C**ardioverter **D**efibrillator

PCNL–**P**er**c**utaneous **N**ephrosto**l**ithotomy

TUNA–**T**rans**u**rethral **N**eedle **A**blation

TURP–**T**rans**u**rethral **R**esection of **P**rostate

VBAC–**V**aginal **B**irth **A**fter **C**esarean

VBACS–**V**aginal **B**irth **A**fter **C**esarean **S**ection

TAKE THE CODING CHALLENGE

Assign the Appropriate Surgical Code

1. Vaginal birth after cesarean section (VBACS), including routine antepartum and postpartum care

2. Radical perineal prostatectomy with complete bilateral pelvic lymph node dissection

3. Arthrocentesis of the left elbow

4. Bronchoscopy with bronchial biopsy and dilation and placement of tracheal stent

5. Repair of a 4.2-cm laceration of the right hand by layered closure

Multiple Choice

1. The largest section of CPT is:
   a. Surgery
   b. Evaluation and Management
   c. Medicine
   d. Radiology

2. A special report should be sent with:
   a. Unlisted codes
   b. Category III codes
   c. CPT codes with modifier 22 appended
   d. All of the above

3. The surgical package always includes:
   a. Surgical supplies
   b. General anesthesia
   c. The preoperative, intraoperative, and postoperative services
   d. Follow-up visits during the postoperative period for complications

4. The multiple surgical rule does not apply to:
   a. Add-on codes
   b. Separate procedures
   c. CPT codes which are modifier 51 exempt
   d. a. and c.

5. When the multiple surgery rule applies, services are reimbursed as follows:
   a. 100% for the highest paying CPT code and 50% for every CPT code thereafter
   b. 100% for all CPT codes
   c. 100% for the highest paying CPT code and 50% for the second through the fifth procedure; any procedure thereafter is considered bundled and therefore not separately reimbursed
   d. 100% for the highest paying CPT code and 50% for the second through the fifth procedure, and any procedure thereafter is reimbursed by report

6. When the multiple endoscopy rule applies, services are reimbursed as follows:
   a. 100% for the highest paying CPT code and 50% for the second through the fifth procedure; any procedure thereafter is considered bundled and therefore not separately reimbursed
   b. Reimbursement is made for the full amount of the higher valued endoscopy and then a percentage of the next highest endoscopy based on the RVU of each CPT code.
   c. Multiple endoscopies are not separately reimbursable.
   d. None of the above

7. Mrs. Barker underwent a hip replacement and presented to the orthopedic surgeon during the postoperative period for a follow-up visit. During the visit, the orthopedic surgeon noted Mrs. Barker's sutures were red, swollen, and oozing pus. The sutures were cleansed and treated to prevent further infection. Mrs. Barker was given a prescription for antibiotics. This postoperative visit is:
   a. Part of the postoperative care and not considered a separate service
   b. Is not part of the postoperative care and may be billed as a separate service
   c. Is not considered postoperative care if modifier 22 is appended
   d. None of the above

8. The following is not included in the global surgical package:
   a. Writing orders
   b. Local infiltration, metacarpal/metatarsal/digital block, or topical anesthesia
   c. Evaluating the patient during the postoperative period
   d. General anesthesia

9. The information in the CPT manual that provides coding guidance is called:
   a. Notes
   b. Guidelines
   c. Index locations
   d. a. and b.

10. CPT codes for unlisted services or procedures may be found:
    a. In the surgery guidelines
    b. In the CPT index
    c. Throughout the surgery section of the CPT manual
    d. All of the above

11. Which is true when coding multiple laceration repairs?
    a. Code only the most complex repair.
    b. Add together the lengths of those in the same classification and located in anatomical sites that are grouped together in the same code descriptor.
    c. Lacerations repaired with tissue adhesive are reported with the appropriate E/M code.
    d. Add together lengths of repairs from different classifications and same anatomical sites, reporting only the most complex repair.

12. Casting and strapping is separately reported:
    a. With all fracture care services
    b. As an initial service performed without a restorative treatment or procedure
    c. Only by the physician who applies the initial cast, strap, or splint
    d. Twice: once when the cast, strap, or splint is applied and again when it is removed

13. Open treatment of a fracture is when:
    a. The fracture is surgically opened and visualized
    b. The bone protrudes from the skin
    c. The fractured bone is opened remote from the fracture site for insertion of an intramedullary nail across the fracture site (the fracture site is not opened and visualized)
    d. a. and c.

14. When the physician utilizes a tongue depressor and a mirror to view the larynx, this is considered to be a(n) _____ type of examination.
    a. Direct
    b. External
    c. Indirect
    d. Common

15. When the battery of a pacemaker or pacing cardioverter-defibrillator is changed, you are changing the:
    a. Electrode
    b. Lead
    c. Pulse generator
    d. Entire system

16. Mr. Jones presented to the ambulatory surgery center for removal of a lesion from his back. With Mr. Jones prepped and draped in the usual sterile fashion, Dr. DiFranco made a 5.0-cm transverse skin incision and excised the lesion. The incision was closed using 3.0 Vicryl for the deep layers and running 3-0 Prolene subcuticular stitch with Steri-Strips for the skin. The pathology report indicated a benign lesion. The correct code(s) would be:
    a. 11406, 12032
    b. 11406, 12002
    c. 11406
    d. 11606, 12032

17. The patient presented to the orthopedist with complaints of pain in his right wrist and thumb. After a problem-focused examination, the physician recommended injections of medication to relieve his pain, to which the patient agreed. The patient was taken to the procedure room. The needle was navigated into the right wrist joint under direct vision, and then a combination of Kenalog 20 mg and lidocaine 1% 2 mL was injected. Then an injection over the distal phalangeal joint of the right thumb was performed, injecting 10 mg Kenalog and lidocaine 1% 1 mL. The patient reported immediate pain improvement after the injection. To report these services, you would select which of the following codes?
    a. 20605-RT, 20600-RT-51, 76942, J3301 × 3
    b. 20605-RT, 20600-RT-51, J3301 × 3
    c. 20605-RT, J3301 × 2
    d. 20605-RT, 76942, J3301 × 2

18. The patient presented for replacement of a single-chamber pacemaker system to a dual-chamber system, including insertion of a new pulse generator and electrodes. The correct code(s) would be:
    a. 33213
    b. 33233, 33214
    c. 33213, 33233
    d. 33214

19. The patient presented with complaints of stomach cramping and diarrhea for several days and reported the cramping and diarrhea was getting worse. The physician performed a sigmoidoscopy and, during the procedure, decided to view the entire colon passing the endoscope through to the cecum. Report the codes for the service(s) provided. The correct code(s) would be:
    a. 45330, 45378-51
    b. 45378, 45330-51
    c. 45330
    d. 45378

20. Four-month-old Michael was brought into the hospital for repair of his unilateral inguinal hernia. His hernia was easily reducible when it was out. The hernia was repaired via a skin incision into the groin at the site of the hernia. All layers of skin and subcutaneous tissue were opened to expose the inguinal canal. The cord contents were dissected, and the vas identified and preserved along with the vessels. The hernia sac was isolated and dissected into the retroperitoneum. The hernia sac was twisted and ligated, and the redundant portion was resected. The floor of the inguinal canal was weak and reinforced with sutures. The testes were placed in the scrotum, and the ilioinguinal and iliohypogastric nerves were infiltrated with local anesthesia. The inguinal canal was reconstructed, and the skin was closed. The patient tolerated the procedure well with no complications during or immediately after the surgery. To report these services, you would select which of the following codes?
    a. 49495
    b. 49491
    c. 49496
    d. 49500

ANSWERS AND RATIONALES

Assign the Appropriate Surgical Code

1. The correct answer is 59610 Routine obstetric care including antepartum care, vaginal delivery (with or without episiotomy, and/or forceps) and postpartum care, after previous cesarean delivery. In the CPT index, you would first look up **Vaginal Delivery.** (*Note:* If you look up the word *delivery,* you will be directed to look under *cesarean* or *vaginal delivery*.) You would then look under "**after previous cesarean delivery.**" This is indicated in the documentation VBACS. You would then be presented with a range of codes: 59610–59612. You would now look up the CPT codes in the Maternity Care and Delivery subsection where your code choices are:
59610 Routine obstetric care including antepartum care, vaginal delivery (with or without episiotomy, and/or forceps) and postpartum care, after previous cesarean delivery
59612 Vaginal delivery only, after previous cesarean delivery (with or without episiotomy and/or forceps)
Because the physician provided the complete global package (antepartum care, delivery, and postpartum care), CPT code 59610 would be the correct choice.

2. The correct answer is 55815 Prostatectomy, perineal radical; with bilateral pelvic lymphadenectomy, including external iliac, hypogastric and obturator nodes. In the CPT index, you would look up **Prostatectomy, Perineal, Radical,** which presents a range of codes: 55810–55815. You would now look up the CPT codes in the Male Genital System subsection, where your code choices are:
55810 Prostatectomy, perineal radical
55812 Prostatectomy, perineal radical; with lymph node biopsy(s) (limited pelvic lymphadenectomy)
55815 Prostatectomy, perineal radical; with bilateral pelvic lymphadenectomy, including external iliac, hypogastric and obturator nodes
The service that was provided included a "complete" lymph node dissection, making CPT code 55815 the correct choice.

3. The correct answer is 20605-LT Arthrocentesis, aspiration and/or injection; intermediate joint or bursa (e.g., temporomandibular, acromioclavicular, wrist, elbow or ankle, olecranon bursa). In the CPT index, you would look up **Arthrocentesis,** which will lead you to **Intermediate Joint 20605, Large Joint 20610,** and **Small Joint 20600.** Because the elbow is considered an intermediate joint, the correct CPT code is 20605.

The LT modifier is appended to show it was the left side. Note: If you are unsure which type of joint the elbow is, you would look up the descriptors of each of the three CPT codes to determine the correct code selection.

4. The correct answer is 31631 Bronchoscopy, rigid or flexible, with or without fluoroscopic guidance; with placement of tracheal stent(s) (includes tracheal/bronchial dilation as required) and 31625 Bronchoscopy, rigid or flexible, with or without fluoroscopic guidance; with bronchial or endobronchial biopsy(s), single or multiple sites. In this case, two CPT codes are required to report the complete service provided. In the CPT index, you would look up **Bronchoscopy,** then **Stent Placement (31631, 31636, 31637)** AND **Biopsy (31625–31629, 31632, 31633).** You would now look up the CPT codes in the Respiratory System subsection, where your code choices are:
31631 Bronchoscopy, rigid or flexible, with or without fluoroscopic guidance; with placement of tracheal stent(s) (includes tracheal/bronchial dilation as required)
31636 Bronchoscopy, rigid or flexible, with or without fluoroscopic guidance; with placement of bronchial stent(s) (includes tracheal/bronchial dilation as required), initial bronchus
31637 Bronchoscopy, rigid or flexible, with or without fluoroscopic guidance; each additional major bronchus stented (List separately in addition to code for primary procedure)
Because the stent placement was in the trachea, the correct CPT code for the stent placement is 31631. The code choices for the biopsy are:
31625 Bronchoscopy, rigid or flexible, with or without fluoroscopic guidance; with bronchial or endobronchial biopsy(s), single or multiple sites
31628 Bronchoscopy, rigid or flexible, with or without fluoroscopic guidance; with transbronchial lung biopsy(s), single lobe
31629 Bronchoscopy, rigid or flexible, with or without fluoroscopic guidance; with transbronchial needle aspiration biopsy(s), trachea, main stem and/or lobar bronchus(i)
31632 Bronchoscopy, rigid or flexible, with or without fluoroscopic guidance; with transbronchial lung biopsy(s), each additional lobe (List separately in addition to code for primary procedure)
31633 Bronchoscopy, rigid or flexible, with or without fluoroscopic guidance; with transbronchial needle aspiration biopsy(s), each additional lobe (List separately in addition to code for primary procedure)
Because the biopsy was bronchial, the correct CPT code for the biopsy is 31625.

5. The correct answer is 12042-RT Repair, intermediate, wounds of neck, hands, feet and/or external genitalia; 2.6 cm to 7.5 cm. You can look this up in the CPT index under **Repair, Skin, Wound.** You are presented with three options: Complex, Intermediate, Simple. The documentation states the wound was closed with layered sutures, making this an intermediate repair; therefore, we would look up the code range 12031–12057. *Note:* If you are unsure of the type of the repair, you would read the instructional notes under Repair (Closure) in the Integumentary subsection, where definitions of the types of repairs are listed. You would now look up the CPT codes in the Integumentary subsection, where your code choices are many. You would narrow down the code selection by the site of the repair, in this case the hand. This narrows the code selection to 12041–12047. The code selection is then determined by the size of the repair, in this case 4.2 cm, which is reported with CPT code 12042.

Multiple Choice Answers

1. The correct answer is **a.** The surgery section is the largest section of the CPT manual.

2. The correct answer is **d.** A special report should accompany any unlisted procedure code, Category III code, or any CPT code with modifier 22. In all of these cases, the special report would provide additional information to the carrier regarding the type of service that was performed, the circumstances surrounding the service performed, or the new technology used to perform the procedure. The information will assist the carrier in determining the appropriate reimbursement rate for the service provided.

3. The correct answer is **c.** The global surgical package includes the preoperative, intraoperative, and postoperative services provided. Answer **a.** is incorrect, as surgical supplies may be reported separately when they are over and above those usually included with the procedure. Answer **b.** is incorrect, as general anesthesia is separately reported. Answer **d.** is incorrect, as complications during the postoperative period are separately reportable.

4. The correct answer is **d.** The multiple surgical rule does not apply to add-on codes and CPT codes that are modifier 51 exempt. It does, however, apply when a physician performs multiple related but separate procedures on the same patient during the same operative session (e.g., surgical procedures that are performed through the same incision).

5. The correct answer is **d.** Services are reimbursed 100% for the highest paying CPT code and 50% for the second through the fifth procedure, and any procedure thereafter is reimbursed by report. Answer **a.** is incorrect, as reimbursement is not made for procedures after the fifth procedure. Answer **b.** is incorrect, as multiple surgical procedures are not all reimbursed at 100%. Answer **c.** is incorrect, as surgical procedures after the fifth procedure are reimbursable by report.

6. The correct answer is **b.** Reimbursement is made for the full amount of the higher valued endoscopy and then a percentage of the next highest endoscopy based on the RVU of each CPT code. Answer **a.** is incorrect, as this is the multiple surgery rule, and endoscopies are not reimbursed according to the multiple surgery rule. Answer **c.** is incorrect, as multiple endoscopies *are* separately reimbursed.

7. The correct answer is **b.** Complications during the postoperative period are not considered part of the global surgical package and may be separately reported. Answer **a.** is incorrect, as complications are not considered "typical" postoperative care. Answer **c.** is incorrect, as modifier 22 is used to report an increased procedural service (e.g., surgical procedure) and would never be appended to an E/M code.

8. The correct answer is **d.** General anesthesia is not included in the surgical package. The following *are* included in the surgical package: writing orders **(a.),** local infiltration, metacarpal/metatarsal/ digital block or topical anesthesia **(b.),** and evaluating the patient in postanesthesia recovery **(c.).** A complete listing and definition of the surgical global package can be found in the Surgery Guidelines.

9. The correct answer is **d.** Both the guidelines located at the beginning of each section and the notes provided within the subsections provide coding guidance.

10. The correct answer is **d.** Unlisted CPT codes can be found in the Surgery Guidelines, in the CPT index, and throughout the Surgery section of the CPT manual.

11. The correct answer is **b.** You would add together the lengths of those in the same classification and located in anatomical sites that are grouped together in the same code descriptor. This coding guidance is located in the CPT manual in the Integumentary subsection under the subheading Repair (Closure). Answer **a.** is incorrect, as you would code all repairs; complex repair would be listed first, but it would not be the only repair coded. Answer **c.** is incorrect, as lacerations that are repaired with tissue adhesive may be coded with *a repair code* and would be added together with the repairs of the same classification and anatomical site as listed in the CPT code descriptor. Answer **d.** is incorrect, as repairs from different classifications (simple, intermediate, complex) would not be added together.

12. The correct answer is **b.** Casting and strapping would be separately reported as an initial service performed without a restorative treatment or procedure. This coding guidance is located in the CPT manual in the Musculoskeletal subsection under the subheading Application of Casts and

Strapping. Answer **a.** is incorrect, as the initial cast application is included with the fracture care and is not separately reportable. Answer **c.** is incorrect, as the physician who is applying the cast, strap, or splint would be able to report the cast, strap, or splint separately only if he were not providing any restorative treatment. Answer **d.** is incorrect, as the procedure listed under application of casts and strapping includes the removal procedure and would only be reported once for both the application and removal.

13. The correct answer is **d.** With open treatment of a fracture, the fracture is surgically opened and visualized, *and* the fractured bone is opened remote from the fracture site for insertion of an intramedullary nail across the fracture site. This coding guidance is located in the Musculoskeletal subsection under the definition "Open Treatment." Answer **b.** is incorrect, as the type of fracture does not have any coding correlation with the type of treatment.

14. The correct answer is **c.** An indirect examination is by tongue depressor and mirror. Answer a is incorrect, as a direct examination is visualization by an endoscope. Answers **b.** and **d.** are incorrect, as external and common are not considered types of examination for the respiratory system.

15. The correct answer is **c.** This coding guidance is located in the Cardiovascular subsection, under the category Pacemaker or Pacing Cardioverter-Defibrillator. CPT states, "When the battery of a pacemaker or pacing cardioverter-defibrillator is changed, it is actually the pulse generator that is changed." Therefore, answers **a., b.,** and **d.** are all incorrect. Additionally, answers **a.** and **b.** are actually the same, as the electrode is considered a lead.

16. The correct answer is **a.** In this scenario, you would need two CPT codes to properly report the services provided. CPT code 11406 represents the benign lesion on the trunk with an excised diameter over 4.0 cm. The wound was closed with layered sutures, which is considered *intermediate repair.* Because only simple repair codes are included with the excision code, you would need to separately report the wound closure with CPT code 12032 Repair, intermediate, wounds of scalp, axillae, trunk and/or extremities (excluding hands and feet); 2.6 cm to 7.5 cm. Answer **b.** is incorrect, as the wound closure repair code 12002 represents a simple repair, and the physician performed a layered closure; furthermore, simple repair codes are included in the excision code and would not be separately reported. Answer **c.** is incorrect, as it does not include the CPT code for the layered closure. Answer **d.** is incorrect, as CPT code 11606 represents a malignant lesion and the lesion was benign.

17. The correct answer is **b.,** 20605-RT (for the arthrocentesis of the right wrist), 20600-RT (for the arthrocentesis of the right thumb), and J3301× 3 for the 30 mg of the Kenalog. Answer **a.** is incorrect, as it includes ultrasonic guidance, which was not used to perform the procedure. Answer **c.** is incorrect, as it does not include the arthrocentesis for the right thumb. Answer **d.** is incorrect, as it does not include the arthrocentesis for the right thumb; it includes ultrasonic guidance, which was not used to perform the procedure; and the Kenalog administered was 30 mg, which is reported as × 3, as J3301 indicates 10 mg of Kenalog.

18. The correct answer is **d.,** 33214 Upgrade of implanted pacemaker system; conversion of single chamber system to dual chamber system (includes removal of previously placed pulse generator, testing of existing lead, insertion of new lead, insertion of new pulse generator). This one CPT code describes the complete procedure performed and includes the *removal* of the previous pulse generator (which is a necessary aspect of *replacement* of the pacemaker system). Answer **a.** is incorrect, as CPT code 33213 includes only the insertion of the dual chamber pacemaker and not the removal. Answer **b.** is incorrect, as the removal of the pulse generator (CPT code 33233) is included in CPT code 33214 and therefore is not separately reported. Answer **c.** is incorrect, as the patient upgraded the pulse generator from a single chamber to a dual chamber, which is represented by CPT code 33214.

19. The correct answer is **d.,** CPT 45378 Colonoscopy, flexible, proximal to splenic flexure; diagnostic, with or without collection of specimen(s) by brushing or washing, with or without colon decompression (separate procedure). Although the documentation states both a sigmoidoscopy and colonoscopy were performed, you would only report one CPT code, as the colonoscopy includes the examination of the rectum and sigmoid colon. When coding endoscopies, you would select the CPT code that describes the fullest extent of the procedure

performed, in this case the entire colon. Answers **a.** and **b.**, although sequenced differently, both include the CPT code for the sigmoidoscopy (45330) and therefore are incorrect. Answer **c.** is incorrect, as it represents the sigmoidoscopy, and the extent of the procedure performed was of the entire colon, represented by the CPT code for the colonoscopy 45378.

20. The correct answer is **a.**, 49495 Repair, initial inguinal hernia, full term infant younger than age 6 months, or preterm infant older than 50 weeks postconception age and younger than age 6 months at the time of surgery, with or without hydrocelectomy; reducible. Answer **b.** is incorrect, as CPT code 49491 is for an infant from birth to 50 weeks postconception. Answer **c.** is incorrect, as this represents an incarcerated or strangulated hernia, and the documentation supports an inguinal hernia. Answer **d.** is incorrect, as CPT code 49500 is for a child 6 months or older. The documentation indicated the child was 4 months old at the time of the procedure.

CHAPTER 11

Radiology

Radiology is the branch of medicine that deals with the study and application of imaging technology, such as radiography, ultrasonography, computed tomography, and magnetic resonance imaging (MRI) for diagnosing and treating disease. The radiation may be either ionizing (as with x-ray) or nonionizing (as with ultrasonography).

A *radiologist* is a *physician* who uses radiation technology for the diagnosis and treatment of disease and *specializes in interpreting radiographs (x-rays) and other imaging scans.*

An *interventional radiologist* is a *physician* whose subspecialty is to *perform minimally invasive procedures.*

Interventional radiology is a subspecialty of radiology that involves the treatment of numerous diseases with minimally invasive, image-guided techniques. An interventional radiologist performs **both** the **surgical procedure** and the **radiological portion** of the procedure. In these cases, codes from both the Surgery section and the Radiology section of the CPT book will be reported.

For example: A breast biopsy is performed by an automated vacuum-assisted or rotating biopsy device using imaging guidance. In this case, the interventional radiologist will perform the surgical procedure (breast biopsy) CPT code 19103 located in the Surgical section of the CPT book and the radiological guidance 77031 located in the Radiology section.

Radiology Planes, Positions, and Projections

Planes

According to *Taber's Cyclopedic Medical Dictionary*, in radiology, "planes are used as points of reference by which positions of parts of the body are indicated. In the human subject, all planes are based on the body being in the upright position." See Figures 11-1 and 11-2.

Coronal plane: Divides the body into front (anterior) and back (posterior).

Midsagittal plane: A vertical plane through the midline of the body dividing the body into right and left halves.

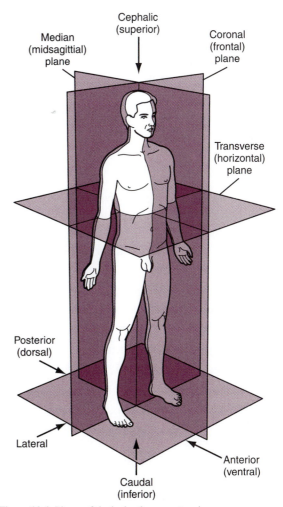

Figure 11-1. Planes of the body: three-quarter view.

173

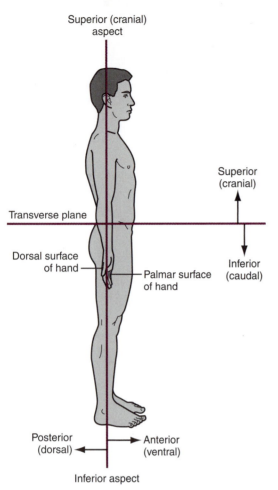

Figure 11-2. Planes of the body: side view.

Sagittal plane: A vertical plane dividing the body into right and left sections.

Transverse plane: A plane that divides the body into top (superior) and bottom (inferior) parts.

Positions

How the patient is placed for the radiographic procedure is called a **position.**

Ventral/prone: Lying facing downward.

Dorsal/supine: Lying on the back, facing upward.

Recumbent: Lying down.

Lateral: Lying on the side (*left lateral recumbent* = lying on the left side; *right lateral recumbent* = lying on the right side).

Oblique: Lying on a slant or diagonally.

Proximal and distal: These terms provide direction or position of one body part in relation to another body part. *Proximal* is nearest to the center of the body, and *distal* is furthest from the center of the body.

For example, the hand is at the distal end of the arm, and the shoulder is at the **proximal** end.

Projections

The path by which the x-ray beam travels through the body is called the **projection.**

Anteroposterior (AP) projection: The x-ray beam travels from the front (anterior) to the back (posterior).

Lateral projection: The x-ray beam travels through the side of the body.

Oblique projection: The x-ray beam travels through the body at an angle.

Posteroanterior (PA): The x-ray beam travels from the back to the front.

Putting It All Together

If a patient is positioned with his or her right side closest to the radiographic camera, this is called **right lateral position,** *and the x-ray beam will travel through the side of the body via a* **lateral projection** (Fig. 11-3).

If the patient is positioned to lie on his or her back (**dorsal** *or* **supine**) *with the front of the body closest to the radiographic camera, the x-ray beam will travel from the front to the back via an* **anteroposterior projection** (Fig. 11-4).

There are various types of radiological procedures. Let's review some of them:

Angiography: A radiographic examination of the arteries in which an injection of a type of dye (contrast) is used to make the arteries easily visible on x-rays.

Aortography: A radiographic examination of the aorta in which an injection of a type of dye (contrast) is used to make the aorta easily visible on x-rays.

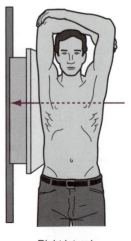

Right lateral projection

Figure 11-3. Right lateral position.

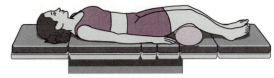

Supine (dorsal decubitus)

Figure 11-4. Supine (dorsal) position.

Arthrography: A radiographic examination of the joints in which an injection of a type of dye (contrast) is used to make the joints easily visible on x-rays.

Computed axial tomography (CT or CAT): A radiographic technique by which detailed images are made by scanning with x-rays that rotate around the patient and using a computer to construct three-dimensional (3D) images of a body structure.

Computed tomography angiography (CTA): A procedure that uses a combination of x-rays and computer technology to produce cross-sectional images of arterial and venous vessels throughout the body.

Cystography: An x-ray visualization of the bladder following injection of contrast material.

Doppler ultrasound: A special form of ultrasound that uses sound waves to measure the velocity of blood flow.

Fluoroscopy: A video x-ray procedure viewed on a monitor that makes it possible to see internal organs in motion.

Interventional radiology: A subspecialty of radiology that performs minimally invasive procedures using image guidance.

Magnetic resonance imaging (MRI): An imaging technique that uses magnetic resonance (the absorption of frequencies of radio and microwave radiation by atoms placed in a magnetic field) to obtain detailed images of the body.

Mammography: Diagnostic procedure to detect breast tumors by the use of x-rays of the soft tissue of the breast.

Nuclear imaging: Noninvasive diagnostic scans that use very small amounts of radioactive materials, or radiopharmaceuticals. Once administered to the patient, these radiopharmaceuticals can localize to specific organs or cellular receptors, allowing the radiologist to diagnose or treat a disease based on cellular function and physiology.

Positron emission tomography (PET): A nuclear medicine imaging procedure that utilizes a short-lived radioactive substance to produce a 3D image of the functional process of the body.

Single-photon emission computerized tomography (SPECT): A nuclear medicine imaging procedure that utilizes a gamma-emitting radioisotope (also

called radionuclide) to produce a 3D image of local metabolic and physiological functions in tissues.

Ultrasonography (ultrasound): The use of ultrasonic waves specifically to image an internal body structure.

Venography: Radiographic examination of the veins of the leg after injection of a contrast dye.

X-ray: Radiographic imaging using high-energy radiation in low doses to visualize and make pictures of the inside of the body.

How the Radiology Section is Organized

The Radiology section is divided into the following subsections:

- Diagnostic Radiology
- Diagnostic Ultrasound
- Radiological Guidance
- Breast Mammography
- Bone/Joint Studies
- Radiation Oncology
- Nuclear Medicine

Before we take a look at the various subsections, let's review some basic coding guidelines, as described in the "Guidelines" given at the beginning of the Radiology section.

Let's Review the Radiology Guidelines

The Professional Component, the Technical Component, and Billing Globally

Radiology procedures are a combination of a physician (professional) component and a technical component. The **technical component** represents the **cost of the equipment, the services of the technician, and the supplies.** The **professional component represents the service provided by the physician.** In the cases where the **physician owns the equipment, employs the technician, and interprets the film,** the physician will bill **globally** (for both the technical and professional components).

Therefore, radiology codes may be reported in various ways (by appending specific modifiers) depending on who provided a specific portion of the service. These modifiers are discussed later in this chapter.

Administration of Contrast Material

Many radiology services (e.g., CT, MRI, angiography) can be performed *"without contrast," "with contrast,"* or **"without contrast followed by contrast material."**

You must carefully read the radiology report to determine what type of contrast, if any, was utilized. For some radiological procedures, this will affect which code you select.

The radiology guidelines state, "The phrase **'with contrast'** used in the codes for procedures performed using contrast for imaging enhancement **represents contrast material administered intravascularly, intra-articularly, or intrathecally (within the spinal canal)."**

Alternately, oral and/or rectal contrast administration alone does not qualify as a study "with contrast."

Codes for radiology services performed with or without contrast or without contrast followed by contrast material will also affect how you locate the CPT code in the index. For example, when looking up a CT, you would first identify if the service included or excluded the use of contrast material and then identify the body area scanned.

CT Scan
with contrast
    Face..........70487
without and with contrast
    Face..........70488
without contrast
    Face..........70486

However, when looking up an MRI code, you would look up the anatomical site, which will provide you with a range of codes. You will find, upon reviewing the CPT codes within the code range, that the CPT code descriptor will include or exclude the mention of the contrast materials. For example, when looking up the CPT code for an MRI of the abdomen, the Alphabetical Index will direct you as follows:

Magnetic Resonance Imaging (MRI)

Abdomen..........74181–74183

You would then look up the code range and find the following choices:

74181 Magnetic resonance (e.g., proton) imaging, abdomen; *without contrast material(s)*

74182 Magnetic resonance (e.g., proton) imaging, abdomen; *with contrast material(s)*

74183 Magnetic resonance (e.g., proton) imaging, abdomen; *without contrast material(s), followed by with contrast material(s) and further sequences*

Separate Procedure

In CPT, the term "separate procedure" is used to designate certain procedures that are integral to a larger service/procedure (bundled). These codes are easily identified in CPT, as the words "separate procedure" are included in their CPT descriptor.

These CPT codes designated as separate procedures identify certain procedures that (1) may be billed by themselves when that is the only service provided, or (as occurs more often) (2) would not be billed because they are performed as part of a larger service or procedure (bundled).

For example, when reporting a splenoportography (by selecting CPT code 76000 Fluoroscopy **[separate procedure],** up to 1 hour physician time, other than 71023 or 71034 [e.g., cardiac fluoroscopy]), fluoroscopy would not need to be reported (i.e., CPT code 75810 Splenoportography, radiologic supervision and interpretation as the fluoroscopy would not need to be reported along with it). This is because code 76000 is considered to be an inclusive component of the splenoportography.

Supervision and Interpretation

Many services, such as interventional procedures (e.g., catheterization, placement of guide wires, injection of contrast material), are reported with a code from the Radiology section in addition to a code from another section of the CPT manual (e.g., Surgery). The reporting of a radiology procedure code and a surgical procedure code is called **"component coding"** or **"combination coding."**

When two separate physicians perform the service (e.g., the surgeon performs the surgical [i.e., interventional] component and the radiologist performs the radiological component), each physician will report the code identifying the procedure (component) performed. In these cases, the radiological component of the procedure is designated as **"radiological supervision and interpretation."**

For example: A hysterosalpingogram (x-ray of the uterus and fallopian tubes; usually performed for diagnosing infertility) consists of an injection of radio-opaque material and fluoroscopy. In this case, the surgeon performs the catheterization and injection of contrast material (58340), whereas the radiologist provides the radiological portion of the procedure (supervision and interpretation [74740]).

In cases where one physician performs both the procedure and the radiological supervision and interpretation, he or she would report the services with both components (surgery and radiology codes).

The injection procedure is coded as:

58340 Catheterization and introduction of saline or contrast material for saline infusion sonohysterography (SIS) or hysterosalpingography

And the radiological supervision and interpretation is coded as:

74740 Hysterosalpingography, radiologic supervision and interpretation

Extent of the Examination

When coding radiology, you must carefully read the radiology report to determine the extent of the procedure before selecting the CPT code.

For example: A *complete ultrasound* of the abdomen consists of ultrasonographic examination of the liver, gallbladder, common bile duct, pancreas, spleen, kidneys, upper abdominal aorta, and inferior vena cava, including any demonstrated abdominal abnormality.

A *limited ultrasound* of the abdomen consists of a single organ, quadrant, or follow-up.

When coding x-rays, you must carefully read the radiology report to determine the number of views taken before selecting the CPT code.

73650 Radiologic examination; calcaneus, **minimum of 2 views**
73630 Radiologic examination, foot; complete, **minimum of 3 views**

The Radiology Codes—and How to Use Them

Diagnostic Radiology
70010–76499

The Diagnostic Radiology subsection is divided according to anatomical site into the following subheadings: Head & Neck, Chest, Spine & Pelvis, Upper Extremities, Lower Extremities, Abdomen, Gastrointestinal Tract, Urinary Tract, Gynecological & Obstetrical, and Heart, followed by the subheadings Vascular Procedures and Other Procedures. Many imaging methods are included, such as radiography, CT, MRI, and MRA.

KEY CODING TIP
To code a diagnostic radiology procedure, you must consider the following:

■ The type of procedure (e.g., x-ray, MRI)
■ The anatomical site (e.g., chest, brain)
■ Number of views (two views, three views, if applicable)
■ Extent of examination (if applicable)
■ Laterality (unilateral or bilateral)
■ Whether contrast material was utilized
■ Whether you are coding for the professional component or technical component, or if the service is being billed globally

When reviewing the radiology report, in addition to the Key Coding Tip, it is helpful to identify within the report information you will need to select the correct CPT code(s) and modifier(s).

A radiology report includes the following documentation:

Heading: Identifies the type of service provided, whether contrast material was utilized, and the anatomical site

of examination (e.g., brain, abdomen, left breast, right foot)—for example, MRI of the Brain With and Without Contrast; CT Scan of the Sinuses With Contrast; Dual-Energy X-ray Absorptiometry (DEXA) Scan, X-Ray of the Right Foot.

Clinical History: Provides the medical history of the patient and/or signs and symptoms. This is where you will indentify why the service(s) was/were ordered. In some cases, such as screenings or routine obstetric ultrasounds, the clinical history may not always be separately stated, as the reason for the examination would be the screening or routine examination.

Protocol: Provides information such as the number of views or images taken and how the contrast was administered (e.g., IV).

Findings: A narrative of the reading provided by the radiologist.

Impression: Contains the conclusion or the diagnosis.

Note: The report will *not include* where the examination takes place (e.g., hospital, radiology facility, physician office). Instead, this information is determined by the location at which the service took place and who provided certain aspects of the service (e.g., technical or professional).

LET'S LET LOOK AT AN EXAMPLE

X-Ray of the **Right Foot** (performed in an orthopedist private office setting)

Clinical History: Pain in foot, injury playing sports, rule out fracture.

Protocol: AP, lateral, and oblique views of the right foot.

Findings: There is plantar spurring of the calcaneus. There is no calcaneal fracture. The tarsal bones are normal. There is no bony spur present in the medial and distal aspects of the right first metatarsal bone. The sesamoid bones are normal. Some bony spurring is also present in the first metatarsophalangeal joint.

There is mild cortical thickening of the distal aspect of the second metatarsal. The third through fifth metatarsals are normal. The second through fifth metatarsal joints are normal. There is no phalangeal fracture.

Impression:
1. Plantar spurring of the calcaneus
2. Medially oriented spur at the distal aspect of the first metatarsal and mild bony spurring of the medial aspect of the first metatarsophalangeal joint
3. No acute fractures

How to Code: We would code this radiology report using the Key Coding Tip and highlighting the key points of

continued

LET'S LET LOOK AT AN EXAMPLE—cont'd

information. The **type of procedure** is an x-ray, the **anatomical site** is the foot, the **number of views** is three (AP, lateral, and oblique), the **laterality** is right, and there was **no contrast material** used. Because the service was performed in an orthopedist's private office, this suggests that the clinician owns the radiological equipment, employs the technician, and has interpreted the film himself or herself—so we would code the service **globally** (i.e., no modifier for a technical or professional component is needed). Therefore, the correct CPT code is:

> **73630-RT** Radiologic examination, foot; complete, minimum of 3 views

The HCPCS modifier RT is appended to indicate the x-ray was of the right foot.

LET'S LOOK AT ANOTHER EXAMPLE

CT Scan of the **Chest With and Without Contrast** (performed in a hospital setting, coding for the physician's interpretation)
Clinical History: Cough.

Protocol: 5-mm axial images apices to adrenal glands pre- and post-100 cc intravenous contrast, coronal reformatted images.

Findings: There are no enlarged mediastinal or hilar lymph nodes. There is no pleural or pericardial effusion. Scanning of the upper abdomen demonstrates the adrenal glands to be within normal limits. Motion artifact degrades several of the slices. There is no gross evidence of pleural or parenchymal mass or abnormal fluid collection.

Impression: Grossly unremarkable CT scan of the chest.

How to Code: We would code this radiology report using the Key Coding Tip and highlighting the key points of information. The **type of procedure** is a CT scan, the **anatomical site** is the chest (thorax), the **number of views** is not applicable to this type of procedure, the **laterality** is not applicable for this procedure, the documentation supports the study as being performed both **without the use of contrast material and with the use of contrast material.** Because the service was performed in a hospital, the facility will code for the technical portion and the physician will code for the professional component. Because we are being asked to code for the physician's interpretation, in this case, we are coding only for the professional component. Therefore, the correct CPT code is:

> **71270–26** Computed tomography, thorax; without contrast material, followed by contrast material(s) and further sections (Modifier 26 is appended to indicate the professional component; see section on modifiers later in this chapter.)

Diagnostic Ultrasound
76506–76999

The Diagnostic Ultrasound subsection is divided by anatomical site (e.g., head and neck, chest). Ultrasonographic procedures are also listed in the Medicine section under Non-Invasive Vascular Diagnostic Studies (e.g., Doppler study of the intracranial arteries) and Echocardiography (e.g., heart).

Diagnostic ultrasound is the use of high-frequency sound to assist in the diagnosis and treatment of patients. Ultrasound can be used to scan any region of the body and as such is used for a variety of reasons. Some of the common uses of ultrasound are for the confirmation and assessment of a pregnancy and the development of the fetus, the diagnosis of disease and/or obstruction, evaluation of blood flow, guidance during surgical procedures, determining abnormal structures (e.g., cyst), and in some cases as a follow-up study.

There are four types of ultrasound display modes listed in the CPT book:

A-mode **(amplitude mode):** A-mode is used to assess an organ's dimensions. This is a one-dimensional measurement procedure.

M-mode **(motion mode):** M-mode is used to analyze moving body parts. With this mode, a single beam is used to produce a one-dimensional M-mode picture, where movement of a structure such as the heart valve can be viewed in a wavelike manner.

B-scan **(brightness mode):** B-mode ultrasound provides a cross-sectional view of tissues that cannot be seen directly. The ultrasound signal produces various points of brightness, which are dependent on the amplitude instead of the spiking movements in the A-mode. B-scans are also referred to as grayscale ultrasounds.

Real-time scan: These scans display a two-dimensional structure and motion in real time. The motion is presented much like a movie of the workings of the inner body.

Limited and Complete Ultrasounds

As mentioned earlier, the **extent of the examination** is a key piece of documentation in determining the correct CPT code selection. One example would be an ultrasound of the retroperitoneum. A complete ultrasound of the retroperitoneum consists of an examination of kidneys, abdominal aorta, common iliac artery origins, and inferior vena cava, including any demonstrated retroperitoneal abnormality. A limited retroperitoneal would represent an ultrasound examination of a single organ (e.g., kidney or urinary bladder). Alternatively, if clinical history suggests urinary tract pathology, complete evaluation of the kidneys and urinary bladder also constitutes a complete retroperitoneal ultrasound.

KEY CODING TIP

To code an ultrasound procedure, you need to consider the following:

- The anatomical site
- The type of mode used to perform the test
- If the ultrasound was complete or limited
- If the ultrasound was obstetric or nonobstetric
- If obstetric, determine the number of gestations; and whether a detailed fetal examination was performed.
- The approach (transvaginal, transrectal, transabdominal)

Obstetric ultrasound procedures require special considerations. In these cases, it is not the extent of the examination but the **number of gestations** (i.e., per pregnancy—for example, in the case of twins), the **trimester** of the pregnancy, and the **approach** that need to be considered.

LET'S LOOK AT AN EXAMPLE

Obstetric Ultrasound (performed in a physician's office)

Protocol: Multiple transabdominal images of the fetus, placenta, and uterus.

Findings: There is a single intrauterine gestation in breech presentation. The cervical length is 4.3 cm. There is a Grade I anterior placenta. There is no placenta previa. The amniotic fluid volume is normal for this stage of gestation. The amniotic fluid index is 8.2 cm.

Fetal Anatomy: The ventricles are normal in caliber and appearance. The posterior fossa, cerebellum, and nuchal areas are normal. The lips and nose are not optimally visualized. The cervical, thoracic, and lumbar spines are normal. There is no open neural tube defect. A four-chamber, left-sided heart is present with 160 beats per minute recorded. There is a left-sided stomach. Normal kidneys, bladder, and anterior abdominal wall with normal cord insertion are noted. Four extremities with motion are noted. The hands and feet areas are normal.

The estimated fetal weight is 230 g, which corresponds with the composite ultrasound gestational age of 18 weeks. The estimated date of delivery based on this examination is 8/19/08.

Impression:

1. Single viable intrauterine gestation in breech presentation dated to 18 weeks gestational age.

2. No fetal abnormalities detected.

3. Estimated date of delivery based on examination is 8/19/08.

How to Code: We would code this ultrasound report using the Key Coding Tip and highlighting the key points of information. The **type of procedure** is an obstetric ultrasound, the **number of gestations** is one, a **detailed fetal anatomy was performed,** and **the approach** was transabdominal. We would therefore select the following CPT code:

76811 Ultrasound, pregnant uterus, real time with image documentation, fetal and maternal evaluation plus detailed fetal anatomic examination, transabdominal approach; single or first gestation

Because the service was provided in the physician's office, we would report globally; therefore, no professional or technical modifier is required.

Radiological Guidance
77001–77032

The codes in this subsection of Radiology are used to report the imaging guidance for various procedures, such as the fluoroscopic guidance for needle placement during a biopsy or aspiration procedure or the mammographic guidance for needle placement for wire localization of the breast.

Breast Mammography
77051–77059

Mammography is a diagnostic procedure to detect breast tumors by the use of x-rays of the soft tissue of the breast. The CPT code descriptors for mammography will state if the mammography was unilateral (77055) or bilateral (77056); or in the case of a screening (77057), the descriptor will indicate not only a bilateral service but also "a two-view film study of each breast." Therefore, if a screening mammography is performed on one breast, or if fewer than two views are taken from each breast, modifier 52 (reduced services) would be appended to CPT code 77057 to show the service was not carried out in its entirety.

When coding for mammograms, you need to consider:

■ If the study is being performed unilaterally or bilaterally.

■ If the test is performed as a screening or diagnostic study.

■ If the study was performed with computer-aided detection (CAD).

CAD is software that acts like a second pair of eyes reviewing the film after the radiologist's initial review. If the computer software detects any breast abnormalities or areas of interest, it marks them, and the radiologist can then go back and look at the areas identified by the CAD.

LET'S LOOK AT AN EXAMPLE

Digital Screening Mammogram With CAD (performed in a physician's office)

Protocol: Bilateral mediolateral oblique and craniocaudal projections of the breasts. The patient had last clinical breast examination in 3/07. Previous mammogram is not available for comparison. Study was performed and interpreted with the use of CAD.

Findings: The examination shows evidence of mature glandular structures. There is no evidence of any nipple retraction or subcutaneous skin thickening noted. There is noted to be fibroglandular parenchyma with mild fatty changes bilaterally. A 1-cm nodule is noted posterior and superior to the left nipple. No suspicious clusters of microcalcifications are seen. The axillary areas are unremarkable.

Impression:

1. Fibroglandular parenchyma

2. Mild fatty changes bilaterally

3. 1-cm irregular nodule just posterior and superior to the left nipple. Spot compression views and biopsy recommended for further evaluation.

How to Code: We would code this mammography report using the Key Coding Tip and highlighting the key points of information. **Two views of each breast were taken** (bilateral mediolateral oblique and craniocaudad projections), the test was **performed as a screening,** and it was **performed with the use of CAD.** We would report two codes: one for the screening mammography and the add-on code for the use of the CAD:

77057 Screening mammography, bilateral (2-view film study of each breast)

77052 Computer-aided detection (computer algorithm analysis of digital image data for lesion detection) with further physician review for interpretation, with or without digitization of film radiographic images; screening mammography (List separately in addition to code for primary procedure)

Because the service was provided in the physician's office, we would report globally; therefore, no professional or technical modifier is required.

Bone/Joint Studies
77071–77084

This subsection of the Radiology section includes studies that evaluate diseases of the bone and joints. DEXA is an imaging study to measure bone density and is primarily used to detect osteoporosis. When coding bone density, you need to determine the bone mass that is being measured. For example, the axial skeleton (hips, pelvis, or spine) or the appendicular skeleton (peripheral; e.g., radius, wrist, heel).

Radiation Oncology
77261–77799

Radiation oncology is the study and treatment of cancers using radiation (x-rays, gamma rays, or electrons). The Radiation Oncology subsection includes services for both the professional component and technical component (i.e., the procedures themselves) and is organized according to the type of treatment provided. You must carefully read all the notes and definitions provided in CPT prior to code selection to assure accurate coding. For example, the notes preceding the CPT codes for clinical treatment planning include definitions of the various types of treatment planning, and the notes preceding radiation treatment management provide information on the manner in which the service is provided.

If a preliminary consultation or evaluation of the patient is provided prior to the decision to treat the patient, this service is reported with the appropriate code from the E/M, Medicine, or Surgery section.

Clinical Treatment Planning (External and Internal Sources). These services represent the **professional component** and include complex **planning services** such as interpretation of special testing, tumor localization, treatment volume determination, treatment time/dosage determination, choice of treatment modality, determination of number and size of treatment ports, and selection of appropriate treatment devices and other procedures. There are three types of clinical treatment plans: simple, intermediate, and complex.

Simulation. Simulation is the process by which the physician can localize, define, and reconstruct a patient's tumor, allowing the physician to define specific treatment fields and the placement of ports for radiation treatment individual to the patient. It is important to note the administration of the radiation is not included and is coded elsewhere with codes from the radiation treatment delivery subsection (77401–77416).

The simulation includes **four levels of service:** simple, intermediate, complex, and 3D.

Medical Radiation Physics, Dosimetry, Treatment Devices, and Special Services. These services describe the decision as to the type of treatment, dose, and the development of the treatment or device. Dosimetry is the measurement of the dose of radiation. For any given service, the codes are divided on the basis of the level of the service (e.g., plan or device): simple, intermediate, and complex.

Radiation Treatment Delivery. These codes represent the technical component of the radiation treatment and are used to report the delivery of the radiation. CPT codes 77402–77416 are reported in units of energy measured in megavolts (MeV) or megaelectron.

KEY CODING TIP

When coding for the radiation treatment delivery, you must consider the following:

■ The amount of radiation delivered (5 MeV, 11–19 MeV)
■ The areas treated (single, two, and so on)
■ The number of ports
■ Use and type of blocks used (simple, multiple)

Radiation Treatment Management. These are *professional services* that represent the *weekly management* of *radiation therapy.* Radiation treatment management services are reported in units of five fractions or treatment sessions (i.e., using the CPT code 77427 Radiation treatment management, 5 treatments). These services are reported in units of five fractions even if the service is not provided on consecutive days. Additionally, multiple services furnished on the same day can be counted separately if there has been a distinct break in the therapy session. If a course of treatment ends with a unit of three or four treatment sessions (i.e., if they are given *in addition* to one or more units of five treatment sessions), this unit of three or four may likewise be reported with CPT code 77427.

For example: A patient who has received 14 treatments during a 4-week period would be reported as CPT code 77427 × **3.** The first two units of five treatments would account for 10 treatments, and the four treatments that were given in addition to these two units of five also would be reported with the code 77427. Therefore, we would report the code three times to account for the total of 14 treatments.

Proton Beam Treatment Delivery. Proton beam treatment delivery uses positively charged atomic particles called protons to deliver radiation to a tumor. There are three levels of service: simple, intermediate, and complex.

Hyperthermia. When we hear the word hyperthermia, we immediately think of a body temperature that is higher than normal, such as a fever. However, hyperthermia can also refer to heat treatment (the carefully controlled use of heat for medical purposes), in this case, in the treatment of cancer. When cells in the body are exposed to higher than normal temperatures, the cells can become more likely to be affected by radiation therapy. When selecting codes for this service, you need to consider if the treatment was externally generated (applied to the skin) or generated by an interstitial probe (a probe that delivers heat directly to the treatment area), and if the treatment was superficial or deep. When the probe is inserted in a body orifice (e.g., rectum, vagina) it would be coded as clinical intracavitary hyperthermia.

Clinical Brachytherapy. Brachytherapy is a type of radiotherapy in which a radioactive source is placed inside or next to the area requiring treatment. Radioactive sources come in different forms (e.g., seeds, ribbon, capsules). The radioactive source may be permanent or temporary, and the placement may be intracavitary or interstitial (within the tissue) or by surface application. The codes are divided according to the number of sources or ribbons at three different levels: simple, intermediate, or complex.

For example: A patient receiving an intermediate application of a radioactive source, interstitial, would be reported with CPT code 77777 Interstitial radiation source application; intermediate.

These codes are easily located in the index under brachytherapy, where you will be directed to a range of codes: 77761–77778 and CPT code 77789.

Nuclear Medicine. Nuclear medicine is the branch of medicine that uses radioactive isotopes (radionuclides) for the diagnosis and treatment of disease. The codes in the nuclear medicine section do not include the provision of the radionuclide; the radionuclide codes are reported as applicable, and they are located in the HCPCS book.

Some of the more common nuclear medicine codes represent nuclear stress tests and bone scans. The nuclear subsection is further divided into two subheadings, Diagnostic and Therapeutic.

Modifiers

As mentioned earlier in this chapter, radiology procedures are a combination of a physician component and a technical component. The technical component represents the cost of the equipment, the services of the technician, and the supplies. The professional component represents the service provided by the physician. To report the technical and professional components, respectively, modifiers (described next) must be appended to the code. (Global reporting, in which case the same physician performs both the technical and professional components and modifiers are therefore not necessary, is described earlier in this chapter.)

Modifier 26—Professional Component. Certain procedures are a combination of a physician component and a technical component. When the physician component is reported separately, the service may be identified by adding modifier 26 to the usual procedure number.

If the physician does not own the equipment and is responsible for the professional component, he or she will append modifier 26 to the CPT code.

TC—Technical Component. Under certain circumstances, a charge may be made for the technical component alone. Under those circumstances, the technical charge is identified by adding modifier "TC" to the usual procedure number.

The technical component will be reported by the facility that owns the equipment and provides the services of the technician and the supplies by appending the HCPCS modifier TC (technical component) to the CPT code.

For example: An orthopedic surgeon seeing a patient in the emergency room for a fractured wrist orders an x-ray of the wrist, and the x-ray is performed in the hospital. Because the hospital owns the equipment, employs the technician, and provides the supplies, the hospital will report the CPT code with the TC modifier (73110-TC). The physician will interpret the film and report his professional component by appending modifier 26 (professional component) to the same CPT code (73110-26).

Other modifiers commonly reported with radiology services include:

Modifier 22 Increased Procedural Services

Modifier 32 Mandated Services

Modifier 52 Reduced Services

Modifier 53 Discontinued Procedure

Modifier 58 Staged or Related Procedure or Service by the Same Physician During the Postoperative Period

Modifier 59 Distinct Procedural Service

Modifier 76 Repeat Procedure or Service by the Same Physician

Modifier 77 Repeat Procedure by Another Physician

Modifier 99 Multiple Modifiers

For complete information regarding modifiers, how and when to use them, along with examples, refer to Chapter 7.

Let's Practice Coding

Now that you have a good understanding of radiology services and have prepared your CPT book, you are ready to code.

To locate a CPT code for an "x-ray" in the CPT book, you would go to the index, look up the word "x-ray," and then look for the anatomical site (chest, abdomen, elbow, and so on). Let's try one.

Let's look up the radiology code for x-ray elbow.
We would first go to the CPT index and look up *x-ray,* and then the subentry *elbow.* When we find *elbow,* we are directed to code range 73070–73080.

   X-ray
      Elbow.................73070–73080
      When we look up the code range 73070–73080 in the Radiology section of the CPT book, the code descriptors read:

73070 Radiologic examination, elbow; 2 views

73080 Radiologic examination, elbow; complete, minimum of 3 views

The determining factor in code selection will be the number of views.
The process is the same for MRAs, MRIs, CTs, and ultrasounds.

For example: To locate a CPT code for an MRI in the CPT book, you would go to the index, look up "Magnetic Resonance Imaging" (note, if you look up the abbreviation "MRI," you are directed to *see Magnetic Resonance Imaging*), and then look for the anatomical site (abdomen, ankle, and so on).

Let's Practice Coding—cont'd

Mammography codes are found by looking up the word "mammography" in the CPT index. Your options will be:

Mammography 77055-77057

Magnetic Resonance Imaging (MRI)

      With Computer-Aided Detection.......................0159T

Screening..77057

With Computer-Aided Detection......................77051–77052

    The determining factor in code selection will be the type of mammography performed.

    Nuclear medicine CPT codes are found by looking up the words "Nuclear Medicine," by anatomical site (brain, esophagus, and so on), and then by type of study (imaging, reflux, and so on). Let's try one.

Let's look up the nuclear medicine code for reflux study of the esophagus.
We would first go to the CPT index and look up *Nuclear Medicine,* the subentry *Esophagus,* followed by *Reflux Study.*

Nuclear Medicine
Esophagus

    Imaging (Motility)................................78258

    Reflux Study...78262

    Radiation oncology codes are found by looking up "Radiation Therapy" in the CPT index. The services are then divided by the type of service provided (e.g., consultation, dose plan, treatment delivery).

Learn More About It

The more you read, the more you know. Increase your knowledge with the following resources.

Recommended Web Sites

American College of Radiology (ACR)

http://www.acr.org/

This site has all of the guidelines and technical standards for each type of radiological procedure.

ACR Radiology Coding Source

http://www.acr.org/SecondaryMainMenuCategories/
    ACRStore/FeaturedCategories/econ/
    TheACRRadiologyCodingSource.aspx

This site has a wealth of information, including current articles, up-to-date Medicare and third-party payer policy and reimbursement, and a Q&A section.

Z Health Publishing

http://www.zhealthpublishing.com/

This site offers specialized books for interventional radiology, cardiology, and vascular surgery coding.

STOP-LOOK-HIGHLIGHT

The key to successfully passing the exam and selecting the correct code lies in your knowing how to use your coding book.

    To help you navigate through your codebook, and to make sure you have the most important information at your fingertips when you take the exam, highlight key text in the chapter guidelines and subheadings, and insert simple notes and coding tips directly into your codebooks.

    When highlighting, use two different color highlighter pens: yellow for standard guidelines and global services and an alternate color for carve-outs and unique notes.

On the Guidelines Page:

■ Under Supervision and Interpretation, write *"(SI)"* as the abbreviation for this terminology and also write *"component or combination coding."*

■ At the bottom of the guidelines page (or wherever there is room on the guidelines page), write the following: *"Modifier 26 is for the professional component, modifier TC is for the technical component, and to bill globally includes both the professional and the technical components."*

■ Depending on your version of the CPT book, if you have the professional edition, **tag the page** that includes the diagrams of the radiology planes.

In the Radiology Guidelines:

■ Under Administration of Contrast Material(s), highlight in yellow the first paragraph, which provides coding guidance on contrast materials: "The phrase 'with contrast' used in the codes for procedures using contrast for imaging enhancement represents contrast material administered intravascularly, intra-articularly, or intrathecally."

■ Also highlight the last paragraph under the same heading, "Oral and/or rectal contrast administration alone does not qualify as a study 'with contrast.'"

In the Subsection Diagnostic Ultrasound:

■ Highlight the definitions for the different modes of ultrasound.

In the Subheading Clinical Treatment Planning (External and Internal Sources):

■ Highlight the definitions for the different types of treatment planning and different types of simulation.

■ At the top of the subheading, write in red ink: "*Professional Component.*"

In the Subheading Radiation Treatment Delivery:

■ At the top of the subheading, write "*Technical Component.*"

In the subheading Radiation Treatment Management:

■ At the top of the subheading, write "*Professional Component.*"

■ Highlight in yellow the first sentence: "*Radiation treatment management is reported in units of five fractions or treatment sessions, regardless of the actual time period in which the services are furnished.*"

In the Subheading Proton Beam Treatment Delivery:

■ Highlight the definitions for the different types of proton beam treatment delivery.

In the Subsection Clinical Brachytherapy:

■ Highlight the definitions for the different types of brachytherapy treatment.

Radiology Vocabulary Words

At the end of the Radiology section, write the vocabulary words listed earlier in this chapter (the radiology planes, positions, and projections listed on pages 171-172 as well as the radiological procedures listed on pages 172–173).

Radiology Acronyms and Abbreviations

At the end of the Radiology section, *write the following acronyms and abbreviations:*

AP–**A**ntero**p**osterior

CAD–**C**omputer-**A**ided **D**etection

CT or CAT–**C**omputed **T**omography

DEXA–**D**ual-**E**nergy **X**-ray **A**bsorptiometry

MRA (MR)–**M**agnetic **R**esonance **A**ngiography

MRI–**M**agnetic **R**esonance **I**maging

PA–**P**ostero**a**nterior

PET–**P**ositron **E**mission **T**omography

TAKE THE CODING CHALLENGE

Assign the Appropriate Radiology Code

1. X-ray of the left knee, four views

2. Diagnostic mammography of the right breast with CAD

3. MRI of the right elbow with contrast

4. Abdominal ultrasound of the left lower quadrant

5. CT of the brain without contrast followed by contrast

Multiple Choice

1. CPT codes that include "with contrast" in their descriptors may be coded when:
   a. The contrast material is administered orally, intravascularly, or intra-articularly
   b. The contrast material is administered by any method
   c. The contrast material is administered intravascularly, intra-articularly, or intrathecally
   d. The contrast material is administered orally and rectally

2. Mrs. Lee presented to the OBGYN's office with irregular menstrual bleeding. Upon examination, Dr. Ng decided to perform a transvaginal pelvic ultrasound to assist with his diagnosis. The code for the ultrasound is:
   a. 76856
   b. 76830
   c. 76817
   d. 76857

3. Mrs. Franken presented for her screening mammography. Upon examination, the breasts were composed of heterogeneously dense fibroglandular tissue bilaterally. No suspicious mass, calcifications, or other findings were noted in either breast. Impression: No mammographic evidence of malignancy. A 1-year screening mammogram was recommended. The correct code(s) are:
   a. 77057-50, 77052
   b. 77057, 77052
   c. 77057-50
   d. 77057

4. Mrs. Jones presented to the general surgeon's office with a complaint of a mass in her right breast. Upon examination, the physician identified a palpable area in the 6:00 position of the right breast and decided to perform an ultrasound. Upon ultrasonic examination, no suspicious mass was seen in the palpable area (6:00–7:00) and 8 cm from the left nipple. Mrs. Jones will return in 3 months for follow-up. The correct code is:
   a. 76645
   b. 76645-RT
   c. 76604
   d. None of the above

5. The standard measurement of energy for radiation treatment is:
   a. Protons
   b. Radionuclide
   c. Megavolts
   d. Dosimetry

6. Services listed in the Radiation Oncology subsection and subheadings are coded depending on which of the following?
   a. Whether the professional or technical component is being reported
   b. The level of service (e.g., simple, intermediate, or complex)
   c. The number of sources
   d. All of the above

7. Mrs. Williams, who is pregnant with twins, presented to a radiology facility for a transabdominal ultrasound during her second trimester. Code for the professional component only. The correct code(s) are:
   a. 76805-26, 76810-26
   b. 76805-26
   c. 76801-26, 76802-26
   d. 76805, 76810

8. Hysterosalpingogram was performed on Mrs. Franklin, who has a history of infertility for 2 years. The patient was prepped and draped in a sterile fashion. A speculum was introduced into the vaginal canal. Contrast material was introduced via a catheter within the uterus, and multiple radiographs were obtained. The uterus was of normal shape, size, and configuration and was anteverted. The right fallopian tube was visualized with distal hydrosalpinx and no spillage seen. The left fallopian tube was also well visualized and showed marked distal hydrosalpinx and no spillage. The patient tolerated the procedure well and left in good condition. Impression: Bilateral distal hydrosalpinx with no spillage noted. The service was provided in the physician office. The correct code(s) are:
   a. 58340
   b. 74740
   c. 58340, 74740
   d. 58340, 74740-26

9. A bone density was performed utilizing the lumbar spine and the right and left hips as sample sites. Impression: Lumbar spine, high fracture risk. Right and left hips, high fracture risk. The correct code(s) are:
   a. 77082
   b. 77079
   c. 77080, 77080-50
   d. 77080

10. Radiation treatment management is reported in units of five fractions or treatment sessions. When there are three or four fractions beyond a multiple of five at the end of the course of treatment, you would:
   a. Report the service as an additional treatment session
   b. Not report the service, as it does not meet the requirements for a treatment session
   c. Report the service with a reduced service modifier (52)
   d. Report the service as an additional treatment only if the additional units were provided as part of a different course of treatment

ANSWERS AND RATIONALES

Assign the Appropriate Radiology Code

1. The correct answer is 73564-LT Radiologic examination, knee; complete, 4 or more views. In the CPT index, you first look up **x-ray,** followed by the subentry **knee.** You are presented with a range of codes: 73560-73564, 73580. You now look up the CPT codes in the Radiology section, where your code choices are:

   73560 Radiologic examination, knee; 1 or 2 views
   73562 Radiologic examination, knee; 3 views
   73564 Radiologic examination, knee; complete, 4 or more views
   73580 Radiologic examination, knee, arthrography, radiologic supervision and interpretation

   The study performed includes four views; therefore, CPT code 73564 is the correct code. Modifier LT is appended to indicate the left knee.

2. The correct answer is 77055-RT Mammography; unilateral. In the CPT index, you first look up **mammography** and are presented with a range of codes: 77055-77057. You now look up these codes in the Radiology section, where your code choices are:

   77055 Mammography; unilateral
   77056 Mammography; bilateral
   77057 Screening mammography, bilateral (2-view film study of each breast)

   Because you know the mammography was diagnostic and was performed only on the right breast, the correct code selection is 77055. You would then append the modifier RT to the mammography code to indicate the study was performed on the right breast. But you are not done coding this scenario yet. You still need to code for the CAD. In the CPT index, once again look up **mammography,** but this time look under mammography for **"with computer-aided detection,"** and you are once again presented with a range of codes: 77051-77052.

   77051 Computer-aided detection diagnostic mammography
   77052 Computer-aided detection (screening mammography)

   Because this was a diagnostic (not a screening) mammography, you would code 77051. The correct answer for this scenario is 77055-RT, 77051. (Note: The modifier RT is appended to the *mammography code,* not to the code for the CAD.)

3. The correct answer is 73222-RT Magnetic resonance (e.g., proton) imaging, any joint of upper extremity; with contrast material. In the CPT index, you first look up **magnetic resonance imaging** (MRI), then the subentry **joint** (because the elbow is a joint), followed by the subentry **upper extremity** (representing the elbow). You are presented with a range of codes: 73221-73223. You now look up the CPT codes in the Radiology section, where your code choices are:

   73221 Magnetic resonance (e.g., proton) imaging, any joint of upper extremity; without contrast material(s)
   73222 Magnetic resonance (e.g., proton) imaging, any joint of upper extremity; with contrast material(s)
   73223 Magnetic resonance (e.g., proton) imaging, any joint of upper extremity; without contrast material(s), followed by contrast material(s) and further sequences

   Because contrast material was utilized, the correct code is 73222. You then append the modifier RT to show that the study was performed on the right elbow. Therefore, the code is 73222-RT.

4. The correct answer is 76705 Ultrasound, abdominal, real time with image documentation; limited (e.g., single organ, quadrant, follow-up). In the CPT index, you first look up **abdomen,** followed by the subentry **ultrasound.** You are presented with a range of codes: 76700-76705. You now look up the CPT codes in the Radiology section, where your code choices are:

   76700 Ultrasound, abdominal, real time with image documentation; complete
   76705 Ultrasound, abdominal, real time with image documentation; limited (e.g., single organ, quadrant, follow-up)

   Although both CPT codes describe the abdominal ultrasound, one is for a *complete* ultrasound and the other is for a *limited* ultrasound (e.g., single organ, quadrant, follow-up). Because this study was of a single quadrant, the extent of the examination is limited; the correct code is therefore 76705 Ultrasound, abdominal, real time with image documentation; limited.

5. The correct answer is 70470 Computed tomography, head or brain; without contrast material, followed by contrast material(s) and further sections. In the CPT index, you look up **computed tomography (CT).** You will be directed to look under **CT scan: specific anatomic site.** Under CT scan, you will look up **without and with contrast,** and you will look up **head.** You will be presented with two choices:

   70470 Computed tomography, head or brain; without contrast material, followed by contrast material(s) and further sections
   70496 Computed tomographic angiography, head, with contrast material(s), including noncontrast images, if performed, and image postprocessing

   Because the study was not performed with image postprocessing, the correct code is 70470.

Multiple Choice Answers

1. The correct answer is **c.** The Radiology Guidelines under Administration of Contrast Material state, "The phrase 'with contrast' used in the codes for procedures using contrast for imaging enhancement represents contrast material administered intravascularly, intra-articularly or intrathecally." Answer **a.** is incorrect, as it includes the administration of oral contrast. Answer **b.** is incorrect, as the guidelines are specific as to what is considered contrast material. Answer **d.** is incorrect, as contrast material administered orally or rectally is not considered contrast material.

2. The correct answer is **b.** Answer **a.** is incorrect because, although CPT code 76856 represents a nonobstetric pelvic ultrasound, it does not represent a transvaginal approach. Answer **c.** is incorrect because, although CPT code 76817 represents a transvaginal approach, it describes an ultrasound for a *pregnant* uterus. Answer **d.** is incorrect because, although code 76857 represents a pelvic ultrasound, it is for a limited study and does not represent a transvaginal approach.

3. The correct answer is **d.** Answer **a.** is incorrect, as there is no need to append the bilateral modifier 50 because CPT code 77057 represents a bilateral procedure and CAD was not utilized. Answer **b.** is incorrect, as CAD was not utilized. Answer **c.** is incorrect, as there is no need to append the bilateral modifier 50 because the CPT code 77057 represents a bilateral procedure.

4. The correct answer is **b.** Answer **a.** is incorrect, as it does not include the RT modifier to indicate the study was performed on the right breast. Answer **c.** is incorrect, as CPT code 76604 is for an ultrasound of the chest. Answer **d.** is incorrect, as the correct answer was listed as answer **b.**

5. The correct answer is **c.** Answer **a.** is incorrect, as protons are positively charged atomic particles and are used for proton beam delivery treatment. Answer **b.** is incorrect, as radionuclides are radioactive isotopes used for nuclear medicine services such as SPECT. Answer **d.** is incorrect, as dosimetry is the measurement of the dose of radiation.

6. The correct answer is **d.** The radiation oncology subsection and subheadings are divided into professional and technical components, the level of service provided, and the number of sources.

7. The correct answer is **a.,** 76805-26 Ultrasound, pregnant uterus, real time with image documentation, fetal and maternal evaluation, after first trimester (> or = 14 weeks 0 days), transabdominal approach; single or first gestation, and 76810-26 Ultrasound, pregnant uterus, real time with image documentation, fetal and maternal evaluation, after first trimester (> or = 14 weeks 0 days), transabdominal approach; each additional gestation. Because Mrs. Williams is pregnant with twins, two codes are used: one for the first gestation (twin A) (76805) and one for the second gestation (twin B) (76810). Because you are coding for the professional component only, you will append CPT modifier 26 to both codes. Answer **b.** is incorrect, as it does not include the add-on code for the additional gestation (twin B). Answer **c.** is incorrect, as this represents the service taking place in the first trimester. Answer **d.** is incorrect, as it does not include the modifier for the professional component (26).

8. The correct answer is **c.,** 58340 Catheterization and introduction of saline or contrast material for saline infusion sonohysterography (SIS) or hysterosalpingography, and 74740 Hysterosalpingography, radiologic supervision and interpretation. Because this service includes an interventional procedure (catheterization and introduction of contrast), two codes are required: one for the interventional component and one for the radiological component. Answer **a.** is incorrect, as it does not include the supervision and interpretation provided for the study. Answer **b.** is incorrect, as it does not include the introduction of the contrast material. Answer **d.** is incorrect, as there is no need to append modifier 26 to the supervision and interpretation because both services were provided globally by the radiologist.

9. The correct answer is **d.,** 77080 Dual-energy x-ray absorptiometry (DEXA), bone density study, 1 or more sites; axial skeleton (e.g., hips, pelvis, spine). Answer **a.** is incorrect, as CPT code 77082 represents a DEXA for a vertebral fracture assessment. Answer **b.** is incorrect, as CPT code 77079 is a CT bone mineral density study. Answer **c.** is incorrect, as CPT code 77080 includes all sites evaluated (spine and hips) and therefore should not be reported twice. Additionally, modifier 50 bilateral procedure would not be appended, as the code includes all sites evaluated.

10. The correct answer is **a.** You would report the service as an additional treatment session. Answer **b.** is incorrect, as the guidelines state, "Code 77427 is also reported if there are three or four fractions beyond a multiple of five at the end of a course of treatment." Answer **c.** is incorrect: as per the guidelines, there is no need to append a reduced service modifier. Answer **d.** is incorrect, as the fraction *would* need to be a part of the course of treatment to be reported.

CHAPTER 12

Pathology

Pathology is the study and diagnosis of disease through the examination of tissues, bodily fluids, organs, and whole bodies (autopsy). Pathology is divided into two major specialties: anatomic (deals with tissue diagnosis) and clinical (deals with laboratory test diagnosis). Additional board-certified subspecialties include dermatopathology (skin pathology), hematopathology (bone marrow and clotting disorders), transfusion medicine (blood banking and donation of blood products), forensic pathology (coroners and medical examiners), and cytopathology (Pap smears and fine-needle aspirations).

Pathologists are physicians who diagnose and treat patients through laboratory medicine. They take at least 4 years of training after medical school to familiarize themselves with the various aspects of the laboratory. Pathologists may also manage the hospital's blood supply to ensure its safety and investigate the cause of unknown deaths.

Most people visit a cardiologist or a neurologist, but **how often has anyone** scheduled an appointment with a pathologist? Usually, pathologists see specimens, not people.

For example, during a routine visit to the gynecologist, a Pap smear might be performed. The gynecologist will send the specimen to the laboratory for examination by a pathologist. The results of this examination by the pathologist are sent back to the treating physician (the gynecologist), who will utilize this information when developing the patient's treatment plan.

Pathologists can analyze a variety of specimens, such as blood, urine, fluid, or a piece of tissue. The specimens may be analyzed for a number of reasons: to confirm a diagnosis, to measure the therapeutic effects of a drug, to determine the absence or presence of a drug, to name a few.

Specimens may be taken in a variety of methods by a variety of health-care providers. A blood specimen might be taken by a technician at a laboratory drawing station, a medical assistant in a physician's office, or even by the physician.

A specimen might be surgically removed, such as fluid aspirated from a breast cyst, a lesion excised from the skin, or a polyp removed from the colon via colonoscopy.

Because pathology deals with specimens, the CPT codes in the Pathology and Laboratory section of the CPT book are codes that describe services that are performed on specimens.

A specimen is a sample of tissue (e.g., urine, blood).

A block is a frozen piece of specimen.

A section is a thinly sliced piece of frozen block which is prepared for rapid microscopic examination while the patient is still on the operating table.

When coding for pathology and laboratory services, it is important to keep the following in mind:

- The *CPT codes in this section describe the laboratory test only.* CPT codes for the collection of specimens (e.g., venipuncture, lumbar puncture) and for the specimen handling are located in other sections of the CPT book. For example, the CPT code for the venipuncture is located in the Surgery section, and the CPT code for the specimen handling is located in the Medicine section.

- Many laboratory CPT codes include a technical and a professional component. The technical component represents the cost of the equipment, the services of the technician, and the supplies. The professional component represents the service provided by the physician.

How the Pathology and Laboratory Section is Organized

The Pathology and Laboratory section is organized according to the type of test performed (e.g., panels, drug testing, therapeutic drug assays)—18 such subsections in all.

Let's take a look at various subsections.

The Pathology and Laboratory Codes—and How to Use Them

Organ or Disease-Oriented Panels
80047–80076

The first subsection is Organ or Disease-Oriented Panels. A panel is a group of tests that are commonly performed together for a specific purpose. (However, the panels described in this section were developed for *ease of coding* only and are not intended to reflect clinical parameters.)

For example: The CPT code 80047 Basic metabolic panel (Calcium, ionized) **must** include the following: Calcium, Ionized (82330), Carbon Dioxide (82374), Chloride (82435), Creatinine (82565), Glucose (82947), Potassium (84132), Sodium (84295), and Blood Urea Nitrogen (BUN) (84520).

Therefore, in order for you to select CPT code 80047, *all of the laboratory tests included in the basic metabolic panel must have been performed.* If even one of the tests listed in the panel is not performed, and all of the other tests are, you would code each test individually.

If any laboratory tests are performed in addition to the tests included in the panel, those tests should be reported separately *in addition* to the panel.

Drug Testing
80100–80104

Drug Testing is the next subsection, which includes CPT codes 80100–80104. These tests are *qualitative,* meaning that the test is performed to determine if the drug is present or absent. If it is determined that the drug is present, a confirmation test (CPT code 80102) may be performed.

LET'S LOOK AT AN EXAMPLE

A 20-year-old female with a history of illegal drug use comes to the emergency room in a coma. The treating physician orders a drug screen for amphetamines, barbiturates, benzodiazepines, cocaine and metabolites, and opiates. The laboratory performs single drug class screening for each analyte using a multiple analyte rapid test immunoassay kit.

How to Code: In this scenario, you would report CPT code 80101 five times because immunoassay single drug class methods would be reported regardless of platform (random access analyzer or multiple analyte test kit). Five units are reported, as each separate drug class is reported separately.

Therapeutic Drug Assays
80150–80299

Therapeutic drug assays are *quantitative* tests, meaning that these tests are performed to determine the exact amount of the drug that is present.

For example: A 52-year-old male with bipolar disorder being treated with the drug lithium presents to the clinic for a follow-up visit. During the examination, the physician draws blood and sends the specimen to the laboratory to be analyzed to determine if the patient's level of lithium meets the therapeutic levels required to effectively treat the patient's condition.

In this scenario you would report CPT code 80178 Lithium.

Evocative/Suppression Testing
80400–80440

These tests involve the administration of evocative or suppressive agents (which are administered by the physician) and the baseline and subsequent measurement of their effects on chemical constituents.

For example: A growth hormone (GH) test measures the amount of human growth hormone in the blood. Too much GH during childhood can cause a child to grow larger than normal, whereas too little GH during childhood can cause a child to grow less than normal. For this test, the patient is given an intravenous solution of insulin or arginine (the evocative agent). At timed intervals, blood samples are drawn, and GH levels are tested in each sample to see if the pituitary gland was stimulated by the insulin (or arginine) to produce expected levels of GH.

This test involves more than just the evaluation of the GH level in the blood (the pathology portion); it also involves a physician component, which consists of the administration of the evocative or suppressive agents, the supplies and drugs, the blood drawings, and the physician monitoring. It is important to note that coding from other sections of the CPT is therefore required to properly report this test. To report the physician's administration of the evocative or suppressive agents, see CPT codes 96360, 96361, 96372–96374, and 96375 in the Medicine section of the CPT book. For the supplies and drugs, see CPT code 99070 (in the Medicine section of the CPT book, under "Miscellaneous Services") or the appropriate HCPCS codes. You would also report the appropriate level of evaluation and management code and the appropriate infusion codes. Prolonged physician attendance codes may also be used if applicable.

Consultations (Clinical Pathology)
80500, 80502

The consultation services described by CPT codes 80500 and 80502 are consultations provided at the request of an attending physician requiring additional medical interpretation of test results. When selecting these codes, it is important to keep in mind the following:

■ The consultation was requested by an attending physician.

■ Additional medical interpretive judgment is required.

■ A written report is required.

CPT code 80500 represents a limited consultation, which does not require a review of the patient's history and medical records. CPT code 80502 is comprehensive and therefore does require a review of the patient's history and medical records.

Urinalysis and Chemistry
Urinalysis Codes: 81000–81099

The urinalysis codes are selected by the method (e.g., dipstick), the purpose (e.g., pregnancy test), or the element evaluated (e.g., bilirubin). The tests can be automated (done by a machine) or nonautomated (done manually) and are coded accordingly.

For example: CPT code 81000 Urinalysis, by dip stick or tablet reagent for bilirubin, glucose, hemoglobin, ketones, leukocytes, nitrite, pH, protein, specific gravity, urobilinogen, any number of these constituents; non-automated, with microscopy.

Chemistry Codes: 82000–84999

The chemistry codes identify specific tests, and the material for examination may come from any source (e.g., breath, feces) unless specified by the code descriptor.

The codes in this subsection are identified by the specific test performed, if the test was automated or nonautomated, the number of tests performed, whether the test was qualitative or quantitative, and the method of testing.

Many common laboratory tests are located in this subsection. For example, at one time or another we may have experienced a burning pain between the breast bone and the belly button when our stomach is empty, between meals, or maybe in the early morning hours. This might be accompanied by nausea, vomiting, and loss of appetite and may be relieved by taking antacids. Your physician might order a *Helicobacter pylori (H. pylori)* breath test analysis (83013) to determine if the cause of the discomfit is due to an *H. pylori* infection.

In this chemistry test, the sample is the air you breathe into a balloon-type bag. Two samples are taken: one as a baseline, and the second is taken after drinking a lemon-flavored solution. The breath samples are tested for an increase in carbon dioxide.

Hematology and Coagulation
85002–85999

Hematology is the study of diseases of the blood and blood-forming tissues. Coagulation is the process by which blood changes from a liquid to a solid (clotting). As such, the codes in this subsection are for services that evaluate blood and blood clotting. Also included in this subsection are codes for bone marrow smear and smear interpretations (85060, 85097). Many of these tests can be easily located in the index by the name of the test performed (e.g., Complete Blood Count (CBC), Bleeding Time). Codes may sometimes be selected on the basis of whether testing is automated or nonautomated.

For example: CPT codes 85044 Blood count; reticulocyte, manual and CPT code 85045 Blood count; reticulocyte, automated both represent the same test (the testing of reticulocytes [immature red blood cells that contain mitochondria and ribosomes] reported as a percentage of total red blood cells). However, one test is performed by a manual method, and the other is automated.

Immunology
8600–86849

Immunology is the study of the immune system (cells and molecules) and its function (protecting the body from infections and diseases). The codes in this section categorize antigen and antibody laboratory services (86000–86804). An antigen is a foreign particle that enters the body. This could be a disease-causing agent such as a virus or a particle of pollen or dust. An antibody is a protein made by the body's immune system. When antigens enter the body, it is the immune system that produces antibodies to fight against the antigens. The CPT codes in this section identify tests used to evaluate conditions of the immune system that have been caused by the action of antibodies (e.g., allergic reactions).

Tissue Typing (CPT codes 86805–86849) is also listed within the Immunology subsection. These codes identify services provided to determine compatibility of a recipient and a donor for organ or bone marrow transplants.

Transfusion Medicine
86850–86999

The CPT codes in this section are most often used by blood banks. The tests in this section include screening tests, compatibility tests, and blood preparation services for transfusions.

Microbiology
87001–87999

Microbiology is the study of microorganisms such as bacteria, viruses, fungi, and parasites. In this section, you will find culture codes that identify not only the organism but also the sensitivities of the organism to an antibiotic. Before selecting the CPT code, read the descriptor carefully, as culture codes may be used for tests in which a specific organism is identified or may involve the sensitivity of the organism to an antibiotic.

For example: CPT code 87070 Culture, bacterial; any other source except urine, blood or stool, aerobic, with isolation and presumptive identification of isolates. This code describes throat culture (growing a culture in a dish, which will allow an infection to grow) through which isolates are identified. CPT code 87184 Susceptibility studies, antimicrobial agent; disk method, per plate (12 or fewer agents) is a sensitivity test to determine the *susceptibility* of a bacterium to an antibiotic.

Anatomic Pathology
88000–88099

The codes in this section represent a postmortem examination by gross (by the naked eye) and/or microscopic viewing. The codes are further determined by the extent of the examination performed.

For example: CPT code 88007 Necropsy (autopsy), gross examination only; with brain and spinal cord describes an examination by sight (gross) and includes the brain and spinal cord, whereas CPT code 88025 Necropsy (autopsy), gross and microscopic; with brain describes a gross and microscopic examination and includes only the brain. Carefully read the code descriptors before making your code selection to ensure you have the correct type of examination and extent of examination.

Cytopathology and Cytogenic Studies
Cytopathology Codes: 88104–88199

Cytopathology is a branch of pathology that studies and diagnoses diseases of the cells. The specimens are obtained by brushing, washing, needle biopsy, or fine-needle aspiration. The most common example is the Pap test. The codes in this section are listed by the method by which the specimen was collected from the patient.

Cytogenic Studies Codes: 88230–88299

Cytogenic studies is the branch of genetics that tests for the structure and function of the cells, in particular the chromosomes.

Surgical Pathology

Surgical pathology is the gross and/or microscopic examination of specimens for the purpose of diagnosis of disease. The surgical pathology codes are divided into six levels according to the type of examination, the type of specimen, and the reason for the examination. Let's look at the different levels.

Level I (CPT code 88300)

This level is reported for any specimen that is examined by gross examination only.

Level II (CPT code 88302)

This level is reported for gross and microscopic examination of specimens that have been removed for a reason other than disease or malignancy—**for example,** a fallopian tube for sterilization, or the removal of skin for a plastic repair. (Hint: When selecting this code, think "normal.")

Level III (CPT code 88304)

This level is reported for gross and microscopic examination of specimens that are *uncomplicated or have a low risk of disease or malignancy*—**for example,** skin cyst/tag/débridement; polyps, inflammatory nasal/sinusoidal.

Level IV (CPT code 88305)

This level is reported for gross and microscopic examination of specimens *having a higher risk of disease or malignancy*—**for example,** skin other than cyst/tag/débridement/plastic repair; kidney biopsy.

Level V (CPT code 88307)

This level is reported for gross and microscopic examination of specimens *of a complex nature*—**for example,** kidney, partial/total nephrectomy; brain, biopsy

Level VI (CPT code 88309)

This level is reported for gross and microscopic examination of specimens of a *very high complexity, multiple complicated* specimens (larynx, partial/total resection with regional lymph nodes), or specimens that are *neoplastic in nature*.

So you can see by the different levels that in some cases the specimen may be the same, but the level of surgical pathology is different. This is because the reason for the surgery was different.

For example:

CPT code 88302 Level II: Surgical pathology, gross and microscopic examination

Skin, *plastic repair*

CPT code 88304 Level III: Surgical pathology, gross and microscopic examination Skin, *cyst/tag/débridement*

Whereas both CPT codes include the gross and microscopic examination of the skin, CPT code 88302 describes the **skin for plastic repair** and CPT code 88304 describes the **skin as cyst/tag/débridement.**

KEY CODING TIP

You can determine the appropriate level of surgical pathology by:

- The type of examination (gross or gross and microscopic)
- The type of specimen (cornea, heart valve, etc.)
- The reason for the surgical procedure (plastic repair, cyst/tag/débridement)

The remaining subsections in the Pathology section are In Vivo, Other Procedures, and Reproductive Medicine Procedures, which represent specialized testing, new technology, and evolving reproductive testing.

Modifiers

Pathologists may use various modifiers as appropriate. Listed below are the most common modifiers applicable to pathology. The CPT modifiers are a two-position numeric code added to the end of a CPT code that alert the insurance carrier that something is different about the CPT code that is being reported (see Chapter 7).

As mentioned earlier in this chapter, the CPT codes in the Pathology and Laboratory section include both the technical and professional components of the service provided. The technical component represents the laboratory equipment, the technician, and supplies, and the professional component represents the skill of the physician in interpreting the test.

If the physician has an in-office laboratory, owns the equipment, and interprets the test, the physician will bill *globally* (i.e., for both the technical and professional components). This is indicated by billing the CPT code without any modifiers. It is also important to note, for physicians to bill for in-office laboratory services, they are required to become certified under the Clinical Laboratory Improvement Amendments of 1988 (CLIA). There are, however, some laboratory tests that are CLIA-waived.

Modifier 26—Professional Component

Certain procedures are a combination of a physician component and a technical component. When the physician component is reported separately, the service may be identified by adding modifier 26 to the usual procedure number.

If the physician does not own the equipment and is responsible for the professional component, he or she will append modifier 26 to the CPT code.

TC—Technical Component

Under certain circumstances, a charge may be made for the technical component alone. Under those circumstances, the technical charge is identified by adding modifier TC to the usual procedure number.

In the same scenario as that in which modifier 26 is used, the laboratory that owned and used the equipment and supplies and provided the technician to run the test will report the same CPT code with modifier TC (which is an **HCPCS modifier**) to indicate the technical portion of the service.

For example, for CPT code 88305 Level IV Surgical Pathology:

88305-26: This would be reported by the physician providing the professional service.

88305-TC: This would be reported by the laboratory providing the technical service.

88305: The CPT code with no modifier would be reported when both the professional and technical (global) services are provided by the same physician/facility.

Modifier 90—Reference (Outside Laboratory)

When laboratory procedures are performed by a party other than the treating or reporting physician, the procedure may be identified by adding modifier 90 to the usual procedure number.

■ Modifier 90 is used when a physician who does not have an in-office laboratory has an arrangement with a laboratory by which the laboratory will bill the physician and in turn the physician will bill the patient or the insurance carrier.

■ It is *not* used for Medicare patients. (The Centers for Medicare and Medicaid Services do not recognize use of this modifier.)

Note: Use of this modifier is carrier-specific. Insurance carriers should be contacted to determine if they recognize use of modifier 90.

Modifier 91—Repeat Clinical Diagnostic Laboratory Test

In the course of treatment of the patient, it may be necessary to repeat the same laboratory test on the same day to obtain subsequent (multiple) test results. Under these circumstances, the laboratory test performed can be identified by its usual procedure number and the addition of modifier 91. Note: This modifier may not be used when tests are rerun to confirm initial results; due to testing problems with specimens or equipment; or for any other reason when a normal, one-time reportable result is all that is required. This modifier may not be used when other code(s) describe a series of test results (e.g., glucose tolerance tests, evocative/suppression testing). This modifier may only be used for laboratory test(s) performed more than once on the same day on the same patient.

■ It is used when a laboratory test needs to be repeated *on the same day* to obtain multiple test results.

■ It is used when the laboratory test is the same (i.e., repeated) and performed on the same patient on the same day.

- It is *not* used to confirm an initial laboratory result.
- It is *not* used when a laboratory test needs to be repeated due to equipment failure or a spoiled specimen.
- It is *not* used when a CPT code describes a *series* of tests (e.g., glucose tolerance tests, evocative/suppression testing).

LET'S LOOK AT AN EXAMPLE

A diabetic patient undergoes a glucose blood test that indicates a high glucose level. The patient is then treated with Glucophage (a drug used to treat high blood sugar) and monitored in the office. A glucose blood test is repeated later that same day, and the results indicate a declining glucose level.

How to Code: In this scenario, CPT code 82962 Glucose, blood by glucose monitoring device(s) would be reported twice (82962, 82962-91).

Modifier 92—Alternative Laboratory Platform Testing

When laboratory testing is being performed using a kit or transportable instrument that wholly or in part consists of a single-use, disposable analytical chamber, the service may be identified by adding modifier 92 to the laboratory procedure code (HIV testing 86701–86703). The test does not require permanent dedicated space; hence by its design, it may be hand carried or transported to the vicinity of the patient for immediate testing at that site, although location of the testing is not in itself determinative of the use of this modifier.

This modifier applies to three codes:

- 86701 Antibody; HIV-1
- 86702 Antibody; HIV-2
- 86703 Antibody; HIV-1 and HIV-2, single assay

This modifier identifies laboratory testing performed by a kit or transportable instrument that wholly or in part consists of a single-use, disposable analytical chamber.

Modifier QW—CLIA Waived Test

This is an HCPCS modifier. It is appended to laboratory tests that have been designated "CLIA waived" (certain laboratory tests may be provided in a physician office without a CLIA certification if the test has been designated as CLIA waived).

Let's Practice Coding

Surgical Pathology

The patient presents with a clinical history of uterine cancer. The patient underwent a total abdominal hysterectomy (corpus and cervix), with the removal of tubes and ovaries. The pathologist performs a gross and microscopic examination of the uterus.

To find the correct CPT code, we would look in the CPT index under Pathology, Surgical, then Gross and Micro Exam. To determine the correct level of surgical pathology, we would need to read the descriptors for CPT code 88302–88309 (Level II–Level VI). We can now apply the Key Coding Tip. We know the specimen is both gross and microscopic (this was narrowed down by the code range 88302–88309), and the type of specimen is the uterus. A review of the CPT codes in our code range narrows the code selection to 88305–88309, as CPT code 88302 and 88304 do not include uterus as a specimen. Next we look for the reason for the procedure, in this case, uterine cancer. A review of CPT code 88305 Surgical Pathology Level IV shows an examination of the uterus, with or without ovaries, for prolapse. Because prolapse is not the reason for the examination of the specimen, we need to look further. CPT code 88307 Surgical Pathology Level V lists uterus with or without tubes and ovaries other than neoplastic/prolapsed. Once again, neither of these reasons describes uterine cancer, so we continue to look further toward CPT code 88309 Surgical Pathology Level VI, which lists uterus, with or without tubes and ovaries, neoplastic, which describes the type of examination (gross and microscopic, the type of specimen [uterus] and the reason for the examination [neoplastic]).

Learn More About It

The more you read, the more you know. Increase your knowledge with the following resources:

Recommended Web Sites

http://www.cms.hhs.gov/clia
The CMS Web site for rules and regulations regarding CLIA certification

http://www.abpath.org/default.aspx
American Board of Pathology

http://www.abpath.org/links.htm
American Board of Pathology List of Links

STOP-LOOK-HIGHLIGHT

The key to successfully passing the exam and selecting the correct code lies in your knowing how to use your coding book.

To help you navigate through your codebook, and to make sure you have the most important information at your fingertips when you take the exam, highlight key text in the chapter guidelines and subheadings, and insert simple notes and coding tips directly into your codebooks.

When highlighting, use two different color highlighter pens: yellow for standard guidelines and global services and an alternate color for carve-outs and unique notes.

Under Pathology and Laboratory on the Guidelines, in red ink, please write the following:

- *Services for the collection of specimens (e.g., venipuncture) are not located in the Pathology/Laboratory section. They are located in their respective sections of CPT.*

- *The CPT code for the handling and/or conveyance of specimen for transfer from the physician's office to a laboratory (99000) is located in the Medicine section.*

In the Subsection Organ or Disease-Oriented Panels:

- *Highlight the first sentence in yellow: "These panels were developed for coding purposes only and should not be interpreted as clinical parameters."*

- *In the second paragraph, please highlight in yellow the second sentence: "If one performs tests in addition to those specifically indicated for a particular panel, those tests should be reported separately in addition to the panel code."*

In the Subsection Drug Testing:

- *In yellow, highlight the word "qualitative" in the first sentence.*

In the Subsection Therapeutic Drug Assays:

- *In yellow, highlight the word "quantitative" in the first sentence.*

In the Subsection Evocative/Suppression Testing:

- *In the subsection guidelines, the fourth sentence down, highlight in yellow: "These codes are to be used for the reporting of the laboratory component of the overall testing protocol. For the physician's administration of the evocative or suppressive agents, see 96360, 96361, 96372–96374, 96375; for the supplies and drugs, see 99070. To report physician attendance and monitoring during the testing, use the appropriate evaluation and management code, including the prolonged physician care codes if required. Prolonged physician care codes are not separately reported when*

evocative/suppression testing involves prolonged infusions reported with 96360, 96361."

In the Subsection Consultations (Clinical Pathology):

- *Highlight in yellow the first paragraph: "A clinical pathology consultation is a service, including a written report, rendered by the pathologist in response to a request from an attending physician in relation to a test result(s) requiring additional medical interpretive judgment."*

- *Using your alternate color highlight the second paragraph: "Reporting of a test result(s) without medical interpretive judgment is not considered a clinical pathology consultation."*

In the Subsection Surgical Pathology:

- *Highlight in yellow the first line of the third paragraph: "Service code 88300 is used for any specimen that in the opinion of the examining pathologist can be accurately diagnosed without microscopic examination."*

- At the bottom of the page, in red ink, please write the following:
  - *Gross—means by sight (examination by the naked eye)*
  - *To select the correct level of surgical pathology, determine:*
    - *The type of examination*
    - *The type of tissue*
    - *The reason for the surgical procedure*

Vocabulary Words

In your CPT book on the blank Note page for Pathology and Laboratory, write the Pathology and Laboratory Vocabulary Words:

Antibodies–Proteins in the body, made by the immune system, that fight infection and disease.

Antigen–Foreign substances that elicit the formation of antibodies.

Assay–The quantitative or qualitative analysis of a substance or mixture.

Automated–A laboratory test performed by a machine.

Block–A frozen piece of specimen.

Coagulation–The process by which blood changes from a liquid to a solid (clotting).

Gross–Examination by the naked eye.

Hematology–The study of diseases of the blood and blood-forming tissues.

Necropsy–Autopsy: an examination and dissection of a dead body to determine cause of death or the changes produced by disease

Nonautomated–A laboratory test performed manually.

Panel–A group of tests that are commonly performed together for a specific purpose.

Qualitative–The performance of a test to determine the presence or absence of a drug.

Quantitative–The performance of a test to determine the exact amount of the drug that is present.

Section–A thinly sliced piece of frozen block, which is prepared for rapid microscopic examination while the patient is still on the operating table.

Specimen–A sample of tissue (e.g., urine, blood).

Acronyms and Abbreviations

In your CPT book on the blank Note page for Pathology and Laboratory, write the following acronyms and abbreviations:

CBC–**C**omplete **B**lood **C**ount

CLIA–**C**linical **L**aboratory **I**mprovement **A**mendments

RBC–**R**ed **B**lood **C**ount

WBC–**W**hite **B**lood **C**ount

TAKE THE CODING CHALLENGE

Assign the Appropriate Pathology and Laboratory Code

1. CPK isoenzymes

2. Lyme disease antibody

3. Bilirubin total transcutaneous

4. Urinalysis pregnancy test

5. Prothrombin time

Multiple Choice

1. Mr. Smith was seen by his primary care physician as a follow-up for his high blood pressure. As part of the examination, the physician performed a basic metabolic panel in his in office laboratory.
   a. 82310, 82374, 82435, 82565, 82947, 84132, 84295
   b. 80048
   c. 80048, 82310, 82374, 82435, 82565, 82947, 84132, 84295
   d. 80048-26

2. Dr. Michaels ran an automated complete blood count (CBC) in his in office laboratory for Mrs. Fredricks. Due to equipment failure, Dr. Michaels had to rerun the test.
   a. 85027
   b. 85027, 85027-91
   c. 82057-52
   d. 82057, 82057-TC

3. When all of the laboratory tests in a panel are performed along with additional laboratory tests not included in the panel, you code:
   a. Only for the panel
   b. Only for the additional tests
   c. Both the panel and the additional tests not included in the panel
   d. The code for the panel with modifier 22 for an increased procedural service

4. Dr. Franklin, who is a pathologist in a hospital setting, provides professional services for surgical pathology specimens. He was asked to provide surgical pathology for the following specimen: an ovary with or without tube, nonneoplastic. Please code for Dr. Franklin's professional service.
   a. 88307
   b. 88307-26
   c. 88305-TC
   d. 88305-26

5. Seven-year-old Gregory presents to his pediatrician, and as part of his routine physical examination, the physician implants a purified protein derivative (PPD). Gregory will return to the physician in 2 days for the PPD reading. Code only for the implant of the PPD.
   a. 86580, 99211
   b. 99393, 86580
   c. 86580
   d. 86580-TC

6. CPT codes listed in the Evocative/Suppression Testing subsection of the Pathology and Laboratory section include the following:
   a. The physician's administration of the evocative or suppressive agents
   b. Prolonged attendance
   c. The supplies and drugs
   d. None of the above

7. Modifier 91 Repeat Clinical Diagnostic Laboratory Test is always appended to the second test when:

a. In the course of treatment of the patient, it may be necessary to repeat the same laboratory test on the same day to obtain subsequent (multiple) results

b. To rerun tests to confirm initial results

c. The specimen becomes tainted or spoiled

d. Both **a.** and **b.**

8. A patient on lithium had her blood sent to the laboratory to determine if the amount of drug in her system is at the therapeutic level.

a. 80176

b. 80103

c. 80178

d. 80102

9. CPT codes in the Pathology and Laboratory section may be billed for:

a. Only the professional component

b. Only the technical component

c. Globally

d. Any of the above

10. CPT codes most often reported by blood banks are located in this subsection:

a. Other Procedures

b. Hematology and Coagulation

c. Microbiology

d. Transfusion Medicine

CODING CHALLENGE ANSWERS AND RATIONALES

Assign the Appropriate Pathology and Laboratory Code

1. The correct answer is 82552 Creative kinase (CK), (CPK); isoenzymes. You will look this up in the CPT index under **CPK,** then **Blood.** You will be presented with a range of codes: 82550–82552. You will now look up the CPT codes in the Pathology section, where your codes choices are:
82550 Creatine kinase (CK), (CPK); total
82552 Creatine kinase (CK), (CPK); *isoenzymes*
The test performed is for isoenzymes; therefore, CPT code 82552 is the correct code.

2. The correct answer is 86618 Antibody; Borrelia burgdorferi (Lyme disease). You will look this up in the CPT index under **Lyme disease.** You are presented with a range of codes: 86617–86618. You will now look up the CPT codes in the pathology section, where your code choices are:
86617 Antibody; Borrelia burgdorferi (Lyme disease) *confirmatory test* (e.g., Western Blot or immunoblot)
86618 Antibody; Borrelia burgdorferi (Lyme disease)
Although both CPT codes describe the test for Lyme disease, CPT code 86617 indicates the test is confirmatory. Because the test we are coding for was not specified as confirmatory, the correct code is 86618.

3. The correct answer is 88720 Bilirubin, total, transcutaneous. You will look this up in the CPT index under **Bilirubin,** then **Total,** then **Transcutaneous.** Although you are given just one code selection, 88720, you should always verify the code by looking it up in the appropriate section of the CPT book, in this case the pathology section, where you can confirm it is the correct code.

4. The correct answer is 81025 Urine pregnancy test, by visual color comparison methods. You will look this up in the CPT index under **Urinalysis,** then **Pregnancy Test.** You will be presented with only one option, 81025. Although you are given just one code selection, you should always verify the code by looking it up in the appropriate section of the CPT book, in this case the pathology section, where you can confirm it is the correct code.

5. The correct answer is 85610 Prothrombin time. You will look this up in the CPT index under **Prothrombin Time.** You will be presented with a

range of codes: 85610–85611. You will now look up the CPT codes in the pathology section, where your code choices are:
85610 Prothrombin time;
85611 Prothrombin time; substitution, plasma fractions, each
Although both CPT codes describe the test for prothrombin time, CPT code 85611 indicates the test is substitution, plasma fractions. Because the test we are coding for only indicates the prothrombin time, the correct code is 85610.

Multiple Choice Answers

1. The correct answer is **b. CPT code 80048** represents the panel that includes CPT codes 82310, 82374, 82435, 82565, 82947, 84132, 84295, and 84520. Answer **a.** is incorrect, as it lists the codes separately. When all the tests in a panel are performed, only the CPT code for the panel should be coded. Answer **c.** is incorrect, as this lists the code for the panel and each code with the panel separately. Answer **d.** is incorrect, as the physician has his own in-office laboratory and provided both the professional and technical components of the service; therefore, he can bill globally, and no modifier is necessary.

2. The correct answer is **a.,** CPT code 85027 Blood count; complete (CBC), automated (Hgb, Hct, RBC, WBC and platelet count). (Note: The tests in the parentheses indicate the tests included in a complete blood count.) You may code the test only once, for the time it was completed. Answer **b.** is incorrect, as modifier 91 may not be used for testing that must be repeated due to testing problems with specimens or equipment. Answer **c.** is incorrect because modifier 52 for reduced services is not applicable, as the test was able to be completed. Answer **d.** is incorrect, as you may code the test once only for the time it was completed, and the HCPCS modifier TC is not applicable, as the physician has an in-office laboratory and will code for the global service.

3. The correct answer is **c.** The subsection guidelines under Organ or Disease-Oriented Panels state, "If one performs tests in addition to those specifically indicated for a particular panel, those tests should be reported separately in addition to the panel code." Answer **a.** is incorrect, as coding only for the panel does not provide reimbursement for the additional tests performed. Answer **b.** is incorrect, as it does not include the CPT code for the panel of tests performed, and answer **d.** is incorrect, as modifier 22 for increased procedural service is not applicable. Each service provided can be represented by a specific CPT code.

4. The correct answer is **d., CPT code 88305 Level IV surgical pathology, gross and microscopic examination, ovary with or without tube, non-neoplastic, with modifier -26.** The scenario indicated Dr. Franklin is providing only the professional service (and not the equipment), which requires modifier 26. Answer **b.** is incorrect because this code is for Level V, surgical pathology, gross and microscopic examination ovary with or without tube, *neoplastic.* Answer **a.** is likewise incorrect, as this code is for Level V, surgical pathology, gross and microscopic examination ovary with or without tube, **neoplastic.** It also does not include modifier 26. Answer **c.** is incorrect because, although the CPT code 88305 is correct, the HCPCS modifier TC is incorrect, as this represents the technical component and not the professional service.

5. The correct answer is **c. CPT code 86580 Skin test; tuberculosis, intradermal,** represents the PPD only. Answer **a.** is incorrect, as it includes a low-level office visit, and we are asked to code only for the implant of the PPD. Answer **b.** is incorrect, as it includes the preventive visit, and we are asked to code only for the implant of the PPD. Answer **d.** is incorrect, as it includes the HCPCS modifier TC, which represents only the technical component, which is not applicable, as the physician who implanted the PPD will also read the results.

6. The correct answer is **d.,** none of the above. The subsection guidelines under Evocative/Suppression Testing state, "These codes are used for the reporting of the laboratory component of the overall testing protocol." Answers **a., b.,** and **c.** represent the physician component of the test and are coded from the appropriate corresponding sections of the CPT book (e.g., Evaluation and Management section, Medicine section).

7. The correct answer is **a.** Appendix A in the CPT provides a complete description of modifier 91 and states this modifier may be used only when "in the course of treatment of the patient, it may be necessary to repeat the same laboratory test on the same day to obtain subsequent (multiple) test results." Answer **b.** is incorrect, as the note included with the full descriptor of modifier 91 states this modifier is not used rerun tests to confirm initial results. It is not the intent of this modifier to allow additional reimbursement for repeat clinical diagnostic laboratory testing without medical necessity. Answer **c.** is incorrect. A specimen that is spoiled or tainted does not provide medical necessity to repeat the test at the cost of the insurance carrier.

8. The correct answer is **c., 80178 Lithium.** This CPT code is from the Therapeutic Drug Assay subsection and is used to report a quantitative examination to test for the amount of drug present—in this case, lithium. Answer **a.** is incorrect, as it is the code for testing lidocaine. Answer **b.** is incorrect, as this is for tissue preparation for drug analysis. Answer **d.** is incorrect, as this is a drug confirmation test.

9. The correct answer is **d.** CPT codes in the Pathology and Laboratory section may be coded for the professional component only, the technical component only, or globally for both the professional and technical components.

10. The correct answer is **d.** The CPT codes in the Transfusion Medicine subsection are most often used by blood banks, as they include services such as blood typing and compatibility tests. Answer **a.** is incorrect, as services in the Other Procedures subsection represent specialized testing, new technology, and evolving reproductive testing. Answer **b.** is incorrect; although hematology is the study of diseases of the blood and coagulation is the process by which blood changes from a liquid into a solid, the CPT codes in the Transfusion subsection represent screening and compatibility tests as well as blood preparation services for transfusions. Answer **c.** is incorrect, as the Microbiology subsection represents culture codes that identify organisms and the sensitivities of the organism to an antibiotic.

CHAPTER 13

Medicine

The Medicine section provides codes for a broad variety of services, including services of all specialties. Most of the services listed in this section are noninvasive or minimally invasive diagnostic and therapeutic procedures. The codes in this section may be reported alone or, as more commonly seen, in addition to CPT codes from other sections of the CPT book, such as office visits, preventive visits, and consultations.

For example, it is quite common to receive a vaccine and/or an electrocardiogram (EKG) when you present for your annual preventive visit. The CPT code for the preventive visit is located in the Evaluation and Management (E/M) section of the CPT manual, and the codes for vaccines, vaccine administration, and EKG are all located in the Medicine section.

Many of the diagnostic tests and procedures performed by specialists during an office visit are also located in the Medicine section. A pulmonologist might perform a spirometry, an allergist might provide allergy testing, and a neurologist might perform a nerve conduction study, all in addition to an office visit. The CPT codes for the spirometry, allergy testing, and nerve conduction are all located in the Medicine section.

The Medicine section also includes CPT codes for other types of health-care professionals, such as physical therapists, occupational therapists, audiologists, and many others.

The Medicine section is utilized by providers as frequently as is the E/M section. Therefore, it is recommended that each year when the new CPT codes come out, the Medicine section should be reviewed along with the E/M section and the specialty-specific section for the physician or group you are coding for.

How the Medicine Section is Organized

Because the Medicine section offers CPT codes for all different specialties, it is organized differently than the other sections of the CPT manual. The Medicine section is organized by the types of services (e.g., biofeedback, dialysis) and by specialty (e.g., gastroenterology, ophthalmology).

In some cases, the subsections are further divided by the tests and services provided.

For example: The Allergy and Clinical Immunology subsection (95004–95199) is further divided into:

Allergy Testing (95004–95075): Testing

Allergen Immunotherapy (95115–95199): Services

Let's Review the Medicine Guidelines

The Medicine section guidelines are similar to those found in the Surgery section, as they once again provide us with the definitions of "separate procedures," "materials supplied by physician," and "special report."

The Medicine section guidelines also provide us with additional coding guidance for "multiple procedures" and "add-on codes."

In the case of multiple procedures, CPT allows for the reporting of separate CPT codes when multiple procedures/services have been provided.

For example: An established 22-year-old patient received an intramuscular flu shot along with his preventive visit. We would report the following CPT codes:

99395 Periodic comprehensive preventive medicine visit, established patient; 18–39 years

90471 Immunization administration (includes percutaneous, intradermal, subcutaneous, or intramuscular injections); 1 vaccine (single or combination vaccine/toxoid)

90658 Influenza virus vaccine, split virus, when administered to individuals 3 years of age and older, for intramuscular use

In this scenario, multiple CPT codes are required to accurately report the services provided.

Add-on codes in the Medicine section have the same definition as those located in the preceding sections of the CPT manual. Because add-on codes are not reported separately and are not considered to be standalone codes, they are exempt from the multiple procedure concept. Therefore, you would never append modifier 51 (multiple procedures) to an add-on code.

For example: Two hours of intravenous hydration would be reported as:

96360 Intravenous infusion, hydration; initial, 31 minutes to 1 hour

+ 96361 Intravenous infusion, hydration; each additional hour *(List separately in addition to code for primary procedure)*

We would report CPT code 96360 for the first hour, whereas the second hour is reported with the add-on code 96361. CPT code 96361 is not considered a standalone code, as you would not be able to report an additional hour of intravenous therapy without having to report the primary procedure (the initial hour) first. You can see how easy it is to identify the add-on code by the plus sign and the terminology "list separately in addition to the code for the primary procedure." Also note there is no need to append modifier 51, as the terminology in the add-on code indicates this is a second procedure.

KEY CODING TIP

Add-on codes:

■ Are never reported alone. They are always reported in addition to the primary procedure code.

■ Are identified by a + sign in front of them.

■ Have descriptors that include terminology such as *"each additional"* or *"list in addition to primary procedure."*

■ Are modifier 51 (multiple procedure) exempt.

Located in the Medicine section guidelines, you will also find a list of unlisted CPT codes that are found in this section.

In addition, the Medicine section guidelines include a list of the Subsection Information. This lists the various subsections of the Medicine section in the order in which they appear and their CPT code ranges. As you can see, this includes everything from immunizations to psychiatry, ophthalmology, dialysis, and allergy, to name just a few. Because the Medicine section is very extensive, we review only some of its more commonly used codes.

The Medicine Codes—and How to Use Them

Immunization Administration for Vaccines/Toxoids
90460–90474

The vaccine administration codes represent the "administration" of the vaccine and are reported in addition to the CPT code for the vaccine that was given to the patient. The vaccine administration codes include:

■ Services provided by the administrative staff, such as preparing the patient's record and scheduling the appointment.

■ Clinical services, such as preparing and administering the vaccine, taking vital signs, reviewing the patient's vaccine history and any past reactions, answering any questions, and documenting the medical record.

Let's Try Another

Jimmy, a 6-year-old established patient, presented to the pediatrician's office for his preventive visit. After a comprehensive history and physical examination and the ordering of the age-appropriate tests, the physician counseled Jimmy's mother on the potential side effects of the MMR, IPV (inactivated poliovirus vaccine), and intranasal flu vaccine that were administered to Jimmy.

Let's highlight the key words necessary to code this service. Using the Key Coding Tip, we would highlight the **age of the patient** (6 years old), **the counseling** (physician counseled Jimmy's mother), and **the vaccines** that were administered (MMR and IPV). In addition, as discussed in the E/M chapter, we would also highlight the status of the patient (established), the type of visit provided (preventive visit), and the supporting documentation for the preventive visit (comprehensive history and physical examination and the ordering of the age-appropriate tests). We already highlighted the age of the patient (6 years old), which is also a key factor in the code selection for a preventive visit.
Jimmy, a 6-year-old established patient *presented to the pediatrician's office for his* preventive visit*. After a* comprehensive history and physical examination, *and the ordering of the age appropriate tests,* the physician counseled Jimmy's mother *on the potential side of effects of the* MMR, and IPV (inactivated poliovirus vaccine), *that were* administered *to Jimmy.*

First, we would code for the E/M service—namely, the office visit and the level of service provided. As

Let's Try Another—cont'd

discussed in Chapter 8, this will include determining the type of office visit provided (in this case, preventive) and patient status (in this case, an established patient). Preventive medicine services for an established patient age 6 years would be reported with CPT code 99393.

99393 Periodic comprehensive established preventive (age 5 through 11 years)

Then we would code for the immunizations:

90460 Immunization administration through 18 years of age via any route of administration, with counseling by physician or other qualified health-care professional; first vaccine/toxoid component

90713 Poliovirus vaccine, inactivated (IPV), for subcutaneous or intramuscular use

90707 Measles, mumps and rubella virus vaccine (MMR), live, for subcutaneous use

+ 90461 × 3 Immunization administration through 18 years of age via any route of administration, with counseling by physician or other qualified health-care professional; each additional vaccine/toxoid component (List separately in addition to code for primary procedure) (The + sign and the words "each additional injection" indicate this is an add-on code.) **Note:** This code would be reported three times, once for each of the vaccine/toxoid components, as the CPT code descriptor states, "each additional **vaccine/toxoid component.**"

KEY CODING TIP

When coding vaccine administration services, consider the following:

- The route of administration (subcutaneous, intranasal, oral, intravesical, intramuscular, or intradermal)
- The age of the patient
- If physician counseling was provided
- The number of vaccine/toxoid components
- Many vaccines are given in combination as one vaccine. For example: measles, mumps, and rubella are all administered in one shot of MMR vaccine. In this case, the vaccine has three components (a component refers to each antigen in a vaccine). Vaccine counseling codes would be reported for each antigen when face-to-face counseling is provided by a physician or other qualified health-care professional. Combination vaccines administered without counseling would be reported with CPT codes 90471–90474, which do not recognize separate vaccine/toxoid components only single or combination vaccines.

KEY CODING TIP

- Report a vaccine administration code for each vaccine provided.
- Only one initial vaccine administration code may be reported. Additional vaccine administrations are reported with the appropriate add-on code for each additional vaccine administration.

As you can see, there is a lot to consider before you can select the vaccine administration code.

Let's Try One Together

An established 19-year-old patient presented to the physician's office for her MMR (measles, mumps, rubella) vaccine.

Let's highlight the key words necessary to code this service. Using the Key Coding Tip, we would highlight the **age of the patient** (19 years old) and the **vaccine(s) administered** (MMR).

Because the documentation does not support a preventive visit (documentation of a comprehensive history, comprehensive physical examination, anticipatory guidance, and ordering of appropriate laboratory tests) or an office visit (documentation of the key components, history, physical, medical decision making), you would code only for the vaccine *administration* and for the vaccine itself. Note: The vaccine administration code was selected on the basis of the age of the patient (19 years old), the route of administration (injectable), and the fact that no physician counseling was provided.

An established 19-year-old patient presented to the physician's office for her MMR (measles, mumps, rubella) vaccine.

The encounter would be coded as follows:

90471 Immunization administration (includes percutaneous, intradermal, subcutaneous, or intramuscular injections); 1 vaccine (single or combination vaccine/toxoid) *Note*: CPT code 90471 is reported only once as the code descriptor states, "**single or combination vaccine/toxoid.**"

90707 Measles, mumps and rubella virus vaccine (MMR), live, for subcutaneous use

Psychiatry

The Medicine section includes specific codes for psychiatry services, such as psychiatric evaluation, psychotherapy, and prescription and review of medications. Psychiatrists may choose to report their services with codes from the E/M section or the codes in this subsection that refer to the specialty-specific services provided by behavioral health providers (psychiatrists, psychologists, and licensed clinical social workers), some of which include psychotherapy services *with* evaluation and management service.

These codes describe many of the patient encounters specific to behavioral health providers. Because they are specific to one specialty, we will notice there is a difference between the E/M code descriptors and the psychiatry code descriptors for the psychiatric diagnostic interview (90801–90802) and the psychotherapy codes (90804–90829).

One of the first differences we notice is that the codes are categorized as either "insight oriented" or "interactive psychotherapy." **Insight-oriented services** are those in which the patient is aware of the character of the illness and verbally communicates during the therapy session. **Interactive psychotherapy** involves the use of physical aids (dolls, drawings) and nonverbal communication during the therapy session.

Next we notice many of the codes are time-based: 20–30 minutes face-to-face with the patient, 45–50 minutes face-to-face, and so on.

The codes are further divided depending on whether a medical evaluation and management service was provided along with the psychotherapy and where the service was provided (outpatient or inpatient hospital, partial hospital, or residential care facility).

As you can see, there are many factors to consider before selecting the appropriate CPT code.

Let's take a closer look at the psychotherapy codes.

Psychiatric Diagnostic Interview 90801, 90802.

The first two codes, 90801 and 90802, represent the psychiatric diagnostic interview. This is a comprehensive examination of the patient, which includes a history and examination, a mental status examination, a patient disposition, communication with family members or other sources, and the medical interpretation and ordering of laboratory and/or diagnostic studies as applicable. The diagnostic interview can be either insight oriented or interactive. These two codes are not time-based.

Time-Based Psychotherapy Codes 90804–90829.

CPT codes 90804–90829 represent time-based psychotherapy codes. They are organized according to whether they are provided in an outpatient setting, inpatient hospital, partial hospital, or residential care facility and are divided depending on whether they are with or without E/M services.

KEY CODING TIP

When coding psychotherapy services, consider the following:

- Where the service was provided (outpatient, inpatient, and so on)
- Whether it was insight-oriented or interactive psychotherapy
- The amount of time documented
- Whether the service was provided with or without an E/M service

---

LET'S LOOK AT AN EXAMPLE

Edward Jones presented for his outpatient psychotherapy session. His main concern was his frequent panic attacks. He denied feeling stressed at this time but admitted to many stressful situations. He states that during these stressful times, he experiences vomiting, loss of appetite, and difficulty breathing. Since the death of his father, he has become fearful of losing his children to death or an accident. He often thinks about missing people or dead people. Mr. Jones agreed to meet again next week for his regular therapy session to work on his issues. The session lasted for 48 minutes.

How to Code: First we determine where the service took place (outpatient). Next we determine the type of therapy; because Mr. Jones was able to verbally communicate his concerns and no interactive aids were utilized, the therapy was insight oriented. Then we note the duration of the therapy (48 minutes). Because no E/M service was documented, the correct CPT code is 90806 Individual psychotherapy, insight oriented, behavior modifying and/or supportive, in an office or outpatient facility, approximately 45 to 50 minutes face-to-face with the patient.

KEY CODING TIP

When looking up psychiatric codes in the CPT index, most of the codes will be listed under **Psychiatric Diagnosis** and **Psychiatric Treatment.**

Other Psychotherapy. These services include *psychoanalysis* (the specific method of psychological therapy developed by Sigmund Freud, which investigates the role of the subconscious mind in mental and emotional disorders) and *family and group therapy services;* these services are *not time-based.*

Other Psychiatric Services or Procedures. These include services such as pharmacological management (management of the patient's prescriptions, including minimal psychotherapy), hypnotherapy, narcosynthesis (a form of psychotherapy provided after the patient has been administered a drug [sedative or narcotic]), and electroconvulsive therapy.

Other services include environmental intervention for medical management; psychiatric evaluation of hospital records; interpretation or explanation of psychiatric records or results of procedures; and the preparation of a report of the patient's psychiatric status for other physicians, agencies, or insurance carriers. *With only one exception, these services are **not time-based.***

The only time-based service in this subheading is represented by the codes 90875 Individual psychophysiological therapy incorporating biofeedback training by any modality (face-to-face with the patient), with psychotherapy (e.g., insight oriented, behavior modifying or supportive psychotherapy); approximately 20–30 minutes and 90876—for approximately 45–50 minutes. These codes are reported when biofeedback is provided at the same time of a psychotherapy session.

Biofeedback. Biofeedback is a technique by which patients are trained to gain some control over certain physiological conditions, such as blood pressure and muscle tension. There are two codes reported for biofeedback: CPT code 90901, which is used to report biofeedback *without* the use of psychophysiological therapy, and CPT code 90911 Biofeedback training, perineal muscles, anorectal or urethral sphincter, including EMG and/or manometry. This is a specific biofeedback method that is more involved than the conventional biofeedback methods identified in CPT code 90901.

Ophthalmology
92002–92499

Like psychiatrists, ophthalmologists may choose to report their services with codes from the E/M section or the codes in this Ophthalmology subsection of the Medicine section.

The notes located at the beginning of the Ophthalmology subsection are key to understanding the different levels of ophthalmology services (intermediate and comprehensive) and the services that are inclusive to these codes.

The ophthalmology visit codes are divided into two categories, new patient (92002–92004) and established patient (92012–92014), and are further divided according to the level of service provided, intermediate or comprehensive.

Comprehensive ophthalmological services include:

■ General evaluation of complete visual system.

■ History, general medical observation, external and ophthalmoscopic examinations, gross visual fields, and basic sensorimotor examination

■ (Often) as indicated: biomicroscopy, examination with cycloplegia or mydriasis, and tonometry

■ (Always): initiation of diagnostic and treatment programs

Intermediate ophthalmological services include:

■ Evaluation of new or existing condition *complicated with a new diagnostic or management problem* not necessarily relating to the primary diagnosis.

■ History, general medical observation, external ocular and adnexal examinations, and other diagnostic procedures as indicated: may include mydriasis for ophthalmoscopy.

KEY CODING TIP

Many services located under Special Ophthalmological Services are for bilateral services. Read the code descriptors carefully. If the service is bilateral but performed on only one eye, you will need to report the service as a *reduced* service by appending modifier 52.

Pulmonary
94002–94799

CPT codes located in this subsection include both diagnostic tests (pulmonary function testing) and therapeutic treatments (nebulizer treatments).

Pulmonary function tests are performed to determine how well the lungs are working. The tests include a **spirometry** (94010–94070) to measure the amount of air the lungs can hold, **lung volume tests (e.g., 94150)** to measure the amount of air remaining in the lungs after exhaling, and lung diffusion tests and pulse oximetry (94760–94762), which measures the amount of oxygen that passes from the lungs to the blood.

Pulmonary stress tests (94620, 94621) are comprehensive tests that include many other tests. When coding for pulmonary stress tests, you need to read the complete code descriptor to determine what is included.

For example: 94620 Pulmonary stress testing; simple (e.g., 6-minute walk test, prolonged exercise test for bronchospasm with *pre- and postspirometry and oximetry)*. This test *includes* the *pulse oximetry* and the *pre- and postspirometry.* Therefore, the pulse oximetry and the spirometry should not be separately reported.

Only one code is used when reporting multiple nebulizer treatments: 94640. If multiple nebulizer treatments are required on the same day, CPT code 94640 should be reported for each treatment provided. For more than 1 inhalation treatment performed on the same date, append modifier 76.

LET'S LOOK AT AN EXAMPLE

An established patient who is a known asthmatic presents to the office with diffuse wheezing and bronchospasm. A nebulizer treatment is administered using a metered-dose inhaler and chamber. After 30 minutes the treatment is repeated with good clinical results and relief for the patient.

How to Code: In this case, CPT code 94640 Pressurized or nonpressurized inhalation treatment for acute airway obstruction or for sputum induction for diagnostic purposes (e.g., with an aerosol generator, nebulizer, metered dose inhaler or intermittent positive pressure breathing [IPPB] device) would be reported twice 94640, 94640-76.

One code that is often confused with CPT code 94640 (the code for nebulizer treatment) is CPT code 94664 Demonstration and/or evaluation of patient utilization of an aerosol generator, nebulizer, metered-dose inhaler or IPPB (intermittent positive pressure breathing).

CPT code 94664 describes the following:

■ Demonstration of a metered-dose inhaler or a nebulizer

■ Bronchodilator administration for the purpose of long-term management of bronchospasm

■ Bronchodilator administration to mobilize sputum for therapeutic purposes (i.e., movement of thick secretions)

■ Bronchodilator administration to mobilize sputum for sputum induction for diagnostic studies (e.g., culture, Gram stain)

LET'S LOOK AT AN EXAMPLE

A 5-year-old patient has been newly diagnosed with asthma. The patient is placed on a metered-dose inhaler with a chamber. The patient's mother is given instruction on how to properly use the device and administer the medication. The patient is observed during the treatment and evaluated for her response, and the mother is evaluated on the proper use of the equipment and medication.

How to Code: In this scenario, the correct CPT code is 94664 for the demonstration and evaluation of the patient utilization of the device. You would not report a nebulizer treatment along with CPT code 94664, as the nebulizer treatment is considered bundled or inclusive with this service.

Physical Medicine and Rehabilitation
97001–97755

Physical medicine and rehabilitation is a branch of medicine that focuses on enhancing and restoring functional ability and the quality of life to those with physical disabilities or impairments.

A *physician* who *specializes in physical medicine and rehabilitation* is called a *physiatrist.* The services in this subsection can be provided by either physicians or qualified therapists.

The services listed in this subsection include therapeutic evaluations and reevaluations, modalities, therapeutic procedures, active wound-care management, tests and measurements and orthotic management, and prosthetic management. Additionally, many of the modalities and the therapeutic procedures are time-based.

Let's take a closer look at some of these services.

Therapeutic Evaluations. The CPT codes for therapy evaluations are divided by the type of evaluation (physical therapy, occupational therapy, or athletic training) and are further divided by evaluation and reevaluation.

The services in this section include both physical and occupational therapy.

Physical therapy (PT) is a rehabilitative process following disease or injury; its purpose is to restore maximum movement and functional ability to individuals by use of specially designed exercises and equipment.

Occupational therapy (OT) is therapy or treatments designed to enable individuals with limitations or impairments to perform or maintain the ability to perform tasks of daily living (e.g., bathing, dressing).

Modalities. Modalities are a variety of treatment tools (e.g., hot and cold packs, whirlpool) used by therapists to decrease pain, inflammation, and muscle strains and sprains. The modalities listed in CPT are further divided according to whether the modality was *"supervised"* (the application of a modality that *does not require direct [one-on-one] patient contact by the provider*) and *"constant attendance"* (the application of a modality that *requires direct [one-on-one] patient contact by the provider).* You will notice the modalities that are *time-based* are listed *under constant attendance* and modalities that are *not time-based* are listed *under supervised.* It is also important to note that in some cases, the same modality is listed under both categories. For example:

97014 Application of a modality to 1 or more areas; electrical stimulation (unattended). *Not time-based and listed under "supervised."*

97032 Application of a modality to 1 or more areas; electrical stimulation (manual), each 15 minutes. *Time-based and listed under "constant attendance."*

Whereas both services appear to be the same, the context in which they are provided is different.

Therapeutic Procedures. Therapeutic services require the physician or the therapist to have direct (one-on-one)

patient contact and as such are time-based. Therefore, time must be documented in the patient's medical record.

LET'S LOOK AT AN EXAMPLE

During Mary Schmidt's physical therapy session for improvement of her left knee pain, she received 6 minutes of unattended electrical stimulation, 30 minutes of therapeutic exercises, and 15 minutes of massage therapy.

How to Code: In this scenario, we would code the following:

97014 Electrical stimulation unattended
97110 x 2 Therapeutic exercises (We would code two units, as 30 minutes of therapeutic exercises was provided.)
97124 Massage therapy

KEY CODING TIP

When coding physical medicine and rehabilitation services, read the code descriptor carefully to determine the following:

- What type of therapy was provided (physical therapy, occupational therapy)
- Whether the modality was supervised (not time-based) or constant attendance (time-based)
- The amount of time spent on providing therapeutic services and/or time-based modalities (necessary to determine the number of units reported)

LET'S LOOK AT AN EXAMPLE

Ernest Williams is a 54-year-old established patient who presented for his physical therapy session for bilateral ankle pain. The therapy session included 30 minutes of therapeutic activities, 15 minutes of ultrasound, and the application of hot and cold packs.

How to Code: Let's highlight the key words necessary to code this service. First, we would highlight the **type of therapy** provided (physical therapy services). Next, we would highlight the **amount of time spent** on the services (30 minutes of therapeutic, 15 minutes of ultrasound). Finally, we would highlight **the hot and cold packs.** Notice the time was not documented for the hot and cold packs, as this is not a time-based CPT code. Therefore, it would be reported only once per treatment session.

In this scenario we would code the following:

97530 × 2	Therapeutic activities (30 minutes, 2 units)
97035	Ultrasound (15 minutes, 1 unit)
97010	Hot and cold packs (supervised, not timed; therefore, it is listed only once)

KEY CODING TIP

CPT codes for modalities 97010–97028 are reported only once per modality per treatment session.

Special Services, Procedures, and Reports
99000–99091

These codes represent the completion of special reports and services that are reported in addition to a basic procedure code. Reimbursement for these services will vary depending on the insurance carrier, and Medicare does not reimburse for these services.

These services are listed under Miscellaneous Services and include services such as specimen handling (99000–99001), services provided on an emergency basis in the office that disrupt other scheduled office services (99058), and special reports (99080) such as insurance forms that provide more information than that conveyed in the usual medical communications or standard reporting form.

Many of the CPT codes in the miscellaneous section are reported *in addition* to the code for the service performed (i.e., the basic procedure code).

LET'S LOOK AT AN EXAMPLE

An established patient presents to the physician's office in respiratory distress, which requires unscheduled emergency care by the physician. The physician was in the process of treating another patient whose care was interrupted by the emergency situation. The physician evaluated the patient in respiratory distress and documented an expanded problem-focused physical examination and medical decision making of high complexity.

How to Code: In this scenario, CPT code 99058 Office services provided on an emergency basis would be reported in addition to the basic procedure code, in this case, the office visit (99213).

Let's Practice Coding

Now that you have a good understanding of services in the Medicine section and have prepared your CPT book, you are ready to code.

Locating Medicine Codes

Because there are many types of services (psychiatry, physical therapy, vaccines, etc.) located in the Medicine section, it is important to remember from the earlier chapter on CPT there are many different ways to look up a CPT code (e.g., procedure, anatomical site).

For example, we can look up the code for "gait training," which is a physical therapy service, by looking up *"gait training"* in the CPT index:

Gait Training..97116

    OR

by looking up *"Physical Medicine/Therapy/Occupational Therapy."* (Note: If we look up Physical Therapy, we are instructed to "See Physical Medicine/Therapy/Occupational Therapy.") The codes are then divided by they type of service (modality, procedure, etc.) and then by specific service. As in the example of gait training:

Physical Medicine/Therapy/Occupational Therapy
Procedures
    Aquatic Therapy......................97113
    Direct.....................................97032–97039
    Gait Training...........................97116

Let's look up the ophthalmology code for an initial eye examination for a new patient.

Ophthalmology codes are located in the CPT index under "Ophthalmology, Diagnostic." The subheading will list the type of service provided (e.g., color vision examination, computerized scanning), in this case, *"eye exam,"* and the subterm, *"New Patient,"* which presents a code range of 92002–92004.

    OR

In the CPT index, we could look up the term *"Eye Exam,"* subheading *"New Patient,"* and be presented with the same code range: 92002–92004.

92002 Ophthalmological services: medical examination and evaluation with initiation of diagnostic and treatment program; intermediate, new patient

92004 Ophthalmological services: medical examination and evaluation with initiation of diagnostic and treatment program; comprehensive, new patient, 1 or more visits

The determining factor for the code selection is the type of examination (intermediate or comprehensive).

The same method of look-up would be applied to most of the services within the Medicine section.

There are a few exceptions. For example, the CPT codes for immunization administrations are located in the CPT index under "Immunization Administration"; however, the CPT codes for the vaccine administered are located in the CPT index under "Vaccines."

Immunization Administration

Each Additional Vaccine/Toxoid.......90472, 90474
    With Counseling...............90461
H1N1...................................90470
One Vaccine/Toxoid..................90471, 90473
    With Counseling...............90460, 90470

Vaccines

Adenovirus...90476–90477

Anthrax..90581

Chickenpox...90716

Learn More About It

The more you read, the more you know. Increase your knowledge with the following Web site:

The Centers for Medicare and Medicaid Services Medical Policy Center

http://www.cms.gov/medicare-coverage-database/overview-and-quick-search.aspx

Once on this site, look for the local coverage determinations (LCDs) for your jurisdiction and search for the LCDs for:

Cataract Extraction

Chiropractic Services

Nerve Conduction Studies

Outpatient Physical and Occupational Therapy Services

Outpatient Psychiatry and Psychology Services

STOP-LOOK-HIGHLIGHT

The key to successfully passing the exam and selecting the correct code lies in your knowing how to use your coding book.

To help you navigate through your codebook, and to make sure you have the most important information at your fingertips when you take the exam, highlight key text in the chapter guidelines and subheadings, and *write* simple notes and coding tips directly into your codebooks.

When highlighting, use two different color highlighter pens: yellow for standard guidelines and global services and an alternate color for carve-outs and unique notes.

In the Subsection Immunization Administration for Vaccines/Toxoids:

- In the description of CPT code 90460, highlight in yellow: *"through 18 years of age," "with counseling by physician or other qualified health care professional" and "vaccine/toxoid component."*
- *In the description of CPT code 90471, highlight the word "injections" and "single or combination vaccine/toxoid."* Also, write in red ink after the code description: *"no age and no counseling."*
- In the description of CPT code 90473, highlight the words "intranasal or oral" and "single or combination vaccine/toxoid." Also write after the code description: *"no age and no counseling."*
- At the bottom of the page write:

The Key Coding Tips for Vaccine Administration:

The route of administration.

The age of the patient.

If physician counseling was provided.

The number of vaccine/toxoid components.

Report a vaccine administration code for each vaccine provided.

Only one initial vaccine administration code may be reported. Additional vaccine administrations are reported with the appropriate add-on code for each additional vaccine administration.

In the Subsection Psychiatric Diagnostic or Evaluative Interview Procedures:

- Highlight in yellow the two paragraphs before CPT code 90801. This provides the definition of what is included in a psychiatric diagnostic interview and interactive psychiatric diagnostic interview.
- At the bottom of the page, write:

Psychiatric Key Coding Tips:

Where the service was provided

Whether it was insight-oriented or interactive psychotherapy

The amount of time documented

Whether it was provided with or without E/M service

- Also, write at the bottom of the page: *"Most, but not all, psychiatry codes are time-based."*
- Under Biofeedback, highlight in yellow: "(For psychophysiological therapy incorporating biofeedback training, see 90875, 90876)."

In the Ophthalmology Section:

- Highlight in yellow the definitions for intermediate ophthalmological services and comprehensive ophthamological services.
- Under Special Ophthalmological Services, write, *"Most of these services are bilateral procedure codes; if performed on one eye, append modifier 52 reduced services."*

In the Physical Medicine and Rehabilitation subsection:

- Under the subheading Modalities, Category, upervised, highlight in yellow the definition of supervised: "the application of a modality that does not require direct (one-on-one) patient contact by the provider."
- Under the subheading Modalities, Category, Constant Attendance, highlight in yellow the definition of constant attendance: "The application of a modality that

requires direct (one-on-one) patient contact by the provider."

■ At the bottom of the page write:

Physical Medicine and Rehabilitation Key Coding Tips:

What type of therapy was provided (physical therapy, occupational therapy)?

Was the modality supervised (not time-based) or constant attendance (time-based)?

What was the amount of time spent on providing therapeutic services and/or time-based modalities (necessary to determine the number of units reported)?

Medicine Section Vocabulary Words

On the blank Note page at the end of the Medicine section, write the following vocabulary words:

Biofeedback–A technique using specialized equipment by which patients are trained to recognize and manipulate signals sent by their bodies and by which they learn to gain some voluntary control over certain physiological conditions, such as muscle tension and involuntary functions such as blood pressure.

Gonioscopy–An examination of the front part of the eye to check the angle where the iris meets the cornea. Gonioscopy is used to distinguish between open-angle glaucoma and closed-angle glaucoma.

Insight-oriented therapy–The patient is aware of the character of the illness and verbally communicates during the therapy session.

Interactive psychotherapy–Involves the use of physical aids (dolls, drawings) and nonverbal communication during the therapy session.

Occupational therapist–A health professional trained to help people who are ill or disabled learn to manage their daily activities.

Physiatrist–A physician who specializes in physical medicine and rehabilitation services.

Physical therapist–A therapist who treats injury or dysfunction with exercises and other physical treatments.

Psychophysiological therapy–A natural way of balancing the mental, emotional, and physical aspects of the body.

Medicine Section Acronyms and Abbreviations

On the blank Note page at the end of the Medicine section, write the following acronyms and abbreviations:

HepB–**Hep**atitis **B**

HIB–**H**emophilus **I**nfluenza **B**

IPPB–**I**ntermittent **P**ositive **P**ressure **B**reathing

IPV–**I**nactivated **P**olio **V**irus

MMR–**M**easles, **M**umps, and **R**ubella

MMRV–**M**easles, **M**umps, **R**ubella, and **V**aricella

OT–**O**ccupational **T**herapy

PFT–**P**ulmonary **F**unction **T**esting

PT–**P**hysical **T**herapy

TAKE THE CODING CHALLENGE

Assign the Appropriate Medicine Code

1. Pharmacological management

2. Gonioscopy

3. Pulse oximetry, single determination

4. Medical testimony

5. Gait training

Multiple Choice

1. Sarah, a 28-year-old established patient, was seen by her primary care physician as a follow-up for her asthma. The physician documented a problem-focused history, an expanded problem-focused physical examination, and medical decision of low complexity. During the examination, the physician also administered an intranasal flu vaccine. The correct codes for *all* services provided by the physician would be:
   a. 99213, 90471, 90660
   b. 90473, 90660
   c. 99213, 90473, 90658
   d. 99213, 90473, 90660

2. An insight-oriented psychiatric diagnostic interview includes:
   a. History, mental health status, disposition, communicating with family or other sources, interpretation of laboratory/diagnostic studies
   b. History, mental health status, disposition, interpretation of laboratory/diagnostic studies
   c. History, mental health status, disposition, communicating with family or other sources, communication with use of physical aids, interpretation of laboratory/diagnostic studies
   d. History, mental health status, disposition, communicating with family or other sources, interpretation of laboratory/diagnostic studies, amount of time documented

3. When an established patient presents to a physician's office for the sole purpose of receiving a vaccine with no other service(s) provided, you would code:
   a. A brief office visit, the appropriate vaccine administration code, and the CPT code for the vaccine administered
   b. The appropriate vaccine administration code and the CPT code for the vaccine administered
   c. The age-appropriate preventive visit code, the appropriate vaccine administration code, and the vaccine administered
   d. A brief office visit (only if the vaccine was administered by the physician), the appropriate vaccine administration code, and the CPT code for the vaccine administered

4. Mrs. Fredericks was in the waiting room area of Dr. Franklin, a cardiologist. While she was waiting to be seen for her complaint of chest pain and tightness, she started to experience shortness of breath and became lightheaded. She immediately informed the front desk staff of her condition and was quickly placed in an examination room. Dr. Franklin was alerted to the emergency and stepped out of the examination room where he was providing follow-up care to another patient to treat Mrs. Fredericks. Dr. Franklin documented a problem-focused history, a detailed examination, and diagnosis of a panic attack with a medical decision of moderate complexity. The total time spent providing emergency care was 40 minutes. The correct code(s) for Dr. Franklin's services would be:
   a. 99291, 99058
   b. 99058
   c. 99214, 99058
   d. 99284, 99058

5. A visual field examination was performed. However, due to recent right eye surgery, the limited visual field was performed on only the left eye. The correct code is:
   a. 92081
   b. 92081-LT, -52
   c. 92082
   d. You would not report a CPT code, as the service was not performed bilaterally.

6. Ophthalmologists may use the following CPT code(s) to report their visits:
   a. Only codes from the Ophthalmology subsection for new and established patients
   b. Consultation codes from the E/M section and codes from the Ophthalmology subsection for new and established patients
   c. Any codes from the E/M section or codes from the Ophthalmology subsection for new and established patients
   d. The CPT codes they select will be insurance-carrier specific.

7. What is the type of procedure provided to a patient after the administration of a drug for psychiatric diagnostic and therapeutic purposes?
   a. Biofeedback
   b. Insight-oriented psychotherapy with E/M
   c. Pharmacological management
   d. Narcosynthesis

8. Mrs. Donaldson received 30 minutes of neuromuscular reeducation of movement, balance, and coordination; electrical stimulation, and 10 minutes of diathermy. Select the correct CPT codes:
   a. 97112 × 2, 97032, 97024
   b. 97112 × 2, 97014, 97024
   c. 97112, 97032, 97024
   d. 97112 × 2, 97014

9. CPT codes in the medicine section include:
   a. CPT codes for all specialties
   b. CPT codes for diagnostic and therapeutic procedures
   c. CPT codes for procedures that are noninvasive or minimally invasive
   d. All of the above

10. A separate procedure is one that:
    a. May never be reported on its own, as it is an integral part of a large procedure
    b. Is always reported on its own; hence the definition "separate"
    c. May be reported by itself when it is not done in conjunction with another larger service or procedure of which it is an integral part
    d. Will only be found in the Medicine section of the CPT manual

ANSWERS AND RATIONALES

Assign the Appropriate Medicine Code

1. The correct answer is 90862 Pharmacologic management, including prescription, use, and review of medication with no more than minimal medical psychotherapy. You will look this up in the CPT index under **Psychiatric Treatment,** and then **Drug Management.** You will be presented with one code: 90862. You would now look up the code in the Medicine section, where you will confirm that the code is correct.

2. The correct answer is 92020 Gonioscopy (separate procedure). You will look this up in the CPT index under **Gonioscopy.** You will be presented with only one code: 92020. You would now look up the CPT code in the Medicine section, where you will confirm that it is correct.

3. The correct answer is 94760 Noninvasive ear or pulse oximetry for oxygen saturation; single determination. You will look this up in the CPT index under **Oximetry,** which will lead you to **Oximetry (Noninvasive).** You will then look for the subentry **Blood O$_2$ Saturation,** and then **Ear or pulse.** You are presented with a range of codes: 94760–94762. You would now look up the CPT codes in the Medicine section, where your code choices are:
   94760 Noninvasive ear or pulse oximetry for oxygen saturation; single determination
   94761 Noninvasive ear or pulse oximetry for oxygen saturation; multiple determinations (e.g., during exercise)
   94762 Noninvasive ear or pulse oximetry for oxygen saturation; by continuous overnight monitoring (separate procedure)
   Although all three codes describe pulse oximetry, only CPT code 94760 describes a single determination and is therefore the correct choice.

4. The correct answer is 99075 Medical testimony. You can look this up in the CPT index under **Testimony,** then **Medical.** You will be presented with only one option: 99075. Although you are given one code selection, you should always verify the code by looking it up in the appropriate section of the CPT book, in this case Medicine, where you will confirm that it is the correct code.

5. The correct answer is 97116 Therapeutic procedures, 1 or more areas, each 15 minutes; gait training (includes stair climbing). You will look this up in the CPT index under **Gait Training.** You will be presented with

only one option: 97116. Although you are given one code selection, you should always verify the code by looking it up in the appropriate section of the CPT book, in this case Medicine, where you will confirm that it is the correct code.

Multiple Choice Answers

1. The correct answer is **d.** First, we would code for the E/M service: CPT code 99213 accurately describes the correct level of service for the office visit. To code for the flu vaccination, we will need to assign two codes—one for the administration of the vaccine and one for the vaccine itself. CPT code 90473 describes the vaccine administration by intranasal route of administration, and CPT code 90660 describes the intranasal flu vaccine. Answer **a.** is incorrect, because although the code for the office visit (99213) and the flu vaccine (90660) are correct, the code for the vaccine administration is wrong, as it describes a vaccine that was administered by injection. Answer **b.** is incorrect, because although the code for the vaccine administration and flu vaccine are correct, it does not include the code for the office visit (99213). Answer **c.** is incorrect, because although the code for the office visit (99213) and the vaccine administration (90473) are correct, the code for the flu vaccine itself (90658) is incorrect; it describes an injectable flu vaccine.

2. The correct answer is **a.,** history, mental health status, disposition, and communication with family or other sources, interpretation of laboratory/diagnostic studies. This answer can be found in the notes preceding CPT code 90801. Answer **b.** is incorrect, as it does not include the communication with family or other sources. Answer **c.** is incorrect, as the service is insight-oriented psychiatric diagnostic, and physical aids are used in interactive psychotherapy and are not applicable to insight-oriented services. Answer **d.** is incorrect, as psychiatric diagnostic interviews are not timed.

3. The correct answer is **b.** We would code the appropriate vaccine administration code and the CPT code for the vaccine administered. Answer **a.** is incorrect, as an office visit is not coded when the sole purpose of the visit is to receive a vaccine; in this case, the vaccine administration codes already include basic administrative and clinical services related to the administration of the vaccine, such as taking vital signs and reviewing the patient's immunization record. Answer **c.** is incorrect, as a preventive visit would be reported only if provided at the time of the vaccine administration and supported by documentation in the patient's

record. Answer **d.** is incorrect; once again, the vaccine administration codes include basic administrative and clinical services.

4. The correct answer is **c.,** level IV office visit (99214) and office services provided on an emergency basis (99058). Answer **a.** is incorrect, as critical care was not provided. Documenting "emergency care for 40 minutes" does not constitute critical care, and the patient's condition was not indicated as critical (impairment of vital organ systems with a high probability of life-threatening deterioration of the patient's condition). Answer **b.** is incorrect, as 99058 represents only the emergency care, and special service codes are billed in *addition* to the basic service provided, in this case, the office visit. Answer **d.** is incorrect, as CPT code 99284 is for a service provided in an emergency room. Although emergency care was provided, the service took place in the physician's office.

5. The correct answer is **a.,** 92081 Visual field examination, *unilateral or bilateral,* with interpretation and report; *limited examination* (e.g., tangent screen, Autoplot, arc perimeter, or single stimulus level automated test, such as Octopus 3 or 7 equivalent). Answer **b.** is incorrect because, as the descriptor of the CPT code 92081 has already allowed for unilateral service, there is no need to append the reduced service modifier 52. Answer **c.** is incorrect, as CPT code 92082 is for an intermediate visual field examination, whereas this patient received a limited examination. Answer **d.** is incorrect, because a code exists (92081) whose descriptor includes both bilateral *and* unilateral service. However, even if a code includes only bilateral procedures, a unilateral procedure could still be reported by appending modifier 52 to the CPT code to show that the service was reduced.

6. The correct answer is **c.** Ophthalmologists may use either the E/M visit codes OR the ophthalmology visit codes to report their visits. Answer **a.** is incorrect, as they may use either E/M or ophthalmology codes to report their visits. Answer **b.** is incorrect, as they may use *any* of the E/M visit codes that are supported by documentation in the patient's medical record, and not just the consultation codes from the E/M section. Answer **d.** is incorrect, as most of the insurance carriers honor both sets of codes. (However, special services, procedures, and reports, codes 99000–99091, reported in addition to a basic procedure code, are insurance-carrier specific.)

7. The correct answer is **d.** With narcosynthesis, a patient will be administered a drug prior to the psychotherapy session. Answer **a.** is incorrect, as biofeedback is a technique by which patients are trained to gain some control over certain physiological conditions (e.g., high blood pressure). Answer **b.** is incorrect, as no drug is administered during an insight-oriented psychotherapy session. Answer **c.** is incorrect, as pharmacological management refers to the physician's review of the patient's medication along with minimal psychotherapy.

8. The correct answer is **b.** CPT code 97112 describes the neuromuscular reeducation for 30 minutes, CPT code 97014 describes the unattended electrical stimulation, and CPT code 97024 represents the diathermy. Answer **a.** is incorrect, as CPT code 97032 represents electrical stimulation, which is provided with constant attendance; because the documentation does not specifically state the service was provided with attendance nor was time indicated, we would select the unattended CPT code. Answer **c.** is incorrect, as it reports only one unit (15 minutes) of neuromuscular reeducation. Answer **d.** is incorrect, as it does not include the diathermy.

9. The correct answer is **d.** The codes in the Medicine section are used by many different physician specialties and ancillary providers, such as physical therapists, audiologists, ophthalmologists, and psychiatrists. Additionally, the codes in the Medicine section represent diagnostic and therapeutic services and procedures as well as noninvasive or minimally invasive procedures.

10. The correct answer is **c.** This information is located in the Medicine guidelines under "Separate Procedure." Answer **a.** is incorrect, because although a "separate procedure" may sometimes be an integral part of a larger service, it may sometimes be performed not in conjunction with that larger procedure—and in that case, it may be reported on its own. Answer **b.** is incorrect. They are ***not always reported.*** Separate procedures may be reported on their own, or they may be bundled into a larger service and not reported, depending on whether or not they are performed in conjunction with that larger service. Answer **d.** is incorrect, as separate procedures are also located throughout the Surgery section of the CPT manual.

Test-Taking Strategies

In preparation for taking the examination, you have been studying and reviewing the complete coding system for some time now. So right now you are the best you can be. I say this because if you have been working in the field of coding, you more than likely have specialized in one field or another (e.g., cardiology, dermatology), but the examination is based on all aspects and specialties within the coding system. When you have been working with one specialty for so long, you tend to forget how to code the other specialties. So by reviewing and studying the entire coding system (CPT, ICD-9-CM, and HCPCS), you are probably the best you can be, as all this knowledge is fresh in your mind.

The examination is open-book, so you have all the answers. If you prepared your coding books (tools) properly, you will know where to look to find the answer to every question on the examination.

Make sure your coding books are the approved versions allowed to be used for the examination. The American Academy of Professional Coders (AAPC) allows the following manuals and supporting material for the CPC examination:

- CPT (AMA Standard or Professional only)
- Your choice of ICD-9-CM (Expert editions are allowed.)
- Your choice of HCPCS (Expert editions are allowed.)
- Any officially published corrections or errata sheets belonging to the three manuals above
- Tabs may be inserted, taped, pasted, glued, or stapled into your coding books as long as the intent of the tab is to bookmark a page. The tabs may not contain any supplemental information. No other information is allowed to be inserted, taped, pasted, or glued into

the manuals, nor are sticky notes allowed to be inserted into the manuals.

- Handwritten notes commonly used in coding activities are permissible.

The examination lasts 5 hours and 40 minutes. This is a considerable amount of time to spend at one sitting, so come prepared to make yourself as comfortable as possible. Dress in layers: some people tend to become hot or cold at different times during the examination, so dressing in layers helps you control your body temperature for maximum comfort.

You are allowed to eat and drink during the examination. Bring plenty of water and snacks to keep your brain powered and your body hydrated.

You are also allowed breaks during the examination; however, the clock will not stop during your break.

The examination is divided into sections and consists of approximately 150 multiple-choice questions. Sections will focus on medical concepts (medical terminology, anatomy, ICD-9-CM, HCPCS, and coding concepts), surgery and modifiers (questions related to the individual body areas and organ systems in the subsection of the Surgery section), Evaluation and Management, Anesthesia, Radiology, Laboratory and Pathology, and Medicine sections. It is advisable to use all the time you are allotted.

Because the test is time based, you do not have to complete the examination in any particular order. It is strongly recommended you first go through the test and quickly answer the questions to which you know the answer. This will allow you more time for questions requiring more time to answer. Additionally, you may find answers to some of the earlier questions in the body of a later question.

When answering your questions, remember to use the process of elimination where applicable. Many of the questions in the Surgery section will include CPT and ICD-9-CM codes and modifiers. If your strong point is ICD-9-CM, focus on eliminating the answers with the incorrect ICD-9-CM codes; by the same token, if your strong point is CPT or modifiers, you can use the process of elimination by eliminating answers with incorrect CPT or modifiers. You will usually be able to narrow down the selection to two potential answers that will require further investigation.

Let's Try One Together

The patient presented for a retroperitoneal ultrasound for complaints of left upper quadrant abdominal pain and hematuria. Upon complete ultrasonic examination of the kidneys and urinary bladder, the patient was diagnosed with renal calculi. Report the professional component for this service.
a. 76775, 592.0
b. 76770, 592.9
c. 76775-26, 592.9
d. 76770-26, 592.0

Let's look at this example and use the process of elimination by modifier. The question asks us to code for the professional component; therefore, we can eliminate answers **a.** and **b.,** as they do not include the 26 modifier for the professional component. That leaves us with two choices: **c.** or **d.** We can now eliminate one answer by the ICD-9-CM codes. The question states the calculi are renal (592.0); therefore, we can eliminate answer **c.,** as the diagnosis code 592.9 unspecified urinary calculus is incorrect (we know specifically it is a renal calculus). Answer **d.** is the correct choice, as it accurately identifies the ultrasound of the retroperitoneum (76770) for the professional component (modifier 26) and the correct diagnosis code for the renal calculi (592.0).

If we were to eliminate one of the two remaining answers by use of CPT, we would eliminate answer **c.,** as the CPT code in answer **c.** describes a limited retroperitoneal ultrasound. The reason we coded a complete retroperitoneal ultrasound (76770) and not a limited retroperitoneal ultrasound (76775) can be found in the coding guidance provided above the CPT codes, which states, "A complete ultrasound examination of the retroperitoneum (76770) consists of real-time scans of the kidneys, abdominal aorta, common iliac artery origins, and inferior vena cava including any demonstrated retroperitoneal abnormality. **Alternatively, if clinical history suggests urinary tract pathology, complete evaluation of the**

kidneys and urinary bladder also comprises a complete retroperitoneal ultrasound." In this example, the hematuria (blood in urine) and the complete ultrasonic examination of the kidneys and urinary bladder meet the criteria of a complete retroperitoneal ultrasound.

Highlighting key words and terms in the question helps, so highlight as you read. In previous chapters, when we practiced coding, we highlighted key words and terms to help identify the services provided (CPT), the reason for the service (ICD-9-CM), supplies utilized (HCPCS), and any modifying factors (modifiers). You are also allowed to write in your examination booklets, using them as you would scrap paper.

It is also important to remember that the examination is based on the coding guidance, rules, and regulations found in the CPT, ICD-9-CM, and HCPCS books and not on specific insurance requirements.

For example, many insurance carriers consider a venipuncture and/or specimen handling to be inclusive with the office visit, and therefore, you may not code those services for that specific carrier. For the examination, however, you would code both the venipuncture and the specimen handling because, according to CPT, they are not considered bundled or packed into the office visit.

When taking the examination, make sure you put all your answers on the answer grid with a number 2 pencil. It is not advisable to write your answers in the question booklet with the intention of entering them on the answer grid after you have answered all the questions. This is an unwise use of your time and usually results in incomplete or inaccurate transfer of data from the question booklet to the answer grid.

When entering your answers on the answer grid, make sure you filled in the circles and do not have any stray marks on the answer grid.

Never leave any question unanswered. If time is running out, remember to go back and review the test for any unanswered questions. If you are still unsure of an answer, guess. This is the time to trust your gut instincts, which will usually guide you to the correct answer.

You should be using the current version of the coding books that match the year of the examination you are taking. So if you are taking a 2011 examination, your CPT, ICD-9-CM, and HCPCS books should all be the 2011 version.

The best advice anyone could offer you is to make sure you get a good night's sleep before the examination, and stay relaxed and confident. Remember, you are allowed two opportunities to take the examination, so there is no need to put unnecessary pressure on yourself.

In Summary

■ Know you are at the top of your game and in the best possible position to take the examination.

■ It is an open-book examination, and you have all the answers!

■ Answer all the questions you know, and then go back to answer those you have left blank. Repeat the process until all questions have been answered.

■ Use all the time allotted.

■ Never leave any question unanswered: guess if you are unsure.

■ Coding for the examination is based on CPT, ICD-9-CM, and HCPCS coding rules and regulations and not those of a specific insurance carrier.

■ Use the process of elimination where applicable.

■ Highlight key words and terms.

■ Enter you answers on the answer grid, and do not make any stray marks on the answer grid.

■ Come prepared with a few sharpened number 2 pencils.

■ Dress comfortably, bring drinks and snacks, and take breaks as needed.

■ Make sure your coding books match the year of the examination you are taking.

■ Get a good night's rest the night before the examination.

Believe in yourself and in your skills, and remember: You only fail when your faith in yourself falters.
Good luck, and I'll see you at the finish line.

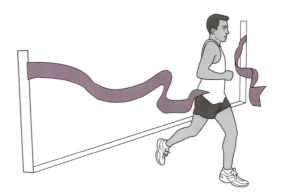

Common Coding Errors

As you go through your coding career, you will hear many different variations on how to code certain scenarios. Please take the information as a grain of salt unless it is backed up with a source document and/or reference material.

A source document and/or reference material is a document from an authoritative source such as the Centers for Medicare and Medicaid Services (CMS); the *CPT Assistant;* or coding guidance on the letterhead, newsletter, or manual from the insurance company.

Source documents and/or reference materials are very important. If you get audited by an insurance carrier, you will need to be able to support your code selection with information from an authoritative source. Simply stating you called the carrier and spoke to Susie or the office manager from another physician's office who told you to code it this way will not help you in an audit situation or provide an authoritative source.

Let's take a look at some of the more common errors made by coders and try to dispel some of the myths that caused the errors.

■ MYTH: Appending Modifier 51 to an add-on code

Modifier 51 is to be appended to multiple procedures other than evaluation and management (E/M) services, physical medicine and rehabilitation services, or provision of supplies that are performed by the same provider at the same session. The modifier is appended to the additional procedure or service.

Add-on codes are used to report additional intraservice work that is related to the primary procedure; therefore, modifier 51 would not be applicable. The Introduction section of the CPT codebook, under Add-on Codes, clearly states: **"All add-on codes found in the CPT codebook are exempt from the multiple procedure concept."**

■ MYTH: Appending Modifier 25 to radiology services

Modifier 25 is a significant, separately identifiable *E/M* service by the same physician on the same day of the procedure or other service. As in the description of this modifier, in the definition of modifier 25 in Appendix A of the CPT codebook, it clearly states: "This circumstance may be reported by adding modifier 25 to the appropriate level of *E/M* service." This indicates you would append modifier 25 only to a code from the E/M section of the CPT codebook.

> **KEY CODING TIP**
> Carefully read the description of the modifier before selection, as some of the modifiers specifically state which type of service the modifier is appended to. In addition to the example we saw previously with modifier 25, modifier 57's description also alerts the coder to append modifier 57 to the appropriate E/M service.

■ MYTH: PPD is a vaccine; therefore, we need to use a vaccine administration code along with each PPD implant

Although the PPD test (a test to screen for tuberculosis) is often given during a preventive visit in conjunction with other immunizations, the code (86580) for the implant of the PPD is located in the Pathology and Laboratory section of the CPT codebook, designating the implant of the PPD as a pathology/laboratory code. As such, it is inappropriate to report a vaccine administration code for the implant of a PPD.

215

■ **MYTH: A low-level E/M visit of 99211 is always reported for patients who present for a vaccine and vaccine administration**

According to the *CPT Assistant,* the following services are included in the vaccine administration codes:

■ Administrative staff services such as making the appointment, preparing the patient chart, billing for the service, and filing the chart

■ Clinical staff services such as greeting the patient, taking routine vital signs, obtaining a vaccine history on past reactions and contraindications, presenting a Vaccine Information Statement (VIS), answering routine vaccine questions, preparing and administering the vaccine with chart documentation, and observing for any immediate reaction

If the only reason for the visit is for the vaccine, you should report only the vaccine and the vaccine administration codes. If, however, the patient is evaluated, documentation must demonstrate the service was separate and significant from the immunization administration, and the service provided must exceed those services included in the vaccine administration.

■ The most common error for new coders is the inability to take the time to fully read the CPT code descriptor, the ICD-9-CM notes, coding guidance, and/or the CPT guidelines located throughout the CPT codebook.

It is exciting to locate the code; however, you must always keep the following in mind:

1. Never select an ICD-9-CM or CPT code from the index of the book.

2. Always verify your code selection from either the Tabular List of the ICD-9-CM or the specific chapter of the CPT codebook.

3. Always read the notes, references, and guidelines in the ICD-9-CM and the CPT. Remember, reading is fundamental, and if you can read you can code.

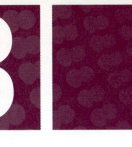

Sample Examination

1. The term auscultation refers to:
   a. The examination by hands or fingers to the external surface of the body
   b. Listening to sounds within the body
   c. High-frequency sounds waves that form an image of the inside of the body
   d. The administration of medication in the form of a mist inhaled into the lungs

2. This suffix means surgical fixation:
   a. -ectomy
   b. -itis
   c. -opexy
   d. -ostomy

3. Policies issued by Medicare Administrative Contractors (MACs) provide coding and utilization guidelines, such as required documentation, how often the service can be performed, and ICD-9-CM codes that provide medical necessity, are located in:
   a. Local Coverage Determination (LCD)
   b. National Coverage Determination (NCD)
   c. *Medicare Carrier Manual* (MCM)
   d. Internet-Only Manual (IOM)

4. A protein made by the body to neutralize or destroy foreign substances is:
   a. Monocyte
   b. Lymphocyte
   c. Interferon
   d. Antibody

5. A grating, clicking, rattling, or crackling sound produced by rubbing bone fragments is called:
   a. Crepitation
   b. Kyphosis
   c. Effusion
   d. Torticollis

6. The epithelium, melanin, and stratum corneum are all located within this organ system:
   a. Musculoskeletal system
   b. Nervous system
   c. Integumentary system
   d. Respiratory system

7. A sigmoidoscopy includes an endoscopic examination of:
   a. The entire rectum and sigmoid colon, and may include examination of a portion of the descending colon
   b. The examination of the rectum and sigmoid colon
   c. The examination of the entire colon, from the rectum to the cecum, and may include the examination of the terminal ileum
   d. An examination of the anal canal

8. The medical term for collarbone is:
   a. Scapula
   b. Humerus
   c. Ulna
   d. Clavicle

9. When you are unable to locate a specific code in CPT to describe the procedure/service performed, you should:
   a. Select the CPT codes whose descriptor comes the closest to the procedure or service performed
   b. Select the CPT codes whose descriptor comes the closest to the procedure or service performed and append a modifier to indicate no specific CPT code was listed in the CPT manual
   c. Select the appropriate unlisted CPT code only if a Category III code is not available
   d. Select the appropriate unlisted CPT code

10. The attempted reduction or restoration of a fracture or joint dislocation to its anatomical alignment by application of manually applied forces is called:
    a. Percutaneous skeletal fixation
    b. Traction
    c. Manipulation
    d. Strapping

11. The time limit associated with coding late effects is:
    a. There is no time limit.
    b. After 6 months of the injury that caused the late effect
    c. After 1 year
    d. The time limit depends on the type of illness/injury that caused the late effect.

12. ICD-9-CM codes classified as Not Otherwise Specified (NOS) are used:
    a. When the ICD-9-CM system does not provide a code specific for the patient's condition
    b. When a definitive diagnosis has not been determined
    c. When the coder lacks the information necessary to code to a more specific four-digit subcategory
    d. Only as a secondary diagnosis code

13. When looking up a code in the ICD-9-CM book, the following is *not* true:
    a. Always consult the Alphabetic Index, Volume 2, before looking up the code in the Tabular List, Volume 1.
    b. Look up and identify all "rule out," "suspected," "probable," or "questionable" diagnoses first.
    c. Interpret abbreviations, cross-references, symbols, and brackets.
    d. Determine if the code is at the highest degree of specificity.

14. In ICD-9-CM, the brackets that appear beneath a code indicate:
    a. Mandatory multiple coding
    b. The fifth digits that are considered valid fifth digits for the code
    c. Synonyms, alternative terminology, or explanatory phrases
    d. Supplementary words, called nonessential modifiers

15. A patient with a cough, fever, and chest pain was sent for a chest x-ray to rule out pneumonia. Select and sequence the correct code(s) for this encounter:
    a. 786.2, 786.50, 780.60
    b. 486
    c. 486, 786.2, 786.50, 780.60
    d. 786.2, 786.50, 780.60, 486

16. Select the correct code for diverticulosis of the colon:
    a. 562.12
    b. 562.10
    c. 562.00
    d. 562.11

17. Due to a fall off a motorcycle, a passenger on the back of the motorcycle was injured, sustaining a fractured ulna. The correct codes are:
    a. 813.82, E818.3
    b. 813.82, E818.8
    c. E818.3, 813.82
    d. 813.83, E818.3

18. Creutzfeldt-Jakob disease with dementia, with behavioral disturbance, is reported with:
    a. One code
    b. Two codes
    c. Three codes
    d. Either one or two codes

19. The following is true about ICD-9-CM nonessential modifiers:
    a. They affect the code assignment.
    b. They do not affect the code assignment.
    c. They are identified by brackets.
    d. They are identified by braces.

20. When a patient presents for chemotherapy, the first listed diagnosis code is:
    a. A "V" code
    b. The primary site of the cancer
    c. The secondary site of the cancer
    d. The site of cancer that is being treated

21. The correct ICD-9-CM code for bloody stool is:
  a. 578.9
  b. 772.4
  c. 578.1
  d. 578.0

22. A Medicare patient presents for trimming of six dystrophic nails. The correct HCPCS code(s) is (are):
  a. G0127, G0127 × 5
  b. G0127
  c. G0127 × 6
  d. 11719

23. During Mrs. Smith's stress test, she was administered two doses of the radiopharmaceutical agent technetium Tc-99 sestamibi, a resting dose of 10.7 mCi, and a stress dose of 33.8 mCi. She also received 32 mg of dipyridamole. The correct HCPCS codes are:
  a. A9500, J1245
  b. A9500 × 2, J1245 × 3
  c. A9502 × 2, J1245
  d. A9502, J1245

24. Due to the patient's inability to operate a manual wheelchair, Dr. Franks ordered a motorized power wheelchair to afford the patient mobility without pain from operating a manual wheelchair. The correct HCPCS code would be:
  a. K0011
  b. K0012
  c. K0006
  d. K0010

25. A totally electric hospital bed without mattress and a power pressure-reducing air mattress for the hospital bed is reported with the following HCPCS code(s):
  a. E0296
  b. E0297, E0277
  c. E0295, E0277
  d. E0277

26. Which of the following HCPCS modifiers would be used to indicate that an Advanced Beneficiary Notice is on file at the physician's office?
  a. GA
  b. GZ
  c. GY
  d. GB

27. A Medicare patient presenting for a screening colonoscopy is reported with the following HCPCS code:
  a. G0121
  b. G0104
  c. G0105
  d. G0122

28. The following is true regarding Category III codes:
  a. Category III codes are endorsed by the Editorial Panel.
  b. Category codes represent services/procedures that are performed by many health-care professionals across the country.
  c. If a Category III code is available, it must be reported instead of a Category I unlisted code.
  d. Unlike Category I codes, Category III codes are updated once every 2 years.

29. According to the CPT Guidelines, a separate procedure:
  a. Identifies procedures that are always reported on their own
  b. Identifies procedures that are never coded, as they are part of another larger procedure
  c. Identifies procedures that are never reported with modifiers
  d. Identifies procedures that may be reported by themselves when the particular procedure is the only service provided or, more often, would not be billed when it is provided as part of a larger service or procedure

30. CPT codes identified by a + sign indicate:
  a. Codes that are always reported first
  b. Codes that are reported in addition to a primary procedure code
  c. Codes that have a decreased reimbursement rate
  d. Codes whose descriptors have been revised

31. CPT codes located in the Musculoskeletal subsection of the CPT manual may be used by:
  a. Orthopedic surgeons
  b. Orthopedic surgeons and spine surgeons
  c. Any physician
  d. Board-certified orthopedic surgeons

32. Specific sections that include instructions and the definition of items that are necessary to interpret and report procedures are called:
  a. Introduction
  b. Index
  c. Guidelines
  d. References

33. CPT codes identified with a full code description are called:
    a. Indented codes
    b. Standalone codes
    c. Complete codes
    d. FDA-approved codes

34. Modifiers are used:
    a. To provide additional information about the service/procedure without changing the description of the service/procedure
    b. To change the description of a procedure/service
    c. Only by surgeons
    d. Only on surgical procedures

35. When a qualified resident or surgeon is not available, and the service of an assistant surgeon is required, which modifier would be appended to the service provided by the assistant surgeon?
    a. 80
    b. 81
    c. 82
    d. 79

36. According to the Radiology Guidelines, for a study to be reported "with contrast," the contrast material is administered:
    a. Orally, rectally, intravascularly, intra-articularly, or intrathecally
    b. Rectally, intravascularly, intra-articularly, or intrathecally
    c. Rectally, intravascularly, or intra-articularly
    d. Intravascularly, intra-articularly, or intrathecally

37. Genetic testing code modifiers are located in:
    a. Appendix A
    b. The Surgery Guidelines
    c. Appendix I
    d. The front flap of the CPT manual

38. Documentation of the duration, severity, timing, and associated signs and symptoms are elements of:
    a. The review of systems (ROS)
    b. The physical examination
    c. The medical decision making (MDM)
    d. The history of presenting illness (HPI)

39. Three of the seven components used in defining the various levels of E/M services are:
    a. History of presenting illness, chief complaint, and review of systems
    b. Past, family, and social history
    c. History, counseling, and time
    d. History, physical examination, and risk

40. Which classification of E/M codes requires the documentation of the three key components (history, physical examination, and medical decision)?
    a. New patients
    b. Consultations
    c. Emergency department services
    d. All of the above

41. Time may be used to determine the level of service:
    a. When counseling and coordination of care dominates (50% or more of the visit) face-to-face time with the physician in the office or floor/unit time in the hospital
    b. When counseling and coordination of care dominates (50% or more of the visit)
    c. Never
    d. When the service is provided by telephone consultation

42. According to the Documentation Guidelines, there are four types of physical examinations:
    a. Limited, extended, detailed, and comprehensive
    b. Problem focused, expanded problem focused, detailed, and comprehensive
    c. Straightforward, low, moderate, and high
    d. Simple, moderate, complex, and extensive

43. According to the E/M and Documentation Guidelines, a concise statement describing the symptom, problem, condition, diagnosis, physician-recommended return, or other factor that is the reason for the encounter is called the:
    a. History
    b. Medical decision
    c. Assessment and plan
    d. Chief complaint

44. Prolonged attendance codes are based on:
    a. Two of the three key components
    b. Three of the three key components
    c. Time
    d. Counseling and coordination of care

45. The CPT codes for preventive care visits are determined on the basis of:
    a. The age of the patient and the status of the patient (new or established)
    b. The age of the patient
    c. Time
    d. The patient's insurance policy

46. A patient received trimethobenzamide (Tigan) capsules for nausea and vomiting. At home, she accidentally left the bottle open on the bathroom counter. Her 2-year-old daughter saw the bottle and, thinking they were candy, ate the pills. Mom found the child unconscious and rushed her to the emergency room. The correct diagnosis code(s) would be:
 a. 963.0, E858.1
 b. E858.1, 963.0
 c. 780.09
 d. 963.0, 780.09, E858.1

47. A pot of boiling water spilled on Stephanie while she was moving it from the stove. She sustained a third-degree burn on the palm of her hand, 3%, and a second-degree burn on the leg, 5%. The correct diagnosis codes would be:
 a. 944.35, 945.20, 948.00, E924.0
 b. 944.36, 945.20, 948.00
 c. 944.35, 945.20
 d. 944.35, 945.20, 948.00, E924.2

48. Mrs. Hancock took her newborn (26 days old) to the pediatrician for his first preventive checkup and a combination vaccine for DTP and polio. The correct diagnosis codes would be:
 a. V20.2, V06.3
 b. V20.32, V06.3
 c. V20.31, V04.0, V06.1
 d. V20.32, V04.0, V06.1

49. Pneumonia due to the RSV organism is coded as:
 a. 486, 079.6
 b. 480.1
 c. 480.1, 079.6
 d. 466.11

50. Consultation, office visit, and admission all describe:
 a. Patient status
 b. Type of service
 c. Place of service
 d. Key components

51. A 6-year-old established patient presented to the pediatrician for his annual examination. During the encounter, the physician also performed a venipuncture, hearing screen, and eye examination (Snellen chart). The child was up to date with his vaccinations, and therefore none were provided. The correct codes would be:
 a. 99393, 36415, 92551, 99173, V20.2
 b. 99393, 36415, 92552, 99173, V20.2, V72.11, V72.0
 c. 99393, 36415, V20.2
 d. 99383, 31645, 99251, 99173, V20.2, V20.11, V72.0

52. A new patient presented to the office with complaints of right-sided facial pain and numbness. His injuries were sustained during an altercation 2 days earlier. He had presented with brief loss of consciousness to the emergency department, where it was thought that he had a right orbital blowout fracture. He denied any visual complaints. He has no known drug allergies, and his past medical history and family history were negative. He denied any use of tobacco, alcohol, and drugs. On examination, there was moderate right-sided facial and periorbital swelling and ecchymosis with flattening of the right cheek that was tender on palpation. Neurologically, there was decreased sensation in the distribution of the infraorbital nerve. Otherwise, there were no deficits. Examination of the eyes showed the extraocular muscles to be intact without any evidence of entrapment. Examination of the ears showed the tympanic membranes were intact and mobile. On examination of the nose, the nasal pyramid was straight and symmetrical in the midline. Intranasally there was moderate mucosal edema, and the right nasal passageway was narrowed due to a deviated septum. The midface and mandible were stable. Palpation of the neck was unremarkable. Based on the history and physical, the moderate decision was made to proceed with an open reduction and internal fixation of the fractures via multiple approaches. The surgery was discussed with the patient and his parents. The correct code(s) would be:
 a. 99205
 b. 99204
 c. 99203
 d. 99243

53. Mary Jones returned to the orthopedic office for a routine follow-up for her hip replacement surgery during the global period. The orthopedist performed a problem-focused history and physical examination, and the wound was healing as expected with no pain or infection, resulting in a minimal medical decision. The correct codes would be:
 a. 99212, V54.81
 b. 99212, 996.42
 c. 99213, 996.42
 d. 99024, V54.81, V43.64

54. A woman presents as a new patient to the gastroenterologist's office, complaining of diarrhea, stomach cramps, and blood in her stool. She states that she has been having symptoms for around 2 weeks, and her loss of 10 pounds brought her into the office today. The physician documents a comprehensive history and physical examination, and due to the severity and duration of the symptoms, the physician performed a colonoscopy at that time. The results of the diagnostic colonoscopy indicated left-sided ulcerative colitis. As part of the moderate medical decision, the patient was given a prescription for prednisone and Asacol and asked to return in a week for a follow-up. The correct codes would be:
   a. 99205-25, 45378, 556.5
   b. 99204, 45378-25, 556.5
   c. 99204-25, 45378, 556.5
   d. 99204-25, 45378, 556.5, 783.21, 787.91, 578.1

55. An established patient returns to the office for the reading of a PPD, which was implanted 2 days earlier. The nurse reading the PPD documented the result as negative. The correct code(s) would be:
   a. 99211, 86580
   b. 86580
   c. 99211
   d. 99212

56. Dr. Jones, a neurologist, saw a patient for an initial inpatient hospital consultation at the request of the patient's primary care physician (PCP). Two days later, the PCP asked Dr. Jones to reevaluate the patient due to a change in her condition. You would report the service with a code from the following code range:
   a. 99221-99223
   b. 99231-99233
   c. 99251-99255
   d. 99238-99239

57. Anticoagulant management services may be reported with an E/M code when:
   a. Adjustment to the dosage for the medication is communicated to the patient
   b. The review and ordering of the tests is necessary
   c. A separately identifiable E/M service is performed
   d. The initial 90 days of therapy have passed

58. Under which circumstances would a new patient visit be reported?
   a. When a patient has not received any professional services from the physician or another physician of the same specialty who belongs to the same group or practice within the past 3 years
   b. When the patient changes his or her insurance coverage
   c. When the patient is first seen in the office, regardless of whether he or she was previously seen for the first time in a different setting (e.g., hospital)
   d. New patients are reported only once, the first time they are seen

59. An 80-year-old man in full arrest was brought into the emergency department by EMS. The patient was allegedly struck by a motor vehicle. The full trauma team was in attendance; they provided CPR and worked on the patient from the time of arrival at 12:15 until 12:50, when vital signs were no longer present and the patient was pronounced dead. The patient was identified by his driver's license. The correct code(s) would be:
   a. 99291, 92950
   b. 99285, 92950
   c. 99291, 99292
   d. 99291

60. Seven-year-old Johnny presented for his second hepatitis B vaccination (three-dose schedule). Mom was counseled regarding the risks and benefits, the vaccine was administered subcutaneously, and Johnny's immunization record was updated. The correct codes would be:
   a. 90471, 90746, V05.3
   b. 99211, 90465, 90746, V05.3
   c. 90460, 90744, V05.3
   d. 90746, V05.3

61. The two organizations responsible for the development of anesthesia codes are:
   a. Centers for Medicare and Medicaid Services and the American Society of Anesthesiologists
   b. Centers for Medicare and Medicaid Services and the American Medical Association
   c. The American Medical Association and the American Society of Anesthesiologists
   d. National Government Services and the American Medical Association

62. Anesthesia time begins when the anesthesiologist begins to prepare the patient for the induction of anesthesia and ends when:
  a. The operation is completed
  b. The anesthesiologist is no longer in personal attendance
  c. The patient may be safely placed under postoperative supervision
  d. Both a and c

63. The following is *not* true regarding qualifying-circumstances anesthesia codes:
  a. They are used in addition to another anesthesia code.
  b. They describe the patient's condition at the time anesthesia was administered.
  c. They describe the administration of anesthesia under difficult circumstances.
  d. They affect the character of the anesthesia services provided.

64. When multiple surgical procedures are performed, you would report:
  a. Only one anesthesia CPT code, the CPT code that represents the most complex procedure
  b. Multiple anesthesia codes, listing the most complex procedure first
  c. Multiple anesthesia codes, listing the most complex procedure first and appending modifier 51 to the additional procedures
  d. Only one anesthesia CPT code, the CPT code that represents the most complex procedure, with modifier 22 appended

65. The type of anesthesia that allows the patient to breathe without assistance and respond to verbal commands is:
  a. General
  b. Local
  c. Moderate conscious sedation
  d. Patient-controlled analgesia (PCA)

66. A healthy 2-year-old patient received anesthesia for a laryngoscopy. The correct code(s) would be:
  a. 00320-P1
  b. 00326-P1
  c. 00320-P1, 99100
  d. 00320, 99100

67. Monitored anesthesia care (MAC) was provided for a 76-year-old patient with severe systemic disease for a colonoscopy. The correct code(s) would be:
  a. 00810, 99100
  b. 00740-P3, 99100
  c. 00810-P3, 99100
  d. 00810

68. Global radiology services are reported:
  a. By appending both the TC and 26 modifiers to the radiology code
  b. By appending the 26 modifier to the radiology code
  c. By appending the TC modifier to the radiology code
  d. By reporting the CPT code without any modifiers

69. A complete ultrasound of the retroperitoneum consists of:
  a. Real-time scans of the kidneys, abdominal aorta, common iliac artery origins, inferior vena cava, and any abnormality
  b. A complete evaluation of the kidneys and urinary bladder when clinical history suggests urinary tract pathology
  c. Real-time scans of the kidneys, abdominal aorta, common iliac artery origins, and any abnormality
  d. Both a and b

70. A patient complaining of severe back pain and blood in the urine presents for an MRI of the abdomen and pelvis without contrast materials, followed by contrast materials and further sequences. The radiology report concluded the patient had several small renal cysts and one kidney stone. The correct codes would be:
  a. 74182, 72196, 593.2, 592.0
  b. 74183, 72197, 593.2, 592.0
  c. 74183, 72197, 724.5, 599.70
  d. 74183, 72197, 724.5, 599.70, 593.2, 592.0

71. **CT Scan of the Chest With and Without Contrast**
  Clinical History: Cough.
  Protocol: 5-mm axial images apices to adrenal glands pre- and post-100 cc intravenous contrast material.
  Findings: There are no enlarged mediastinal or hilar lymph nodes. There is no pleural or pericardial effusion. Scanning of the upper abdomen demonstrates the adrenal glands to be within normal limits. Motion artifact degrades several of the slices. There is no gross evidence of pleural or parenchymal mass or abnormal fluid collection.
  Impression: Grossly unremarkable CT of the chest.
  Based on this report, the correct codes would be:
  a. 71270, V70.0
  b. 71270, 786.2
  c. 71270-52, V70.0
  d. 71250, 786.2

72. **Right Lower Extremity Venous Duplex Doppler Sonogram**
    Clinical History: Right leg swollen. Ulcer in the right ankle.
    Protocol: Real-time images, spectral analysis, and graded compression.
    Findings: The right lower extremity venous structures were evaluated from the level of the common femoral vein in the groin to the popliteal vein. The vessel walls appear normal. There is no evidence of wall thickening. Normal phasic venous flow was observed in each of the visualized venous vessels. The vessel walls are completely compressible, and there is no evidence of intraluminal thrombus. Normal augmentation of flow was observed in each of the visualized areas. There is no evidence of retrograde flow or reflux noted.
    Impression: No evidence of deep vein thrombosis. No evidence of reflux or valvular incompetence.
    Based on this report, the correct codes would be:
    a. 93970-RT, 729.81, 707.10
    b. 93971-RT, 453.40
    c. 93971-RT, 729.81, 707.10
    d. 93970-RT, 453.40

73. Radiation treatment delivery codes (77401-77416) represent what type of component?
    a. Global
    b. Professional
    c. Technical
    d. Complete

74. Clinical brachytherapy requires the use of radioelements applied into or around a treatment field. An intermediate application includes how many sources/ribbons?
    a. Greater than 10
    b. One to four
    c. Five to 10
    d. None; an intermediate application refers to the insertion of Heyman capsules.

75. A patient complaining of sore throat pain with fever for several days presented to the clinic. The laboratory at the clinic performed a rapid strep test and a throat culture with susceptibility studies, antimicrobial agent, disk method. The correct codes would be:
    a. 87880, 87070, 87184
    b. 87880, 87070
    c. 87880, 87070, 87185
    d. 87046, 87070, 87184

76. The following is true about organ- or disease-oriented panels:
    a. They are developed as clinical guidelines for physicians.
    b. They may be reported in addition to a test that is not included in the panel.
    c. They are developed to limit the performance of other laboratory tests.
    d. A panel may be reported when 50% or more of the tests listed in the panel are performed.

77. The physician ordered an electrolyte panel and a calcium total. The correct code(s) for the laboratory tests would be:
    a. 82374, 82435, 84132, 84295, 82310
    b. 80051, 82330
    c. 80051, 82310
    d. 80051

78. While running the blood for a basic metabolic panel, the machine jammed. The blood sample taken included a sufficient amount to rerun the test. The correct code(s) would be:
    a. 80047-52, 80047-91
    b. 80047-91
    c. 80047
    d. 80047-52

79. The following is not true when providing evocative/suppression testing:
    a. The codes for the physician's administration of the evocative or suppressive agents are separately reportable.
    b. The codes for the supplies and drugs are not separately reported.
    c. Prolonged physician attendance and monitoring during the testing is separately reported.
    d. Prolonged physician care codes are not separately reported when evocative/suppression testing involves prolonged infusions.

80. A 52-year-old male, with an onset of neck pain, severity 4/9, and left upper extremity radiating pain to dorsal elbow and dorsal wrist pain, underwent a needle EMG and nerve conduction study of the median motor nerve with F wave and two sensory nerves.
    The correct codes would be:
    a. 95860, 95900, 95904
    b. 95860, 95903, 95904
    c. 95860, 95903, 95904 × 2
    d. 95860, 95903 × 2, 95904

81. A patient was seen for osteopathic manipulation for the following regions: lumbar spine, right and left hip, right and left knee, and sacrum. According to the CPT Guidelines for osteopathic manipulation, how many regions were treated?
    a. Six
    b. Four
    c. Three
    d. One; doctors of osteopathic medicine treat the body as a whole

82. A patient presented to the psychiatrist's office for minimal psychotherapy and for a review and refill of his prescription medications. The correct code(s) would be:
    a. 90862
    b. 90805
    c. There is no documentation of time; since psychotherapy is a timed service, no CPT code should be reported.
    d. 90804, 90862

83. A patient with dysphagia presented to the outpatient clinic for an evaluation of swallowing by flexible fiberoptic endoscopy. The correct codes would be:
    a. 92613, 787.20
    b. 92613, 787.29
    c. 92612, 787.20
    d. 92612, 787.29

84. A patient received 15 minutes of manual electrical stimulation and anorectal manometry as treatment for her urge incontinence and anal spasms. The correct codes would be:
    a. 97014, 91122, 788.31, 564.6
    b. 97014, 91122, 788.31, 728.85
    c. 97032, 91122, 788.31, 564.6
    d. 97032, 91122, 788.31, 728.85

85. A patient presented to the audiologist for a binaural hearing aid examination and selection. During the encounter, the audiologist performed a comprehensive audiometry, a tympanogram, and acoustic reflex testing. The correct codes would be:
    a. 92591, 92557, 92567, 92568
    b. 92590, 92557, 92567, 92568
    c. 92591, 92557, 92550, 92568
    d. 92590, 92557, 92550, 92568

86. A special report:
    a. Is routinely provided
    b. Includes the credentials of the physician providing the service
    c. Should be submitted when reporting unlisted CPT codes, modifier 22, and Category III codes
    d. Should be submitted only when reporting unlisted CPT codes

87. When reporting repair codes from the Integumentary section, the following is true:
    a. When multiple wounds are repaired, you would report a complex wound repair code.
    b. Wounds that are repaired with only adhesive strips or a tissue adhesive would be reported with an E/M code.
    c. Débridement would be separately reported when gross contamination requires prolonged cleansing.
    d. Simple ligation of vessels in an open wound is separately reported.

88. A Mohs' surgeon refers to a surgeon who has two separate, distinct roles:
    a. A surgeon and a radiologist
    b. An assistant surgeon and a pathologist
    c. A surgeon and a pathologist
    d. An assistant surgeon and a radiologist

89. The application of casts and strapping may not be reported when:
    a. The cast application or strapping is a replacement procedure
    b. The cast application or strapping is the initial service performed without a restorative treatment
    c. The cast application or strapping is provided to stabilize or protect a fracture/injury
    d. The physician who applies the initial cast, strap, or splint assumes all of the subsequent fracture care

90. The global surgical package includes:
    a. Preoperative, intraoperative, and postoperative services
    b. Preoperative, intraoperative, and postoperative services and complications within the global period
    c. Preoperative and postoperative services
    d. Preoperative and intraoperative services

91. A patient presents for treatment of basal cell carcinoma and actinic keratosis. A 3.5-cm malignant lesion was excised from the patient's trunk, and four premalignant lesions (actinic keratosis) on the shoulder were destroyed by cryosurgery. The correct codes would be:
    a. 17000, 17003, 11604, 702.0, 173.5
    b. 11604, 17000, 17003, 173.5, 702.0
    c. 11604, 17000-59-51, 17003, 173.5, 702.0
    d. 11604, 17000-59-51, 17003-59-51, 173.5, 702.0

92. **Preoperative Diagnosis:** Left neck adenopathy.
Postoperative Diagnosis: Same.
Nature of Operation: Biopsy of deep level II cervical lymph node.
Anesthesia: General with laryngeal mask.
Operative Findings: The patient had an enlarged level II left neck adenopathy.
Operative Procedure: The patient was brought into the operating room and was laid in supine position. He was given general anesthesia by laryngeal mask. Neck was distended from the chest by placement of a shoulder roll. The left neck was prepped and draped in the usual sterile technique. A skin crease incision was taken. After going through skin and subcutaneous tissue, the platysma was opened and the lymph node was identified in the level II region anterior to the jugular vein. The lymph node was gently dissected away from the jugular vein. Hemostasis was achieved by Bovie and ligation with 3-0 Vicryl. Once the lymph node was withdrawn, hemostasis was complete. The lymph node was sent fresh for evaluation. Closure was done with 3-0 Vicryl for platysma and 4-0 Biosyn for skin. Dressing was done.
The patient was extubated and brought to the recovery room in stable condition.
Based on this report, the correct codes would be:
a. 38500, 785.6
b. 38510, 785.6
c. 38505, 785.6
d. 38520, 785.6

93. Mrs. Peters returned to the clinic for a bilateral nasal endoscopy. On endoscopic examination of the nose, there was minimal mucosa edema with thick mucoid secretions. There was persistent synechiae and scarring on the right obstructing the ostiomeatal complex on the right. The recurrent headaches are a component and related to chronic sinusitis.
The correct codes would be:
a. 31233, 473.9
b. 31235, 473.9
c. 31231, 473.9
d. 31231-50, 473.9

94. A patient presents with low back pain radiating to the bilateral leg areas; the pain increases with walking or bending. The physician performed multiple trigger-point injections into the left gluteus medius, injecting 10 mL of mepivacaine to alleviate the patient's pain and to improve her activities of daily living. The correct codes would be:
a. 20552, J0670
b. 20552 × 2, J0670 × 2
c. 20553, J0670
d. 20550, J0670

95. Select the CPT code(s) for extracapsular cataract extraction by phacoemulsification with placement of posterior chamber IOL:
a. 66982, 66985
b. 66984, 66985
c. 66985
d. 66984

96. Select the codes for placement of a left chest wall central venous access device with subcutaneous port performed with intraoperative fluoroscopy on a 73-year-old patient:
a. 36570, 77001
b. 36570-LT, 77002
c. 36571-LT, 77001
d. 36571, 77002

97. A patient underwent a therapeutic nonobstetrical dilation and curettage (D&C) for pyometrium and stenosis of the cervix. The correct codes would be:
a. 58120, 615.0, 622.4
b. 59160, 615.9, 622.4
c. 57558, 615.9, 622.4
d. 58120, 615.9, 622.4

98. **Preoperative Diagnosis:** Endometrial hyperplasia with atypia and polyp, postmenopausal bleeding.
Postoperative Diagnosis: Same.
Nature of Operation: Gynecological oncology standby for 1 hour time.
Operative Indications: The patient is an 83-year-old female who was brought into the operating room by Dr. Niece and Dr. Michaels. I was asked to stand by in the event malignancy was diagnosed on frozen section.
Operative Procedure: The patient was brought to the operating room; she underwent a total abdominal hysterectomy (TAH) bilateral salpingo-oophorectomy (BSO) with frozen section that revealed no carcinoma.
The total standby time was 1 hour. During this time, I [the surgeon] was available solely for the purpose of this patient with no other patient care activities.
Based on this report, the correct codes would be:
a. 99360, 621.33
b. No codes should be reported, as the physician did not provide any service during the surgical procedure.
c. 99360 × 2, 621.33
d. 99360, 621.33, 627.1

99. A 58-year-old patient with a strangulated umbilical hernia underwent a hernia repair with mesh. The correct codes would be:
a. 49582, 49568
b. 49582, 49568-51
c. 49587, 49568
d. 49587, 49568-51

100. The following code represents a repeat transurethral resection of prostate tissue 3 years post–original procedure:
a. 52500
b. 52630
c. 52601
d. 52640

101. A patient presented to the gastroenterologist complaining of weight loss and of blood in his stool. The physician performed a colonoscopy with removal of three colon polyps using hot biopsy forceps. The correct codes would be:
a. 45384, 569.0
b. 45384 × 3, 569.0
c. 45384, 783.21, 578.1, 569.0
d. 45384 × 3, 783.21, 578.1, 569.0

102. Select the correct code for a laparoscopic cholecystectomy with exploration of common duct:
a. 47570
b. 47563
c. 47564
d. 47610

103. A diagnostic endoscopy is:
a. Always reported as the primary procedure
b. Designated as an add-on code
c. Always included in the surgical endoscopy
d. Never reported alone

104. A 55-year-old male new patient presented to the urologist for evaluation of dysuria. The physician documented an expanded problem-focused history and, during the comprehensive examination, performed a venipuncture for PSA and testosterone total. The postvoid residual by ultrasound revealed 22 mL, the automated urine dipstick was positive for ketones and protein, specific gravity was 1.020, and pH was 7.0. A simple uroflow showed voided time 66 sec, straining to urinate present, prolonged urination time present, intermittency present, split stream absent, and hesitancy absent. The assessment and plan included a diagnosis of benign prostatic hyperplasia (BPH) without significant obstruction, a transrectal ultrasound was ordered to measure the prostate size, and a prescription for Cialis was given for erectile dysfunction (moderate medical decision).
The correct codes would be:
a. 99202-25, 51736, 51798, 36415, 81003, 600.00, 788.1, 788.21
b. 99202-25, 51736, 51798, 36415, 81003, 600.00, 788.1, 607.84
c. 99202-25, 51736, 51798, 36415, 81002, 600.00, 788.1, 607.84
d. 99204-25, 51736, 51798, 36415, 81003, 600.00, 788.1, 607.84

105. **Preoperative Diagnosis:** Hematuria.
Postoperative Diagnosis: Hematuria.
Patient presents for a cystourethroscopy. Flexible cystoscopy was performed with the 16-Fr flexible cystoscope after obtaining consent and explaining risks such as bleeding, dysuria, and infection. Patient was prepped with Betadine, and lidocaine jelly was instilled. The examination was done supine in the lithotomy position. The urethra was normal. Bladder examination reveals completely normal mucosa with normal ureteral orifices. Procedure was tolerated well. The patient was given an antibiotic after the procedure.
Based on this report, the correct code(s) would be:
a. 52000, 96372, J1580
b. 52000-25, 96372, J1580
c. 52000, 96372
d. 52000

106. The study of the motion and flow of urine is called:
a. Urodynamics
b. Urology
c. Uromotion
d. Uroflowology

107. Under fluoroscopic guidance, Mr. Smith underwent a subcutaneous permanent pacemaker placement with transvenous placement of electrodes in the right atrium and right ventricle. The correct code(s) would be:
a. 33206, 71090
b. 33207, 71090
c. 33208, 71090
d. 33210

108. Coronary artery bypass procedures using both venous grafts and arterial grafts during the same procedure are reported:
   a. Alone, as they represent both the arterial and venous grafting
   b. In combination with the appropriate arterial graft code and the appropriate combined arterial-venous graft code
   c. Using a code from the coronary artery bypass–venous graft codes and a code from the arterial graft code
   d. Using a code from the coronary artery bypass–venous graft codes and a code from the arterial graft code and the appropriate combined arterial-venous graft code

109. Mrs. Escobar had continuous complaints of syncope and palpitations. Her cardiologist suspected arrhythmia and implanted a patient-activated cardiac event recorder with looping memory. The correct codes would be:
   a. 33282, 780.2, 785.1
   b. 33284, 780.2, 785.1
   c. 33282, 785.1, 780.4
   d. 33828, 427.9

110. Travis, a 2-year-old boy, was born with an a trioventricular canal defect. Due to the child's inability to gain weight and dyspnea, Dr. Jones ordered a transesophageal echocardiogram to evaluate the defect. The correct codes would be:
   a. 93315, 783.41, 786.09
   b. 93315, 745.69
   c. 93312, 745.69
   d. 99312, 783.41, 786.09

111. When a catheter is placed into an artery or vein and moved or manipulated from the original artery/vein punctured or from an artery that branches off the aorta, it is called:
   a. Nonselective catheter placement
   b. Aorta catheter placement
   c. Branch catheter placement
   d. Selective catheter placement

112. A patient underwent a right arthroscopic anterior Bankart repair with a right posterior Bankart repair and a SLAP repair of the right shoulder with extensive débridement of degenerative joint disease and rotator cuff tear with a partial posterior superior synovectomy during one operative session. The correct codes would be:
   a. 29806-RT, 29806-59-RT, 29823-59-RT, 29820-59
   b. 29806-RT, 29807-51-RT
   c. 29806-RT, 29807-51-RT, 29823-59-51-RT
   d. 29806-RT, 29807-51-RT, 29820-51

113. A patient diagnosed with myalgia received bilateral trigger-point injections into the trapezius muscle. The correct code(s) would be:
   a. 20552
   b. 20552 × 2
   c. 20551 × 2
   d. 20553

114. A complete ultrasound examination of the retroperitoneum may be reported when documentation includes the following:
   a. Real-time scans of the kidneys, abdominal aorta, common iliac artery origins, and inferior vena cava, including any demonstrated retroperitoneal abnormality
   b. Complete evaluation of the kidneys and urinary bladder, along with clinical history, suggests urinary tract pathology
   c. Complete single-organ evaluation with clinical history suggests urinary tract pathology
   d. Both **a.** and **b.**

115. Radiology Report
   Bone age: Single AP view of the left wrist and hand was obtained. The patient is 9 years of age. This was compared with the hand of a patient 8 years and 10 months from the standard Greulich and Pyle atlas of skeletal development of the hand and wrist. Although the carpal bones, navicular lunate, triquetrum, greater multangular, lesser multangular, capitate, and hamate are all present in the patient's wrist, the standard shows moderately more maturation formation of these carpal bones, which would indicate some degree of retardation.
   Impression: There is some degree of retardation in the growth and development of the bones of the wrist in this patient when compared to the standard.
   Based on this report, the correct codes would be:
   a. 77072, 783.40
   b. 77072, 783.42
   c. 77073, 783.40
   d. 77073, 783.42

116. An asymptomatic postmenopausal patient was sent for a bone density DEXA of the axial skeleton. The study showed the patient to have osteopenia of the lumbar spine. The correct codes would be:
   a. 77081, 733.90, V49.81
   b. 77080, 733.90
   c. 77082, 733.90, V49.81
   d. 77082, 733.90

117. Mrs. Kramer presented to the mental health clinic to see Dr. Felix for minimal psychotherapy and pharmacological management. The correct code(s) would be:
    a. 90862, 90804
    b. 90805
    c. 90862
    d. 90845

118. The appropriate psychotherapy code is determined by:
    a. The type of psychotherapy provided, the place of service, face-to-face time, and if E/M services were also provided
    b. The type of psychotherapy provided, the status of the patient, face-to-face time, and if E/M services were also provided
    c. The type of psychotherapy provided, the place of service, face-to-face time, and if pharmacological management was provided
    d. The type of psychotherapy provided, who provided the service (e.g., MD or clinical social worker), face-to-face time, and if E/M services were also provided

119. An intermediate ophthalmological service is described as:
    a. A general evaluation of the complete visual system
    b. A low-level evaluation and management service
    c. An evaluation of a new or existing condition complicated with a new diagnostic or management problem, not necessarily relating to the primary diagnosis
    d. A midlevel E/M service

120. Dr. Franklin ordered an intermediate visual field examination for Mary Jones. During the examination, Mary was called away, and only one eye was tested. The correct code would be:
    a. 92083
    b. 92083-52
    c. 92082
    d. 92082-52

121. **Radiology Report:** Right lower extremity venous duplex Doppler sonogram.
    Clinical History: Right leg swollen, ulcer in right ankle.
    Protocol: Real-time images, spectral analysis, and graded compressions.
    Findings: The right lower extremity venous structures were evaluated from the level of the common femoral vein in the groin to the popliteal vein. The vessel walls appear normal. There is no evidence of wall thickening. Normal phasic venous flow was observed in each of the visualized venous vessels. The vessel walls are completely compressible, and there is no evidence of intraluminal thrombus. Normal augmentation of flow was observed in each of the visualized areas. There is no evidence of retrograde flow or reflux noted.
    Impression: No evidence of acute deep vein thrombosis.
    Based on this report, the correct codes would be:
    a. 93971-RT, 451.19
    b. 93970-RT-52, 451.19
    c. 93970-RT, 729.81, 707.13
    d. 93971-RT, 729.81, 707.13

122. A patient with mastodynia presented for a bilateral mammogram with CAD (computer-aided detection). The correct codes would be:
    a. 77056, 77051, 611.71
    b. 77057, 77052, 611.71
    c. 77055, 77051, 611.71
    d. 77056, 77052, 611.71

123. An 89-year-old male (new patient) presented to the physician's office for evaluation of scrotal discomfort, testicular tenderness, and urinary frequency. The patient never had this condition before and complains the symptoms are worse at night. He denies fever, chills, gross hematuria, nausea, or vomiting. The patient reports a bothersome testicular mass. He has no known drug allergies. A complete past, family, and social history was documented and reviewed with the patient along with a complete review of systems. A comprehensive physical examination was documented. A venipuncture and prostate-specific antigen (PSA) and testosterone total was performed. The patient was diagnosed with hypertrophy of prostate, hydrocele, and impotence of organic origin. The patient was sent to a radiology facility for a scrotal ultrasound. The medical decision was of moderate complexity. The correct codes would be:
    a. 99204, 84403, 36415, 84153, 76870
    b. 99204, 84403, 36415, 84153
    c. 99203, 84403, 36416, 84153
    d. 99204, 84403, 36416, 84153, 76870

124. Context, duration, location, and associated signs and symptoms are all considered as elements of:
    a. The medical decision
    b. The physical examination
    c. The history of presenting illness
    d. The review of systems

125. A concise statement describing the symptom, problem, condition, diagnosis, or other factor that is the reason for the encounter is called:
a. Chief complaint
b. Referral
c. Risk factor reduction
d. Prognosis

126. A patient underwent an excision of a subcutaneous right chest wall mass, 2.9 cm. The correct code would be:
a. 21552
b. 21555
c. 21556
d. 21557

127. Jackie Franklin presented to the physician complaining of neck pain that radiated down her arms. To relieve her pain, the physician provided osteopathic manipulation to the following regions: cranial head, cervical spine, left hip, left and right shoulders, and left and right hands. According to the guidelines in CPT for osteopathic manipulative treatment (OMT), how many body regions were treated?
a. Seven
b. Three
c. Five
d. Four

128. Ben Smith, 54 years old, underwent a flexible colonoscopy with polyp removal by snare technique under moderate conscious sedation; the procedure time was 25 minutes. The correct code(s) would be:
a. 45385
b. 45385, 99148
c. 45384, 99148
d. 45385, 99143

129. The codes in Chapter 11 of the ICD-9-CM Manual are to be used:
a. For both the mother's and the child's record
b. Only for the child's record
c. Only for the mother's record
d. In the mother's record; recording the codes in the child's record is optional

130. The fifth digit in ICD-9-CM category 948 Burns classified according to extent of body surface represents:
a. The percentage of body surface burned
b. The percentage of body surface with third-degree burn
c. The percentage of body surface with second-degree burn
d. The percentage of body surface with deep third-degree burn with loss of body part

131. ICD-9-CM describes coding to the highest degree of specificity as:
a. Coding signs and symptoms along with definitive diagnosis codes
b. The inclusion of rule-out codes when a physician is formulating his or her diagnosis
c. The coding of a diagnosis code to the highest number of digits available
d. Multiple coding for a single condition

132. A patient received 30 minutes of acupuncture without electrical stimulation. The acupuncturist removed the needles and reinserted the needles to provide an additional 15 minutes of acupuncture with electrical stimulation. The correct codes would be:
a. 97810 × 2, 97813
b. 97810, 97811, 97813
c. 97810, 97811, 97814
d. 97810, 97814

133. Select the code for Graves' disease with thyrotoxic crisis or storm:
a. 242.01
b. 242.00
c. 242.90
d. 242.91

134. To treat 7-year-old Johnny's continuous ear infections, Dr. Kildare inserted bilateral ventilating tubes. The service was provided under general anesthesia. The correct code would be:
a. 69436
b. 69436-50
c. 69433
d. 69433-50

135. A patient diagnosed with hypertensive retinopathy underwent an intracapsular cataract extraction with insertion of intraocular lens prosthesis. The correct codes would be:
a. 66983, 362.11
b. 66983, 362.12
c. 66982, 362.11
d. 66982, 362.12

136. The patient (post–Mohs' surgery) presented to the plastic surgeon for a reconstruction of a defect in the left lateral lower lid and canthus repaired with an orbicularis myocutaneous flap. The correct code(s) would be:
a. 17311, 15732
b. 17311, 14060
c. 15732
d. 13150

137. According to the CPT Guidelines for Critical Care Services, the following is not true:
   a. Services for a patient who is not critically ill but is located in a critical care unit are reported using other appropriate E/M codes.
   b. Critical care time provided by the physician does not have to be continuous.
   c. Time spent in activities that occur outside of the unit or off the floor may be reported as critical care time as long as the time spent directly contributes to the treatment of the patient.
   d. Time spent on the floor/unit documenting critical care services in the medical record may be counted as critical care time.

138. CPT codes for anticoagulant management (99363-99364) may be reported:
   a. Only in the outpatient setting
   b. Only in the hospital setting
   c. In any setting the service takes place
   d. In the hospital setting for the first time, followed by outpatient setting thereafter

139. Mrs. Jones was seen by her primary care physician for strep throat. She was given amoxicillin. Three days later, she called the doctor's office and asked to speak to her physician, as she was not feeling any relief from the antibiotic. The physician spent 15 minutes on the phone with Mrs. Jones, reassuring her that she needed to give the antibiotic time to work and to set a return appointment to the office upon completion of her prescription if she did not feel better at that time. The correct code would be:
   a. 99441
   b. 99442
   c. 99443
   d. No CPT code should be reported

140. Mrs. Peters was followed in the clinic for her antepartum and postpartum care by Dr. Michaels. Her 6 lb 3 oz baby boy was delivered by cesarean by Dr. Franklin, a hospital physician who was not affiliated with Dr. Michaels's practice. Code for the services of Dr. Franklin would be:
   a. 59400
   b. 59409
   c. 59510
   d. 59514

141. A condition in which gastric juices containing acid travel back from the stomach up into the esophagus is called:
   a. Gastroesophageal reflux disease (GERD)
   b. Diverticulosis
   c. Diverticulitis
   d. Ulcerative colitis

142. A patient presenting for a radiological procedure was positioned, lying on the right side. This is called:
   a. Right recumbent
   b. Right lateral recumbent
   c. Right prone
   d. Right supine

143. In radiology, the term "projection" refers to:
   a. How the patient is placed for the examination
   b. The path the x-ray beam travels
   c. The various planes of the body
   d. The radiological technique

144. CPT defines code 88300 as level 1–Surgical pathology, gross examination only. The term "gross" for this purpose is defined as:
   a. Examination of the specimen by site
   b. A disgusting specimen
   c. Examination of the specimen before removal
   d. A unit amount

145. Mrs. Brown, a 68-year-old established Medicare patient, presented to the gynecologist for her routine preventive Pap test and breast examination. The physician sent the specimen out to the laboratory for testing. The correct codes would be:
   a. G0101, Q0091
   b. 99397, 99000
   c. 99397, 88164
   d. G0101, P3000

146. Diagnosis codes for sunburns are located in which chapter of the ICD-9-CM?
   a. Injury and Poisoning
   b. Skin and Subcutaneous Tissue
   c. External Causes
   d. Symptoms, Signs, and Ill-Defined Conditions

147. According to the ICD-9-CM Coding Guidelines, how many codes are required to completely describe a pressure ulcer?
   a. One
   b. Two
   c. Three
   d. One, with an additional code if applicable

148. Wound closure utilizing adhesive strips as the sole method of repair is coded by using:
   a. The appropriate E/M code
   b. The appropriate classification of repair code
   c. A simple repair code
   d. An E/M code with modifier 22

149. A patient encounter for the complaint of headache, diagnosis given as probable migraine headache, possible gastroenteritis, would be coded as:
a. 784.0
b. 346.90
c. 346.90, 558.9
d. 558.9

150. The term "metastatic" is used to indicate:
a. The site mentioned is the secondary site
b. The site is not specific to primary or secondary
c. The site mentioned is the primary site
d. The site mentioned is for carcinoma in situ

Sample Test Answers and Rationale

1. The term auscultation refers to:
   a. The examination by hands or fingers to the external surface of the body—*Incorrect*
   This refers to refers to palpation.
   b. **Listening to sounds within the body—Correct Answer**
   c. High-frequency sound waves that form an image of the inside of the body—*Incorrect*
   This refers to an ultrasound.
   d. The administration of medication in the form of a mist inhaled into the lungs—*Incorrect*
   This refers to a nebulizer treatment.

2. This suffix means surgical fixation:
   a. -ectomy—*Incorrect*
   This refers to a surgical removal.
   b. -itis—*Incorrect*
   This refers to an inflammation.
   c. **-opexy—Correct Answer**
   d. -ostomy—*Incorrect*
   This refers to a new, permanent opening.

   Note: Some versions of the CPT books (Professional Edition) include a section in the front of the book called "Illustrated Anatomical and Procedural Review," which includes some common suffixes and prefixes.

3. Policies issued by Medicare Administrative Contractors (MACs) provide coding and utilization guidelines, such as required documentation, how often the service can be performed, and ICD-9-CM codes that provide medical necessity, are located in:
   a. **Local Coverage Determination (LCD)— Correct Answer**
   The LCD is a policy provided by Medicare Administrative Contractors at the local level.
   b. National Coverage Determination (NCD)—*Incorrect*
   This is a policy developed by the Centers for Medicare and Medicaid Services at the national level.
   c. *Medicare Carrier Manual* (MCM)—*Incorrect*
   The CMS Online Manual System is used by CMS program components, partners, contractors, and state survey agencies to administer CMS programs. It offers day-to-day operating instructions, policies, and procedures based on statutes and regulations; guidelines; models; and directives.
   d. Internet-Only Manual (IOM)—*Incorrect*
   The Internet-Only Manuals (IOMs) are a replication of the Agency's official record copy. They are CMS's program issuances, day-to-day operating instructions, policies, and procedures. The CMS program components, providers, contractors, Medicare Advantage organizations, and state survey agencies use the IOMs to administer CMS programs. They are also a good source of Medicare and Medicaid information for the general public.

4. A protein made by the body to neutralize or destroy foreign substances is called:

  a. Monocyte—*Incorrect*

  Large, circulating white blood cells that are formed in the bone marrow and fight against fungi and bacteria.

  b. Lymphocyte—*Incorrect*

  A type of white blood cell that produces antibodies.

  c. Interferon—*Incorrect*

  Proteins released by cells to stimulate the immune response.

  d. Antibody—Correct Answer

5. A grating, clicking, rattling or crackling sound produced by rubbing bone fragments is called:

  a. Crepitation—Correct Answer

  b. Kyphosis—*Incorrect*

  The abnormal backward curve of the vertebral column (hunchback).

  c. Effusion—*Incorrect*

  An abnormal collection of fluid in various spaces of the body (e.g., the knee).

  d. Torticollis—*Incorrect*

  Spasms in the neck muscles causing the head to tilt to one side and causing difficulty in rotating the head (stiff neck).

6. The epithelium, melanin, and stratum corneum are all located within this organ system:

  c. Integumentary system—Correct Answer

  The epithelium is a membranous tissue that lines the internal organs, cavities, and surfaces of structures throughout the body. Melanin is a pigment that gives the skin and hair their natural color, and the stratum corneum is a layer of dead cells in the epidermis that forms a barrier to keep moisture in.

7. A sigmoidoscopy includes an endoscopic examination of:

  a. The entire rectum and sigmoid colon, and may include examination of a portion of the descending colon—Correct Answer

  This information is located in your CPT book in the Digestive System subsection of the Surgery section under the definitions of endoscopy.

  b. The examination of the rectum and sigmoid colon—*Incorrect*

  This defines a proctosigmoidoscopy.

  c. The examination of the entire colon, from the rectum to the cecum, and may include the examination of the terminal ileum—*Incorrect*

  This defines a colonoscopy.

  d. An examination of the anal canal—*Incorrect*

  This defines an anoscopy.

8. The medical term for collarbone is:

  a. Scapula—*Incorrect*

  The scapula, or shoulder blade, is the bone that connects the humerus (arm bone) with the clavicle (collar bone).

  b. Humerus—*Incorrect*

  This is the bone extending from the shoulder to the elbow.

  c. Ulna—*Incorrect*

  This is the forearm bone between the elbow and wrist.

  d. Clavicle—Correct Answer

  Note: Some versions of the CPT books (Professional Edition) include anatomical diagrams. *This information is located in your CPT book in the beginning pages of the Musculoskeletal subsection of the Surgery section.*

9. When you are unable to locate a specific code in CPT to describe the procedure/service performed, you should:

  a. Select the CPT codes whose descriptor comes the closest to the procedure or service performed—*Incorrect*

  In the CPT manual, under instructions for use of the CPT Codebook, it is clearly stated, "Do not select a CPT code that merely approximates the service provided."

  b. Select the CPT codes whose descriptor comes the closest to the procedure or service performed, and append a modifier to indicate no specific CPT code was listed in the CPT manual—*Incorrect*

  No modifier exists to indicate that no specific CPT code was available.

  c. Select the appropriate unlisted CPT code only if a Category III code is not available—Correct Answer

  This information can be found in your CPT book under Category III codes, first paragraph.

  d. Select the appropriate unlisted CPT code—*Incorrect*

  The appropriate unlisted CPT codes should be selected only if no Category III code exists.

10. The attempted reduction or restoration of a fracture or joint dislocation to its anatomical alignment by application of manually applied forces is called:
- **a.** Percutaneous skeletal fixation—*Incorrect* **This describes a method of immobilizing fracture fragments with fixation (pins) placed across the fracture site.**
- **b.** Traction—*Incorrect* **This describes the use of weights and pulleys to gradually change the position of a bone.**
- **c.** Manipulation—Correct Answer This information is located in the CPT book in the Surgery section under the musculoskeletal subsection guidelines.
- **d.** Strapping—*Incorrect* **This describes the taping of a body part to provide support and stability.**

11. The time limit associated with coding late effects is:
- **a.** There is no time limit—Correct Answer This information is located in the ICD-9-CM Coding Guidelines under Late Effects.
- **b.** After 6 months of the injury that caused the late effect—*Incorrect* **There is no time limit associated with late effects, as per the ICD-9-CM Guidelines.**
- **c.** After 1 year—*Incorrect* **There is no time limit associated with late effects, as per the ICD-9-CM Guidelines.**
- **d.** The time limit depends on the type of illness/injury that caused the late effect—*Incorrect* **There is no time limit associated with late effects, as per the ICD-9-CM Guidelines.**

12. ICD-9-CM codes classified as Not Otherwise Specified (NOS) are used:
- **a.** When the ICD-9-CM system does not provide a code specific for the patient's condition—*Incorrect* **In these cases, an ICD-9-CM code classified as Not Elsewhere Classifiable (NEC) would be used.**
- **b.** When a definitive diagnosis has not been determined—*Incorrect* **In these cases, you would code the signs and symptoms.**
- **c.** **When the coder lacks the information necessary to code to a more specific four-digit subcategory**—Correct Answer This information is located in the ICD-9-CM book under ICD-9-CM Official Conventions.
- **d.** Only as a secondary diagnosis code—*Incorrect* **ICD-9-CM codes that are classified as NOS may be used as a primary diagnosis code.**

13. When looking up a code in the ICD-9-CM book, the following is ***not*** true:
- **a.** Always consult the Alphabetic Index, Volume 2, before looking up the code in the Tabular List, Volume 1—*Incorrect* **This statement is true and is mentioned in the ICD-9-CM book under "How to Use the ICD-9-CM for Physicians" under the correct steps to coding.**
- **b.** Look up and identify all "rule-out," "suspected," "probable," or "questionable" diagnoses first—Correct Answer **The key to determining the correct answer is to properly read the question. In this question, you are to identify what is *not* true.** This information is located in the ICD-9-CM book under "How to Use the ICD-9-CM for Physicians." **Here you will find the steps to correct coding.**
- **c.** Interpret abbreviations, cross-references, symbols, and brackets—*Incorrect* **This statement is true and is mentioned in the ICD-9-CM book under "How to Use the ICD-9-CM for Physicians" under the correct steps to coding.**
- **d.** Determine if the code is at the highest degree of specificity—*Incorrect* **This statement is true and is mentioned in the ICD-9-CM book under "How to Use the ICD-9-CM for Physicians" under the correct steps to coding.**

14. In ICD-9-CM, the brackets that appear beneath a code indicate:
- **a.** Mandatory multiple coding—*Incorrect* **Slanted brackets indicate mandatory multiple coding.**
- **b.** **The fifth digits that are considered valid fifth digits for the code**—Correct Answer This information is located in the ICD-9-CM book under ICD-9-CM Official Conventions.
- **c.** Synonyms, alternative terminology, or explanatory phrases—*Incorrect* **These are identified by brackets, which are located after the description of the code.**
- **d.** Supplementary words, called nonessential modifiers—*Incorrect* **These are identified by parentheses.**

15. A patient with a cough, fever, and chest pain was sent for a chest x-ray to rule out pneumonia. Select and sequence the correct code(s) for this encounter:

a. **786.2, 786.50, 780.60—Correct Answer**
Because a definitive diagnosis has not been determined, and there is no rule-out diagnosis code, you would code the signs and symptoms that prompted the diagnostic test.

b. 486—*Incorrect*
The pneumonia should not be coded, as the definitive diagnosis has not yet been determined.

c. 486, 786.2, 786.50, 780.60—*Incorrect*
You would not code the pneumonia (because the diagnosis has not been determined) along with the signs and symptoms.

d. 786.2, 786.50, 780.60, 486—*Incorrect*
You would not code the pneumonia (because the diagnosis has not been determined) along with the signs and symptoms.

16. Select the correct code for diverticulosis of the colon:

a. 562.12—*Incorrect*
This is the code for diverticulosis of the colon *with hemorrhage.*

b. **562.10—Correct Answer**

c. 562.00—*Incorrect*
This code describes diverticulosis of the *small intestine.*

d. 562.11—*Incorrect*
This code describes diverticulitis of the colon.

17. Due to a fall off a motorcycle, a passenger on the back of the motorcycle was injured, sustaining a fractured ulna. The correct codes are:

a. **813.82, E818.3—Correct Answer**

b. 813.82, E818.8—*Incorrect*
The E code is incorrect, as the fourth digit in this E code describes "other specified person." Our diagnostic statement clearly states the passenger was injured.

c. E818.3, 813.82—*Incorrect*
These are the correct ICD-9-CM codes; however, they are not properly sequenced. E codes are never listed as primary diagnosis codes.

d. 813.83, E818.3—*Incorrect*
The E code is correct; however, the diagnosis code for the fracture represents a fracture of *the radius* and ulna. Our diagnostic statement mentions only a fracture of the ulna.

18. Creutzfeldt-Jakob disease with dementia, with behavioral disturbance, is reported with:

a. One code—*Incorrect*
Two codes are required to fully describe this mental disorder.

b. Two codes—Correct answer
In the Alphabetic Index under the main term *Disease*, subterm *Jacob-Creutzfeldt,* subterm *with dementia,* subterm *with behavioral disturbance,* you will find 046.19, *[294.11]. Remember that the ICD-9-CM Official Conventions state that slanted brackets that appear in the Alphabetical Index indicate mandatory multiple coding.*

c. Three codes—*Incorrect*
Three codes are not needed, as ICD-9-CM code 046.19 describes the Creutzfeldt-Jakob disease, and 294.11 describes the dementia with the behavioral disturbance.

d. Either one or two codes—*Incorrect*
The slanted brackets appearing in the Alphabetic Index indicate mandatory multiple coding.

19. The following is true about ICD-9-CM nonessential modifiers:

a. They affect the code assignment—*Incorrect*
Essential modifiers affect the code assignment.

b. **They do not affect the code assignment—Correct Answer**
Nonessential modifiers are identified by parentheses enclosing supplementary words that may be present in the description of the disease. This information is found in the ICD-9-CM Official Conventions.

c. They are identified by brackets—*Incorrect*
Brackets are located under codes to indicate the fifth digits that are considered valid fifth digits for the code.

d. They are identified by braces—*Incorrect*
Braces enclose terms each of which is modified by the statement appearing to the right of the brace.

20. When a patient presents for chemotherapy, the first listed diagnosis code is:
    a. **A "V" code—Correct Answer**
       This information is located in the ICD-9-CM Coding Guidelines, Chapter 18, number 7, Aftercare, **which states that when a patient's encounter is solely to receive radiation or chemotherapy for the treatment of a neoplasm, the V code is to be listed first, followed by the diagnosis code.**
    b. The primary site of the cancer—*Incorrect*
       The aftercare code (V) code is listed first to describe the specific reason for the encounter.
    c. The secondary site of the cancer—*Incorrect*
       The aftercare code (V) code is listed first to describe the specific reason for the encounter.
    d. The site of cancer that is being treated—*Incorrect*
       This would be listed as the secondary diagnosis code.

21. The correct ICD-9-CM code for bloody stool is:
    a. 578.9—*Incorrect*
       This code describes a gastric hemorrhage.
    b. 772.4—*Incorrect*
       This code describes gastric hemorrhage in a fetus or neonate.
    c. **578.1—Correct Answer**
    d. 578.0—*Incorrect*
       This code describes hematemesis (vomiting of blood).

22. A Medicare patient presents for trimming of six dystrophic nails. The correct HCPCS code(s) is (are):
    a. G0127, G0127 × 5—*Incorrect*
       The code descriptor indicates "any number of nails"; therefore, HCPCS code G0127 should be reported only once regardless of the number of nails trimmed.
    b. **G0127—Correct Answer**
       The code descriptor includes any number of nails; therefore, it is reported only once regardless of the number of nails trimmed.
    c. G0127 × 6—*Incorrect*
       The code descriptor indicates "any number of nails"; therefore, HCPCS code G0127 should be reported only once regardless of the number of nails trimmed.
    d. 11719—*Incorrect*
       This is a CPT code, and it represents *nondystrophic* nails.

23. During Mrs. Smith's stress test, she was administered two doses of the radiopharmaceutical agent technetium Tc-99 sestamibi, a resting dose of 10.7 mCi, and a stress dose of 33.8 mCi. She also received 30 mg of dipyridamole. The correct HCPCS codes are:
    a. A9500, J1245—*Incorrect*
       These codes are incorrect, as they do not include the total amount of the drugs administered in units.
    b. **A9500 × 2, J1245 × 3—Correct Answer**
       The technetium Tc-99 sestamibi is listed as per study dose. Because two doses were administered, you would code A9500 twice. The dipyridamole is listed as per 10 mg; because 30 mg was administered, you would report J1245 three times.
    c. A9502 × 2, J1245—*Incorrect*
       HCPCS code A9502 is for technetium Tc-99m *tetrofosmin,* diagnostic, per study dose, and the patient received *sestamibi;* the HCPCS code for the dipyridamole did not include the number of units for the drug administered.
    d. A5902, J1245—*Incorrect*
       A9502 is an incorrect HCPCS code, as indicated previously, and there are no units listed with either code to identify the correct amount of the drugs administered.

24. Due to the patient's inability to operate a manual wheelchair, Dr. Franks ordered a motorized power wheelchair to afford the patient mobility without pain from operating a manual wheelchair. The correct HCPCS code would be:
    a. K0011—*Incorrect*
       This code describes a wheelchair that includes programmable control parameters for speed adjustment, tremor dampening, acceleration control, and braking.
    b. K0012—*Incorrect*
       This code describes a lightweight, portable, motorized/power wheelchair.
    c. K0006—*Incorrect*
       This code describes a heavy-duty wheelchair that is not motorized.
    d. **K0010—Correct Answer**
       This code describes a standard-weight frame motorized/power wheelchair.

25. A totally electric hospital bed without mattress and a power pressure-reducing air mattress for the hospital bed is reported with the following HCPCS code(s):
  a. E0296—*Incorrect*
  This code describes the correct type of hospital bed, but the mattress included is not a power pressure-reducing air mattress.
  b. E0297, E0277—**Correct Answer**
  You will need two HCPCS codes to correctly identify the equipment. E0297 describes the correct type of hospital bed without mattress, and E0277 identifies the mattress as a power pressure-reducing air mattress.
  c. E0295, E0277—*Incorrect*
  E0295 describes a *semi-electric* hospital bed without a mattress, and E0277 is the correct code for the power pressure-reducing air mattress.
  d. E0277—*Incorrect*
  This code is incorrect, as it lists only the mattress and not the bed.

26. Which of the following HCPCS modifiers would be used to indicate that an Advanced Beneficiary Notice is on file at the physician's office?
  a. **GA—Correct Answer**
  This information is located in Appendix 2, Modifiers, of the HCPCS book.
  b. GZ—*Incorrect*
  This modifier indicates an item or service is expected to be denied as not reasonable or necessary.
  c. GY—*Incorrect*
  This modifier indicates a service is statutorily excluded, does not meet the definition of any Medicare benefit, or, for non-Medicare insurers, is not a contract benefit.
  d. GB—*Incorrect*
  This modifier indicates a claim is being resubmitted for payment because it is no longer covered under a global payment demonstration.

27. A Medicare patient presenting for a screening colonoscopy is reported with the following HCPCS code:
  a. **G0121—Correct Answer**
  This code identifies a patient presenting for a screening colonoscopy who is not at high risk.
  b. G0104—*Incorrect*
  This code represents a screening by flexible sigmoidoscopy.
  c. G0105—*Incorrect*
  This codes represents the correct service (screening colonoscopy); however, it is *specific for a high-risk patient*.
  d. G0122—*Incorrect*
  This code represents screening by barium enema.

28. The following is true regarding Category III codes:
  a. Category III codes are endorsed by the Editorial Panel—*Incorrect*
  This statement is false: Category III codes do not conform to the usual requirements for CPT Category I codes and therefore are not endorsed by the Editorial Panel.
  b. Category codes represent services/procedures that are performed by many health-care professionals across the country—*Incorrect*
  This statement is false: These codes represent temporary codes for emerging technology, services, and procedures.
  c. If a Category III code is available, it must be reported instead of a Category I unlisted code—**Correct Answer**
  This statement is true. This information is located in the CPT Manual under the Coding Guidelines for Category III codes.
  d. Unlike Category I codes, Category III codes are updated once every 2 years—*Incorrect*
  This statement is false: Category III codes are made available on a semi-annual basis via electronic distribution on the AMA website, and the full set of Category III codes will be included in the next published edition for that CPT cycle.

29. According to the CPT Guidelines, a separate procedure:
  a. Identifies procedures that are always reported on their own—*Incorrect*
  Separate procedures may be reported on their own only when they are not part of a more global procedure.
  b. Identifies procedures that are never coded, as they are part of another larger procedure—*Incorrect*
  When a separate procedure code is not part of a more global procedure, it may be reported on its own.
  c. Identifies procedures that are never reported with modifiers—*Incorrect*
  Modifiers may be appended to separate procedure codes when applicable.
  d. Identifies procedures that may be reported by themselves when the particular procedure is the only service provided or, more often, would not be billed when it is provided as part of a larger service or procedure—**Correct Answer**

30. CPT codes identified by a + sign indicate:
    a. Codes that are always reported first—*Incorrect*
    Add-on codes would always be reported in addition to the primary procedure code.
    b. Codes that are reported in addition to a primary procedure code—**Correct Answer**
    Add-on codes are always reported in addition to a primary procedure.
    c. Codes that have a decreased reimbursement rate—*Incorrect*
    When reported, add-on codes do not have a reduced reimbursement rate.
    d. Codes whose descriptors have been revised—*Incorrect*
    Codes with revised descriptors are identified in CPT with a triangle.

31. CPT codes located in the Musculoskeletal subsection of the CPT manual may be used by:
    a. Orthopedic surgeons—*Incorrect*
    CPT codes located in the Musculoskeletal subsection are not limited to orthopedic surgeons. Any CPT code may be reported by any qualified physician or health-care professional.
    b. Orthopedic surgeons and spine surgeons—*Incorrect*
    CPT codes located in the Musculoskeletal subsection are not limited to orthopedic surgeons and spine surgeons. Any CPT code may be reported by any qualified physician or health-care professional.
    c. Any physician—**Correct Answer**
    This information is located in the Introduction of the CPT manual under Instructions for Use of the CPT book. **CPT states any procedure or service in any section of the CPT manual may be reported by any qualified physician or health-care professional.**
    d. Board-certified orthopedic surgeons—*Incorrect*
    CPT codes located in the Musculoskeletal subsection are not limited to board-certified orthopedic surgeons. Any CPT code may be reported by any qualified physician or health-care professional.

32. Specific sections that include instructions and the definition of items that are necessary to interpret and report procedures are called:
    a. Introduction—*Incorrect*
    The Introduction provides instructions on how to use the CPT.
    b. Index—*Incorrect*
    The Index is where we begin our search to locate a CPT code.
    c. Guidelines—**Correct Answer**
    Section-specific instructions are provided in the section guidelines of the CPT book. **For example, the Radiology guidelines include guidelines specific to codes in the Radiology section.**
    d. References—*Incorrect*
    References in the CPT are identified by green and red arrows and refer to additional coding guidance located in either the CPT Changes, An Insider's View, or *CPT Assistant*.

33. CPT codes identified with a full code description are called:
    a. Indented codes—*Incorrect*
    These codes do not include the complete code descriptor.
    b. Standalone codes—**Correct Answer**
    This information is located in your CPT book in the Introduction under Format of the Terminology.
    c. Complete codes—*Incorrect*
    This terminology is not used in CPT.
    d. FDA-approved codes—*Incorrect*
    FDA-approved codes are identified in the CPT manual by the flash/lightning bolt symbol.

34. Modifiers are used:
    a. **To provide additional information about the service/procedure without changing the description of the service/procedure—Correct Answer**
    b. To change the description of a procedure/service—*Incorrect*
    Modifiers do not change the description of a service/procedure; they provide additional information about the service/procedure.
    c. Only by surgeons—*Incorrect*
    All qualified professionals may use modifiers.
    d. Only on surgical procedures—*Incorrect*
    Modifiers are reported on all types of CPT codes, such as E/M and Physical Therapy.

35. When a qualified resident or surgeon is not available, and the services of an assistant surgeon are required, which modifier would be appended to the service provided by the assistant surgeon?

 a. 80—*Incorrect*
 This modifier identifies an assistant surgeon.

 b. 81—*Incorrect*
 This modifier identifies a minimum assistant surgeon.

 c. **82—Correct Answer**
 This modifier identifies an assistant surgeon who provided the services due to the unavailability of a qualified resident surgeon.

 d. 79—*Incorrect*
 This modifier identifies an unrelated procedure or service by the same physician during the postoperative period.

36. According to the Radiology Guidelines, for a study to be reported "with contrast," the contrast material is administered:

 a. Orally, rectally, intravascularly, intra-articularly, or intrathecally—*Incorrect*
 According to the Radiology Guidelines, oral and/or rectal contrast administration does not qualify as a study "with contrast."

 b. Rectally, intravascularly, intra-articularly, or intrathecally—*Incorrect*
 According to the Radiology Guidelines, rectal contrast administration does not qualify as a study "with contrast."

 c. Rectally, intravascularly, or intra-articularly—*Incorrect*
 According to the Radiology Guidelines, rectal contrast administration does not qualify as a study "with contrast," and intrathecally also qualifies as "with contrast."

 d. **Intravascularly, intra-articularly, or intrathecally—Correct Answer**
 This information is located in your CPT book in the Radiology Guidelines under Administration of Contrast Materials.

37. Genetic testing code modifiers are located in:

 a. Appendix A—*Incorrect*
 This appendix includes a list of all modifiers with the exception of genetic testing modifiers, which are located in Appendix I.

 b. The Surgery Guidelines—*Incorrect*
 The Surgery Guidelines do not include any listings of modifiers.

 c. **Appendix I—Correct Answer**

 d. The front flap of the CPT manual—*Incorrect*
 Some CPT manuals include a quick listing of modifiers on the front flap of the manual; however, the genetic testing modifiers are not included in the quick listing.

38. Documentation of the duration, severity, timing, and associated signs and symptoms are elements of:

 a. The review of systems (ROS)—*Incorrect*
 This is an inventory of body systems (e.g., constitutional, cardiovascular) obtained through a series of questions in an effort to identify the signs/symptoms of the patient.

 b. The physical examination—*Incorrect*
 This is the hands-on physical examination by the physician.

 c. The medical decision making (MDM)—*Incorrect*
 This is the physician's assessment and plan for the patient based on the history and physical examination.

 d. **The history of presenting illness (HPI)—Correct Answer**
 This is a chronological description of the development of the patient's present illness. This information is located in the CPT manual in the E/M Guidelines under History of Presenting Illness.

39. Three of the seven components used in defining the various levels of E/M services are:

 a. History of presenting illness, chief complaint, and review of systems—*Incorrect*
 These are all elements of the history component.

 b. Past, family, and social history—*Incorrect*
 This is an element of the history component.

 c. **History, counseling, and time—Correct Answer**
 The seven components are history, examination, medical decision making, counseling, coordination of care, nature of presenting problem, and time. This information is located in your CPT book in the E/M Guidelines under Levels of Service.

 d. History, physical examination, and risk—*Incorrect*
 The history and the physical examination are two of the seven components; however, risk is an element of the medical decision making.

40. Which of the classification of E/M codes requires the documentation of the three key components (history, physical examination, and medical decision)?

 a. New patients

 b. Consultations

 c. Emergency department services

 d. **All of the above—Correct Answer**
 The descriptors for each of these types of service require the documentation of all three key components.

41. Time may be used to determine the level of service:
    a. **When counseling and coordination of care dominates (50% or more of the visit) face-to-face time with the physician in the office or floor/unit time in the hospital— Correct Answer** This information is located in your CPT book in the E/M Guidelines under Select the Appropriate Level of E/M Services.
    b. When counseling and coordination of care dominates (50% or more of the visit)— *Incorrect* **The counseling and coordination of care needs to be provided at a face-to-face encounter in the office or floor-unit time in the hospital setting.**
    c. Never—*Incorrect* **Time may be used to determine the level of service when counseling and coordination of care dominates (more than 50% of the visit) face-to face time with the physician in the office or floor/unit time in the hospital.**
    d. When the service is provided by telephone consultation—*Incorrect* **The counseling and coordination of care must be provided at a face-to-face encounter. CPT has specific codes for telephone services.**

42. According to the Documentation Guidelines, there are four types of physical examinations:
    a. Limited, extended, detailed, and comprehensive—*Incorrect* **Limited and extended are not terms used to describe the types of physical examinations.**
    b. **Problem-focused, expanded problem-focused, detailed, and comprehensive— Correct Answer** This information is located in your CPT book in the E/M Guidelines under Determine the Extent of Examination Performed.
    c. Straightforward, low, moderate, and high— *Incorrect* **This describes the types of medical decision making.**
    d. Simple, moderate, complex, and extensive— *Incorrect* **These are not terms used to describe the types of physical examinations.**

43. According to the E/M and Documentation Guidelines, a concise statement describing the symptom, problem, condition, diagnosis, physician-recommended return, or other factor that is the reason for the encounter is called the:
    a. History—*Incorrect* **This is separate from the chief complaint and includes the history of presenting illness; the review of systems; and the past, family, and social history.**
    b. Medical decision—*Incorrect* **This describes the physician assessment and plan after taking the patient's history and physical examination.**
    c. Assessment and plan—*Incorrect* **This is part of the medical decision-making process.**
    d. **Chief complaint—Correct Answer** **The chief complaint provides the reason for the visit.** This information is located in the E/M Guidelines under Chief Complaint.

44. Prolonged attendance codes are based on:
    a. Two of the three key components—*Incorrect* **The code descriptors for prolonged attendance codes are based on time.**
    b. Three of the three key components—*Incorrect* **The code descriptors for prolonged attendance codes are based on time.**
    c. **Time—Correct Answer** **CPT codes 99354–99357 and 99358–99359 are all based on time.**
    d. Counseling and coordination of care—*Incorrect* **The code descriptors for prolonged attendance codes are based on time.**

45. The CPT codes for preventive care visits are determined on the basis of:
    a. **The age of the patient and the status of the patient (new or established)—Correct Answer** **Once you determine if the patient is new or established and the age of the patient, you can select the appropriate preventive visit code.**
    b. The age of the patient—*Incorrect* **This is only one factor in determining the correct preventive visit code. You also need to know if the patient was new or established.**
    c. Time—*Incorrect* **Time is not a factor in determining the preventive visit codes.**
    d. The patient's insurance policy—*Incorrect* **Although some policies may not cover preventive visits, from a coding and billing point of view, you should always base coding and billing on the documentation.**

46. A patient received trimethobenzamide (Tigan) capsules for nausea and vomiting. At home, she accidentally left the bottle open on the bathroom counter. Her 2-year-old daughter saw the bottle and, thinking they were candy, ate the pills. Mom found the child unconscious and rushed her to the emergency room. The correct diagnosis code(s) would be:

   a. 963.0, E858.1—*Incorrect*
     This answer is missing the diagnosis code for the condition of the patient.

   b. E858.1, 963.0—*Incorrect*
     This answer is missing the diagnosis code for the condition of the patient and is sequenced incorrectly.

   c. 780.09—*Incorrect*
     This answer doesn't include the code for the poison and how the poisoning occurred.

   d. 963.0, 780.09, E858.1—Correct Answer
     The first code describes the drug (Tigan), the second code describes the condition of the patient, and the third code describes how the poisoning occurred.

47. A pot of boiling water spilled on Stephanie while she was moving it from the stove. She sustained a third-degree burn on the palm of her hand, 3%, and a second-degree burn on the leg, 5%. The correct diagnosis codes would be:

   a. 944.35, 945.20, 948.00, E924.0—Correct Answer
     The first code describes the third-degree burn of the palm of the hand, the second code describes the second-degree burn, the third code describes the total body surface area (TBSA), and the fourth code describes the burn from boiling water.

   b. 944.36, 945.20, 948.00—*Incorrect*
     The first code describes a third-degree burn of the back of the hand and does not include the E code.

   c. 944.35, 945.20—*Incorrect*
     This selection does not include the code for the TBSA, and it does not include the E code.

   d. 944.35, 945.20, 948.00, E924.2—*Incorrect*
     The E code in this selection describes a burn by hot, boiling *tap water*.

48. Mrs. Hancock took her newborn (26 days old) to the pediatrician for his first preventive checkup and a combination vaccine for DTP and polio. The correct diagnosis codes would be:

   a. V20.2, V06.3—*Incorrect*
     The first diagnosis code describes a healthy-baby checkup for a baby over 28 days old.

   b. V20.32, V06.3—Correct Answer
     The first code describes a healthy-baby check-up for a baby 8 to 28 days old, and the second code describes the combination vaccine for DTP and polio.

   c. V20.31, V04.0, V06.1—*Incorrect*
     The first diagnosis code describes a healthy-baby checkup for a baby under 8 days old, and the remaining diagnosis codes are for separate vaccines for polio and DTP.

   d. V20.32, V04.0, V06.1—*Incorrect*
     This is incorrect, as the last two diagnosis codes are for separate vaccines for polio and DTP and not the combination vaccine.

49. Pneumonia due to the RSV organism is coded as:

   a. 486, 079.6—*Incorrect*
     In this code selection, the pneumonia and the RSV are separately listed, and the pneumonia is not described as being due to the RSV.

   b. 480.1—Correct Answer
     This one code describes the pneumonia due to respiratory syncytial virus (RSV).

   c. 480.1, 079.6—*Incorrect*
     The ICD-9-CM code 079.6 would not be reported to identify the organism, as it is specified in code 480.1.

   d. 466.11—*Incorrect*
     This code describes bronchiolitis due to RSV.

50. Consultation, office visit, and admission all describe:

   a. Patient status—*Incorrect*
     Describes if the patient is new, established, an inpatient, or an outpatient.

   b. Type of service—Correct Answer
     This describes the reason the service was performed.

   c. Place of service—*Incorrect*
     This describes the setting where the service was performed (e.g., physician's office, emergency department).

   d. Key components—*Incorrect*
     This refers to E/M visits.

51. A 6-year-old established patient presented to the pediatrician for his annual examination. During the encounter, the physician also performed a venipuncture, hearing screen, and eye examination (Snellen chart). The child was up to date with his vaccinations, and therefore none were provided. The correct codes would be:

a. **99393, 36415, 92551, 99173, V20.2—Correct Answer**

b. 99393, 36415, 92552, 99173, V20.2, V72.11, and V72.0—*Incorrect*
The hearing test represented by this code selection is not specifically described as a screening hearing examination. ICD-9-CM code V20.2 includes the routine vision and hearing testing.

c. 99393, 36415, V20.2—*Incorrect*
This code selection does not include the hearing and vision screen (these are not inclusive to a preventive visit).

d. 99383, 31645, 99251, 99173, V20.2, V70.0, V72.0—*Incorrect*
With this code selection, the preventive visit is for an *established patient* and not a new patient.

52. A new patient presented to the office with complaints of right-sided facial pain and numbness. His injuries were sustained during an altercation 2 days earlier. He had presented with brief loss of consciousness to the emergency department, where it was thought that he had a right orbital blowout fracture. He denied any visual complaints. He has no known drug allergies, and his past medical history and family history were negative. He denied any use of tobacco, alcohol, and drugs. On examination, there was moderate right-sided facial and periorbital swelling and ecchymosis with flattening of the right cheek that was tender on palpation. Neurologically, there was decreased sensation in the distribution of the infraorbital nerve. Otherwise, there were no deficits. Examination of the eyes showed the extraocular muscles to be intact without any evidence of entrapment. Examination of the ears showed the tympanic membranes were intact and mobile. On examination of the nose, the nasal pyramid was straight and symmetrical in the midline. Intranasally there was moderate mucosal edema, and the right nasal passageway was narrowed due to a deviated septum. The midface and mandible were stable. Palpation of the neck was unremarkable. Based on the history and physical, the moderate decision was made to proceed with an open reduction and internal fixation of the fractures via multiple approaches. The surgery was discussed with the patient and his parents. The correct code would be:

a. 99205—*Incorrect*
The three key components (history, physical, and medical decision) do not support a level 5 encounter.

b. 99204—*Incorrect*
The three key components (history, physical, and medical decision) do not support a level 4 encounter. New patients require all three key components to be at the same level, or the level of service is determined by the lowest component.

c. 99203—Correct Answer
Documentation of the history supported a level 3 history (four of the HPI, two of the ROS, and all three PFSH), the documentation of the physical examination supported a detailed level 3 examination (head [including face], neck, eyes, skin, ear/nose/throat, neurological), and the medical decision was at moderate complexity level 4. New patients require three of three components are met; therefore, this is a level 3 new patient visit.

d. 99243—*Incorrect*
Although the level of service is correct, the documentation supported a new patient visit and not a consultation (there was no request from a physician/provider for an opinion or evaluation, and there was no documentation of a letter or report being sent back to a requesting physician/provider).

53. Mary Jones returned to the orthopedic office for a routine follow-up for her hip replacement surgery during the global period. The orthopedist performed a problem-focused history and physical examination, and the wound was healing as expected with no pain or infection, resulting in a minimal medical decision. The correct codes would be:

a. 99212, V54.81—*Incorrect*
An E/M visit would not be reported for a routine follow-up with no complications during the global surgical period.

b. 99212, 996.42—*Incorrect*
An E/M visit would not be reported for a routine follow-up with no complications during the global surgical period. Additionally, the diagnosis code describes the dislocation of a prosthetic joint.

c. 99213, 996.42—*Incorrect*
An E/M visit would not be reported for a routine follow-up with no complications during the global surgical period. Additionally, the diagnosis code describes the dislocation of a prosthetic joint.

d. **99024, V54.81, V43.64—Correct Answer**
The patient was seen for routine follow-up with no complications during the global surgical period.

54. A woman presents as a new patient to the gastroenterologist's office, complaining of diarrhea, stomach cramps, and blood in her stool. She states that she has been having symptoms for around 2 weeks, and her loss of 10 pounds brought her into the office today. The physician documents a comprehensive history and physical examination, and due to the severity and duration of the symptoms the physician performed a colonoscopy at that time. The results of the diagnostic colonoscopy indicated left-sided ulcerative colitis. As part of the moderate medical decision the patient was given a prescription for prednisone and Asacol and asked to return in a week for a follow-up. The correct codes would be:

   a. 99205-25, 45378, 556.5—*Incorrect*
The documentation does not support a level 5 new patient visit.

   b. 99204, 45378-25, 556.5—*Incorrect*
This is incorrect, as the modifier 25 is appended to the E/M and not the surgical procedure.

   c. **99204-25, 45378, 556.5—Correct Answer**
Documentation supports a level 4 new patient visit (comprehensive history and physical are both level 5, and the medical decision was level 4). New patients require all three key components be at the same level; therefore, this is a level 4 new patient visit. Modifier 25 is appended to the E/M to indicate a separately identifiable E/M was provided by the same physician on the same day of the procedure within 0 to 10 global days. The left-sided ulcerative colitis would be the only diagnosis reported, as the loss of weight, blood in stool, and diarrhea are all signs and symptoms of a definitive diagnosis of left-sided colitis.

   d. 99204-25, 45378, 556.5, 783.21, 787.91, 578.1—*Incorrect*
There is no need to report the signs and symptoms when they are part of a definitive diagnosis.

55. An established patient returns to the office for the reading of a PPD, which was implanted 2 days earlier. The nurse reading the PPD documented the result as negative. The correct code(s) would be:

   a. 99211, 86580—*Incorrect*
You would not report the PPD, as it was previously implanted. The patient was returning only for the reading of the PPD.

   b. 86580—*Incorrect*
This code describes the implant of the PPD.

   c. **99211—Correct Answer**
The reason for the visit was for the reading of the PPD. Because this was performed and documented by the nurse, 99211 would be selected.

   d. 99212—*Incorrect*
This code describes a *physician encounter*, whereas this scenario describes a *nurse encounter*. Additionally, the documentation did not support a level 2 visit.

56. Dr. Jones, a neurologist, saw a patient for an initial inpatient hospital consultation at the request of the patient's primary care physician (PCP). Two days later, the PCP asked Dr. Jones to reevaluate the patient due to a change in her condition. You would report the service with a code from the following code range:

   a. 99221–99223—*Incorrect*
These codes describe hospital admission codes.

   b. **99231–99233—Correct Answer**
This service would be reported with a subsequent hospital care code. CPT no longer has codes for follow-up consultations.

   c. 99251–99255—*Incorrect*
These codes describe consultations. The CPT Inpatient Consultation Guidelines state, "Only one consultation should be reported by a consultant per admission. Subsequent services during the same admission are reported using subsequent hospital care codes (99231-99233)."

   d. 99238–99239—*Incorrect*
These codes describe hospital discharge codes.

57. Anticoagulant management services may be reported with an E/M code when:
   a. Adjustment to the dosage for the medication is communicated to the patient—*Incorrect*
   This service is included in the anticoagulant management codes and would not be separately reported.
   b. The review and ordering of the tests is necessary—*Incorrect*
   This service is included in the anticoagulant management codes and would not be separately reported.
   c. A separately identifiable E/M service is performed—Correct Answer
   This information is located in the CPT manual's Anticoagulant Management Guidelines.
   d. The initial 90 days of therapy have passed—*Incorrect*
   After the first 90 days of therapy, CPT code 99364 would be reported for each subsequent 90 days of therapy.

58. Under which circumstances would a new patient visit be reported?
   a. When a patient has not received any professional services from the physician or another physician of the same specialty who belongs to the same group or practice within the past 3 years—Correct Answer
   This information is located in your CPT book in the E/M Guidelines.
   b. When the patient changes his or her insurance coverage—*Incorrect*
   The patient's insurance coverage is not a determining factor as to the status of the patient.
   c. When the patient is first seen in the office, regardless of whether he or she was previously seen for the first time in a different setting (e.g., hospital)—*Incorrect*
   Because the patient was previously seen by the physician, he or she would be an established patient. The place of service is not the determining factor for a new or established patient.
   d. New patients are reported only once, the first time they are seen—*Incorrect*
   This statement applies to how the facility will code for its services.

59. An 80-year-old man in full arrest was brought into the emergency department by EMS. The patient was allegedly struck by a motor vehicle. The full trauma team was in attendance; they provided CPR and worked on the patient from the time of arrival at 12:15 until 12:50 when vital signs were no longer present and the patient was pronounced dead. The patient was identified by his driver's license. The correct code(s) would be:
   a. 99291, 92950—Correct Answer
   This code selection meets the definition of critical care, the direct delivery by a physician(s) for a critically ill or injured patient. Because the CPR (92950) is not a bundled service with critical care, it is separately reported.
   b. 99285, 92950—*Incorrect*
   The first code represents an emergency department visit. Although the patient was seen in the emergency department, *critical care services were provided.*
   c. 99291, 99292—*Incorrect*
   This code selection represents 75 to 104 minutes of critical care and does not include the CPR.
   d. 99291—*Incorrect*
   This code does not include the CPR, which is separately reportable.

60. Seven-year-old Johnny presented for his second hepatitis B vaccination (three-dose schedule). Mom was counseled regarding the risks and benefits, the vaccine was administered subcutaneously, and Johnny's immunization record was updated. The correct codes would be:
   a. 90471, 90746, V05.3—*Incorrect*
   CPT code 90471 describes a vaccine administration code when no counseling is provided.
   b. 99211, 90465, 90746, V05.3—*Incorrect*
   Documentation does not support an E/M service.
   c. 90460, 90744, V05.3—Correct Answer
   CPT code 90460 describes the vaccine administration for a child younger than 18 years of age where counseling is provided. CPT codes 90744 and V05.3 correctly identify the vaccine and the diagnosis code.
   d. 90746, V05.3—*Incorrect*
   This code selection does not include the vaccine administration code.

61. The two organizations responsible for the development of anesthesia codes are:

a. Centers for Medicare and Medicaid Services and the American Society of Anesthesiologists—*Incorrect*
The Centers for Medicare and Medicaid Services (CMS) does not develop the anesthesia codes.

b. Centers for Medicare and Medicaid Services and the American Medical Association—*Incorrect*
The Centers for Medicare and Medicaid Services (CMS) does not develop the anesthesia codes.

c. **The American Medical Association and the American Society of Anesthesiologists—Correct Answer**

d. National Government Services and the American Medical Association—*Incorrect*
National Government Services does not develop the anesthesia codes.

62. Anesthesia time begins when the anesthesiologist begins to prepare the patient for the induction of anesthesia and ends when:

a. The operation is completed—*Incorrect*
The anesthesiologist will still be attending to the patient upon completion of the operation.

b. The anesthesiologist is no longer in personal attendance—*Incorrect*
Although it is correct that anesthesia time ends when the anesthesiologist is no longer in personal attendance, this selection is incorrect *because it is incomplete:* the other condition that indicates anesthesia time has ended is that the patient may be safely placed under postoperative supervision (option *c*). For this reason, option *d* is correct, as it includes *both* options *b* and *c*.

c. The patient may be safely placed under postoperative supervision—*Incorrect*
Although it is correct that anesthesia time ends when the patient may be safely placed under postoperative supervision, this selection is incorrect *because it is incomplete:* the other condition that indicates anesthesia time has ended is that the anesthesiologist is no longer in personal attendance (option *b*). For this reason, option *d* is correct, as it includes *both* options *b* and *c*.

d. **Both b and c—Correct Answer**
This information is located in the Anesthesia Guidelines under Time Reporting.

63. The following is *not* true regarding qualifying-circumstances anesthesia codes:

a. They are used in addition to another anesthesia code—*Incorrect*
Qualifying-circumstances anesthesia codes *are* used in addition to another anesthesia code; the question asked what is *not true* regarding qualifying-circumstances anesthesia codes.

b. **They describe the patient's condition at the time anesthesia was administered—Correct Answer**
Physical status modifiers are used to indicate the patient's condition at the time the anesthesia was administered, and this is *not* true of qualifying-circumstances anesthesia codes. This information is located in your CPT manual in the Anesthesia Guidelines under Physical Status Modifiers. Note: You should also review the guidelines under Qualifying Circumstances.

c. They describe the administration of anesthesia under difficult circumstances—*Incorrect*
Qualifying-circumstances anesthesia codes *are* used to report anesthesia administered under difficult circumstances.
The question asked what is *not true* regarding qualifying-circumstances anesthesia codes.

d. They affect the character of the anesthesia services provided—*Incorrect*
Qualifying-circumstances anesthesia codes *do* provide additional information about the administration of the anesthesia services; the question asked what is *not true* regarding qualifying-circumstances anesthesia codes. This information is located in your CPT manual in the Anesthesia Guidelines under Qualifying Circumstances.

64. When multiple surgical procedures are performed, you would report:

    a. **Only one anesthesia CPT code, the CPT code that represents the most complex procedure—Correct Answer**
    This information is located in your CPT manual in the Anesthesia Guidelines under Separate or Multiple Procedures.

    b. Multiple anesthesia codes, listing the most complex procedure first—*Incorrect*
    Multiple anesthesia codes are not reported.

    c. Multiple anesthesia codes, listing the most complex procedure first and appending modifier 51 to the additional procedures—*Incorrect*
    Because multiple anesthesia codes are not reported, modifier 51 would not be applicable.

    d. Only one anesthesia CPT code, the CPT code that represents the most complex procedure, with modifier 22 appended—*Incorrect*
    Modifier 22 describes increased procedural services and does not describe the reporting of multiple procedures regarding anesthesia services.

65. The type of anesthesia that allows the patient to breathe without assistance and respond to verbal commands is:

    a. General—*Incorrect*
    General anesthesia provides a state of unconsciousness.

    b. Local—*Incorrect*
    Local anesthesia is the application of an anesthetic directly into the area involved.

    c. **Moderate conscious sedation—Correct Answer**

    d. Patient-controlled analgesia (PCA)—*Incorrect*
    PCA is a system that allows the patient to administer pain medication.

66. A healthy 2-year-old patient received anesthesia for a laryngoscopy. The correct CPT code(s) would be:

    a. **00320-P1—Correct Answer**
    P1 modifier would be appended to indicate the status of the patient.

    b. 00326-P1—*Incorrect*
    CPT code 00326 describes anesthesia services for patients younger than 1 year of age.

    c. 00320-P1, 99100—*Incorrect*
    Qualifying-circumstances code 99100 would not be reported, as the patient was over 1 year of age.

    d. 00320, 99100—*Incorrect*
    Qualifying-circumstances code 99100 would not be reported, as the patient was over 1 year of age. In addition, the physical status modifier P1 needs to be appended to indicate this was a normal, healthy patient.

67 Monitored anesthesia care (MAC) was provided for a 76-year-old patient with severe systemic disease for a colonoscopy. The correct CPT code(s) would be:

    a. 00810, 99100—*Incorrect*
    This code selection does not include the physical status modifier to describe the severe systemic disease.

    b. 00740-P3, 99100—*Incorrect*
    The anesthesia code 00740 is for an upper endoscopy.

    c. **00810-P3, 99100—Correct Answer**

    d. 00810—*Incorrect*
    This code selection does not include the physical status modifier for the severe systemic disease and does not include the code for the qualifying circumstance due to the age of the patient.

68. Global radiology services are reported:

    a. By appending both the TC and 26 modifiers to the radiology code—*Incorrect*
    The TC and 26 modifiers would never be appended to the same code, as these modifiers are used to define the separate components of the radiology service.

    b. By appending the 26 modifier to the radiology code—*Incorrect*
    The 26 modifier is used to report the professional component of the radiology service.

    c. By appending the TC modifier to the radiology code—*Incorrect*
    The TC modifier is used to report the technical component of the radiology service.

    d. **By reporting the CPT code without any modifiers—Correct Answer**

69. A complete ultrasound of the retroperitoneum consists of:

    a. Real-time scans of the kidneys, abdominal aorta, common iliac artery origins, inferior vena cava, and any abnormality—*Incorrect*
    A complete ultrasound of the retroperitoneum *also consists* of a complete evaluation of the kidneys and urinary bladder when clinical history suggests urinary tract pathology.

    b. A complete evaluation of the kidneys and urinary bladder when clinical history suggests urinary tract pathology—*Incorrect*
    This does not include the real-time scans of the body areas/organs listed in answer a.

    c. Real-time scans of the kidneys, abdominal aorta, common iliac artery origins, and any abnormality—*Incorrect*
    This answer is missing the scans of the inferior vena cava and the complete evaluation of the kidneys and urinary bladder when indicated by urinary tract pathology.

    d. Both a and b—Correct Answer
    This information is located in the CPT manual in the Radiology Guidelines under Diagnostic Ultrasound, Abdomen and Retroperitoneum.

70. A patient complaining of severe back pain and blood in the urine presents for an MRI of the abdomen and pelvis without contrast materials, followed by contrast materials and further sequences. The radiology report concluded the patient had several small renal cysts and one kidney stone. The correct codes would be:

    a. 74182, 72196, 593.2, 592.0—*Incorrect*
    The MRI codes describe the study as with contrast only.

    b. 74183, 72197, 593.2, 592.0—Correct Answer

    c. 74183, 72197, 724.5, 599.70—*Incorrect*
    The CPT codes are correct; however, the ICD-9-CM codes describe the signs and symptoms of the renal cysts and kidney stone and therefore would not be reported.

    d. 74183, 72197, 724.5, 599.70, 593.2, 592.0—*Incorrect*
    You would not report the signs and symptoms, which are part of the definitive illness—in this case, the renal cysts and the renal stone.

71. **CT Scan of the Chest With and Without Contrast**
Clinical History: Cough.
Protocol: 5-mm axial images apices to adrenal glands pre- and post-100 cc intravenous contrast material.
Findings: There are no enlarged mediastinal or hilar lymph nodes. There is no pleural or pericardial effusion. Scanning of the upper abdomen demonstrates the adrenal glands to be within normal limits. Motion artifact degrades several of the slices. There is no gross evidence of pleural or parenchymal mass or abnormal fluid collection.
Impression: Grossly unremarkable CT of the chest.

    Based on this report, the correct codes would be:

    a. 71270, V70.0—*Incorrect*
    When there is no definitive diagnosis, you would code the signs and symptoms that prompted the study—in this case, the cough.

    b. 71270, 786.2—Correct Answer
    Because there was no definitive diagnosis, you would code the signs and symptoms that prompted the study, in this case the cough (ICD-9 code 786.2). The CPT code 71270 correctly describes the CT of the chest (thorax) without and with contrast material.

    c. 71270-52, V70.0—*Incorrect*
    You would not use modifier 52 to reduce the service if the study was normal. The signs and symptoms would be listed as the diagnosis code, as no definitive diagnosis was documented.

    d. 71250, 786.2—*Incorrect*
    The CPT code 71250 describes a CT of the chest *without* any contrast material.

72. Right Lower Extremity Venous Duplex Doppler Sonogram
Clinical History: Right leg swollen. Ulcer in the right ankle.
Protocol: Real-time images, spectral analysis, and graded compression.
Findings: The right lower extremity venous structures were evaluated from the level of the common femoral vein in the groin to the popliteal vein. The vessel walls appear normal. There is no evidence of wall thickening. Normal phasic venous flow was observed in each of the visualized venous vessels. The vessel walls are completely compressible and there is no evidence of intraluminal thrombus. Normal augmentation of flow was observed in each of the visualized areas. There is no evidence of retrograde flow or reflux noted.
Impression: No evidence of deep vein thrombosis. No evidence of reflux or valvular incompetence.
Based on this report, the correct codes would be:
a. 93970-RT, 729.81, 707.10—*Incorrect*
The CPT code 93970 describes a bilateral study; therefore, appending the RT modifier is inappropriate.
b. 93971-RT, 453.40—*Incorrect*
The CPT code 93971 and modifier are correct; however, no diagnosis of deep vein thrombosis was made, and therefore the signs and symptoms that prompted the study would be reported.
c. **93971-RT, 729.81, 707.10—Correct Answer**
The CPT code 93971 describes the Doppler of one lower extremity and the RT modifier identifies the right leg. The signs and symptoms of leg swelling and ulcer provide the medical necessity for the study, because there was no definitive diagnosis.
d. 93970-RT, 453.40—*Incorrect*
The CPT code 93970 describes a bilateral study, and the diagnosis code of deep vein thrombosis was not documented.

73. Radiation treatment delivery codes (77401–77416) represent what type of component?
a. Global—*Incorrect*
These codes are not reported globally.
b. Professional—*Incorrect*
The professional component is reported with radiation treatment management codes.
c. **Technical—Correct Answer**
This answer is located right underneath the heading of Radiation Treatment Delivery: CPT states that radiation therapy (77401–77416) recognizes the technical component and the various energy levels.
d. Complete—*Incorrect*
This is not a component type.

74. Clinical brachytherapy requires the use of radioelements applied into or around a treatment field. An intermediate application includes how many sources/ribbons?
a. Greater than 10—*Incorrect*
This represents a complex application.
b. One to four—*Incorrect*
This represents a simple application.
c. **Five to 10—Correct Answer**
This information is located in the CPT manual in the Radiology section, Clinical Brachytherapy Guidelines, under definitions.
d. None; an intermediate application refers to the insertion of Heyman capsules—*Incorrect*
This does not refer to sources or ribbons.

75. A patient complaining of sore throat pain with fever for several days presented to the clinic. The laboratory at the clinic performed a rapid strep test and a throat culture with susceptibility studies, antimicrobial agent, disk method. The correct codes would be:
a. **87880, 87070, 87184—Correct Answer**
b. 87880, 87070—*Incorrect*
This does not include the CPT code for the susceptibility studies.
c. 87880, 87070, 87185—*Incorrect*
This includes the susceptibility by enzyme method.
d. 87046, 87070, 87184—*Incorrect*
The first CPT code describes a stool culture.

76. The following is true about organ- or disease-oriented panels:
a. They are developed as clinical guidelines for physicians—*Incorrect*
These panels were developed for coding purposes only.
b. **They may be reported in addition to a test that is not included in the panel—Correct Answer**
This information is located in the CPT Manual in the Pathology Guidelines under Organ- or Disease-Related Panels.
c. They are developed to limit the performance of other laboratory tests—*Incorrect*
They are not intended to limit the performance of others laboratory tests.
d. A panel may be reported when 50% or more of the tests listed in the panel are performed—*Incorrect*
All the tests included in the panel must be performed to use the code for the panel.

77. The physician ordered an electrolyte panel and a calcium total. The correct code(s) for the laboratory tests would be:

a. 82374, 82435, 84132, 84295, 82310—*Incorrect* **You would not list the codes individually if there is a panel code that includes all the tests provided. The additional code for the calcium total was correct.**

b. 80051, 82330—*Incorrect* **This code selection includes the correct CPT code for the panel; however, the code for the calcium (82330) is ionized and not total.**

c. **80051, 82310—Correct Answer This selection includes the one CPT code for the electrolyte panel and the additional code for the calcium total.**

d. 80051—*Incorrect* **This code selection does not include the additional code for the calcium total.**

78. While running the blood for a basic metabolic panel, the machine jammed. The blood sample taken included a sufficient amount to rerun the test. The correct code(s) would be:

a. 80047-52, 80047-91—*Incorrect* **You would not report the code twice, and modifier 91 would not be appended to show it was a repeat clinical test, as the description of the modifier clearly states this modifier is not to be used to rerun or confirm initial results due to testing problems with the specimens or the equipment.**

b. 80047-91—*Incorrect* **Modifier 91 would not be appended when the test is rerun due to difficulties with the specimen or equipment.**

c. **80047—Correct Answer No modifier is appended, as you are able to report the code only once.**

d. 80047-52—*Incorrect* **A reduced service modifier would not be appended, as the second test was completed.**

79. The following is not true when providing evocative/suppression testing:

a. The codes for the physician's administration of the evocative or suppressive agents are separately reportable—*Incorrect* **According to the evocative/suppression guidelines, these services are separately reported.**

b. **The codes for the supplies and drugs are not separately reported—Correct Answer You may report the codes for the supplies and drugs separately.** This information is located in the CPT Manual in the Pathology section under the Evocative/Suppression Guidelines.

c. Prolonged physician attendance and monitoring during the testing is separately reported—*Incorrect* **According to the Evocative/Suppression Guidelines, these services are separately reported.**

d. Prolonged physician care codes are not separately reported when evocative/suppression testing involves prolonged infusions—*Incorrect* **According to the Evocative/Suppression Guidelines, these services would not be reported separately when the prolonged infusion services are provided.**

80. A 52-year-old male, with an onset of neck pain, severity 4/9, and left upper extremity radiating pain to dorsal elbow and dorsal wrist pain, underwent a needle EMG and nerve conduction study of the median motor nerve with F wave and two sensory nerves. The correct codes would be:

a. 95860, 95900, 95904—*Incorrect* **CPT code 95900 describes the nerve conduction study for a motor nerve without the F wave. Additionally, two sensory nerves were tested; therefore, CPT code 95904 should be reported twice.**

b. 95860, 95903, 95904—*Incorrect* **Two sensory nerves were tested; therefore, CPT code 95904 should be reported twice.**

c. **95860, 95903, 95904 × 2—Correct Answer CPT code 95860 describes the needle EMG, CPT code 95903 describes the nerve conduction study for the one motor nerve with the F-wave, and CPT code 95904 describes the nerve conduction study for the two sensory nerves.**

d. 95860, 95903 × 2, 95904—*Incorrect* **Only one motor nerve was tested; therefore, CPT code 95903 should be reported only once.**

81. A patient was seen for osteopathic manipulation for the following regions: lumbar spine, right and left hip, right and left knee, and sacrum. According to the CPT Guidelines for osteopathic manipulation, how many regions were treated?

   a. Six—*Incorrect*
     The right and left hip and knees are not counted as separate regions.

   b. Four—**Correct Answer**
     In the CPT Manual in the Osteopathic Manipulative Treatment Guidelines, **the regions are defined as head, cervical, thoracic, lumbar, sacral, pelvic, lower extremities, upper extremities, rib cage, abdomen, and viscera. In this case, there are four regions: lumbar, pelvis (hip), lower extremities (both knees), and the sacrum.**

   c. Three—*Incorrect*
     The lumbar spine and sacrum are counted separately.

   d. One; doctors of osteopathic medicine treat the body as a whole—*Incorrect*
     While this is a true statement, it does not refer to the regions treated by osteopathic manipulation.

82. A patient presented to the psychiatrist's office for minimal psychotherapy and for a review and refill of his prescription medications. The correct code(s) would be:

   a. 90862—**Correct Answer**
     Pharmacological management includes minimal psychotherapy and is not a time-based code.

   b. 90805—*Incorrect*
     This code describes 20 to 30 minutes of psychotherapy with a medical E/M service.

   c. There is no documentation of time; because psychotherapy is a timed service, no CPT code should be reported—*Incorrect*
     Pharmacological management, which describes the service, is not a time-based CPT code.

   d. 90804, 90862—*Incorrect*
     The documentation does not support 20 to 30 minutes of psychotherapy services in addition to the pharmacologic management.

83. A patient with dysphagia presented to the outpatient clinic for an evaluation of swallowing by flexible fiberoptic endoscopy. The correct codes would be:

   a. 92613, 787.20—*Incorrect*
     The CPT code 92613 describes the physician interpretation and report only.

   b. 92613, 787.29—*Incorrect*
     This CPT code describes the physician interpretation and report only, and the diagnosis code describes the dysphagia as other and not unspecified.

   c. 92612, 787.20—**Correct Answer**

   d. 92612, 787.29—*Incorrect*
     The CPT code 92612 is correct; however, the diagnosis code describes the dysphagia as other and not unspecified.

84. A patient received 15 minutes of manual electrical stimulation and anorectal manometry as treatment for her urge incontinence and anal spasms. The correct codes would be:

   a. 97014, 91122, 788.31, 564.6—*Incorrect*
     The physical therapy code (97014) describes electrical stimulation that is *unattended*.

   b. 97014, 91122, 788.31, 728.85—*Incorrect*
     This physical therapy code (97014) describes electrical stimulation that is unattended, and the diagnosis code 728.85 is not specific to an anal spasm.

   c. 97032, 91122, 788.31, 564.6—**Correct Answer**

   d. 97032, 91122, 788.31, 728.85—*Incorrect*
     Although the CPT codes in this selection are correct, the diagnosis code is not specific to an anal spasm.

85. A patient presented to the audiologist for a binaural hearing aid examination and selection. During the encounter, the audiologist performed a comprehensive audiometry, a tympanogram, and acoustic reflex testing. The correct codes would be:

   a. 92591, 92557, 92567, 92568—**Correct Answer**

   b. 92590, 92557, 92567, 92568—*Incorrect*
     CPT code 92590 describes a monaural hearing aid examination.

   c. 92591, 92557, 92550, 92568—*Incorrect*
     CPT code 92550 describes a tympanogram with reflex threshold measurements.

   d. 92590, 92557, 92550, 92568—*Incorrect*
     This sequence of codes includes an incorrect code for the hearing aid examination (monaural) and tympanogram (includes reflex threshold measurements).

86. A special report:
   a. Is routinely provided—*Incorrect*
   Special reports are rarely provided.
   b. Includes the credentials of the physician providing the service—*Incorrect*
   This is not a required item for a special report (refer to the Surgery Guidelines under Special Report).
   c. Should be submitted when reporting unlisted CPT codes, modifier 22, and Category III codes—Correct Answer
   These three circumstances would require a special report to inform the insurance company of the service provided (unlisted CPT code), the unusual service or additional time and/or amount of work (modifier 22) provided, or new technology (Category III codes).
   d. Should be submitted only when reporting unlisted CPT codes—*Incorrect*
   A special report should also be submitted when appending modifier 22 or when reporting a Category III code.

87. When reporting repair codes from the Integumentary section, the following is true:
   a. When multiple wounds are repaired, you would report a complex wound repair code—*Incorrect*
   When multiple wounds are repaired, you would add together the lengths of the wounds with the same classification.
   b. Wounds that are repaired with only adhesive strips or a tissue adhesive would be reported with an E/M code—*Incorrect*
   Wounds that are repaired with tissue adhesive may be reported with a CPT code from the wound repair section.
   c. Débridement would be separately reported when gross contamination requires prolonged cleansing—Correct Answer
   This information is located in the CPT Manual in the Integumentary section within the Repair (closure) guidelines.
   d. Simple ligation of vessels in an open wound is separately reported—*Incorrect*
   This is considered part of any wound closure.

88. A Mohs' surgeon refers to a surgeon who has two separate, distinct roles:
   a. A surgeon and a radiologist—*Incorrect*
   Mohs' surgery does not include a radiological component.
   b. An assistant surgeon and a pathologist—*Incorrect*
   The Mohs' physician acts as the surgeon and the pathologist.
   c. A surgeon and a pathologist—Correct Answer
   This information is located in the CPT Manual in the Integumentary section in the Mohs' Micrographic Surgery guidelines.
   d. An assistant surgeon and a radiologist—*Incorrect*
   The Mohs' physician acts as the surgeon, and the surgery does not include a radiological component.

89. The application of casts and strapping may not be reported when:
   a. The cast application or strapping is a replacement procedure—*Incorrect*
   The cast application or strapping *may* be reported when it is a replacement procedure. This information is located in the CPT Manual in the Musculoskeletal section in the Application of Casts and Strapping guidelines.
   b. The cast application or strapping is the initial service performed without a restorative treatment—*Incorrect*
   The cast application or strapping *may* be reported when it is the initial service performed without a restorative treatment. This information is located in the CPT Manual in the Musculoskeletal section in the Application of Casts and Strapping guidelines.
   c. The cast application or strapping is provided to stabilize or protect a fracture/injury—*Incorrect*
   The cast application or strapping *may* be reported when it is provided to stabilize or protect a fracture/injury. This information is located in the Musculoskeletal section in the Application of Casts and Strapping guidelines.
   d. The physician who applies the initial cast, strap, or splint assumes all of the subsequent fracture care—Correct Answer
   When the physician who applies the initial cast, strap, or splint assumes all of the subsequent fracture care, this is *not* reported, as the initial cast, splint, or strapping application is included in the treatment of fracture and/or dislocation codes. This information is located in the CPT Manual in the Musculoskeletal section in the Application of Casts and Strapping guidelines.

90. The global surgical package includes:
  a. **Preoperative, intraoperative, and postoperative services—Correct Answer**
  b. Preoperative, intraoperative, and postoperative services and complications within the global period—*Incorrect*
  Complications during the global surgical period are separately reported.
  c. Preoperative and postoperative services—*Incorrect*
  The global surgical package also includes the intraoperative services.
  d. Preoperative and intraoperative services—*Incorrect*
  The global surgical package includes the postoperative services.

91. A patient presents for treatment of basal cell carcinoma and actinic keratosis. A 3.5-cm malignant lesion was excised from the patient's trunk, and four premalignant lesions (actinic keratosis) on the shoulder were destroyed by cryosurgery. The correct codes would be:
  a. 17000, 17003, 11604, 702.0, 173.5—*Incorrect*
  In this code selection, the surgeries are not sequenced with the most complex surgery listed first, and the modifiers are not appended.
  b. 11604, 17000, 17003, 173.5, 702.0—*Incorrect*
  Although with this code selection, the surgeries are properly sequenced, without appending modifier 59, the destruction of the premalignant lesions would be considered bundled.
  c. **11604, 17000-59-51, 17003, 173.5, 702.0— Correct Answer**
  In this code selection, the CPT codes are sequenced with the most complex surgery listed first. CPT code 17000 requires modifiers 59 to indicate the service was provided on a separate site and 51 to indicate multiple surgeries. CPT code 17003 does not require a modifier, as it is an add-on code.
  d. 11604, 17000-59-51, 17003-59-51, 173.5, 702.0—*Incorrect*
  Modifiers 59 and 51 do not need to be appended to CPT code 17003, as it is an add-on code.

92. Preoperative Diagnosis: Left neck adenopathy.
Postoperative Diagnosis: Same.
Nature of Operation: Biopsy of deep level II cervical lymph node.
Anesthesia: General with laryngeal mask.
Operative Findings: The patient had an enlarged level II left neck adenopathy.
Operative Procedure: The patient was brought into the operating room and was laid in supine position. He was given general anesthesia by laryngeal mask. Neck was distended from the chest by placement of a shoulder roll. The left neck was prepped and draped in the usual sterile technique.

A skin crease incision was taken. After going through skin and subcutaneous tissue, the platysma was opened and the lymph node was identified in the level II region anterior to the jugular vein. The lymph node was gently dissected away from the jugular vein. Hemostasis was achieved by Bovie and ligation with 3-0 Vicryl. Once the lymph node was withdrawn, hemostasis was complete. The lymph node was sent fresh for evaluation. Closure was done with 3-0 Vicryl for platysma and 4-0 Biosyn for skin. Dressing was done.

The patient was extubated and brought to the recovery room in stable condition.

Based on this report, the correct codes would be:
  a. 38500, 785.6—*Incorrect*
  The CPT code 38500 describes an open superficial lymph node biopsy.
  b. **38510, 785.6—Correct Answer**
  c. 38505, 785.6—*Incorrect*
  The CPT code 38505 describes a superficial lymph node needle biopsy.
  d. 38520, 785.6—*Incorrect*
  The CPT code 38520 describes the correct type of procedure for a cervical lymph node; however, it includes the excision of scalene fat pad.

93. Mrs. Peters returned to the clinic for a bilateral nasal endoscopy. On endoscopic examination of the nose, there was minimal mucosa edema with thick mucoid secretions. There was persistent synechiae and scarring on the right, obstructing the ostiomeatal complex on the right. The recurrent headaches are a component and related to chronic sinusitis. The correct codes would be:

a. 31233, 473.9—*Incorrect*
The CPT code 31233 describes a nasal endoscopy with maxillary sinoscopy.

b. 31235, 473.9—*Incorrect*
The CPT code 31235 describes a nasal endoscopy with sphenoid sinoscopy.

c. **31231, 473.9—Correct Answer**
No modifier is necessary, as the code descriptor states unilateral or bilateral.

d. 31231-50, 473.9—*Incorrect*
No modifier is necessary, as the code descriptor states unilateral or bilateral.

94. A patient presents with low back pain radiating to the bilateral leg areas. The pain increases with walking or bending. The physician performed multiple trigger-point injections into the left gluteus medius, injecting 10 mL of mepivacaine to alleviate the patient's pain and to improve her activities of daily living. The correct codes would be:

a. **20552, J0670—Correct Answer**
The description of this code includes single or multiple injections into one or two muscles and therefore would be reported only once. The drug injected is reported with the HCPCS code J0670.

b. 20552 × 2, J0670 × 2—*Incorrect*
CPT code 20552 would not be reported twice, as the code descriptor includes multiple injections into one or two muscles. The drug code would be reported only once, as it lists the amount per 10 mL.

c. 20553, J0670—*Incorrect*
The CPT code 20553 describes multiple injections into three or more muscles.

d. 20550, J0670—*Incorrect*
The CPT code 20550 describes an injection into a tendon sheath and not a muscle.

95. Select the CPT code(s) for extracapsular cataract extraction by phacoemulsification with placement of posterior chamber IOL:

a. 66982, 66985—*Incorrect*
The CPT code 66982 describes the correct procedure; however, it includes the use of special equipment. CPT code 66985 for the insertion of the IOL would not be separately reported, as it is included in the surgical procedure.

b. 66984, 66985—*Incorrect*
The CPT code 66984 correctly describes the surgical procedure; however, you would not report 66985 separately, as it is included in the surgical procedure.

c. 66985—*Incorrect*
This code describes only the placement of the IOL not associated with a concurrent cataract removal.

d. **66984—Correct Answer**
This one CPT code describes the surgical procedure and the placement of the IOL.

96. Select the codes for placement of a left chest wall central venous access device with subcutaneous port performed with intraoperative fluoroscopy on a 73-year-old patient.

a. 36570, 77001—*Incorrect*
CPT code 36570 describes the port placement for patients younger than 5 years of age. No modifier was appended to indicate the left side.

b. 36570-LT, 77002—*Incorrect*
CPT code 36570 describes the port placement for patients younger than 5 years of age. The fluoroscopy code 77002 describes fluoroscopy for needle placement.

c. **36571-LT, 77001—Correct Answer**
CPT code 36571 describes the port placement for patients 5 years and older. The fluoroscopy code is specific for a central venous access device placement. The LT modifier would be appended to indicate the left side.

d. 36571, 77002—*Incorrect*
The fluoroscopy code 77002 describes fluoroscopy for needle placement. No modifier was appended to indicate the left side.

97. A patient underwent a therapeutic nonobstetrical dilation and curettage (D&C) for pyometrium and stenosis of the cervix. The correct codes would be:

  a. 58120, 615.0, 622.4—*Incorrect*
  The diagnosis code 615.0 does not describe the pyometra.

  b. 59160, 615.9, 622.4—*Incorrect*
  The CPT code 59160 describes a D&C that is performed postpartum.

  c. 57558, 615.9, 622.4—*Incorrect*
  This CPT code 57558 describes a D&C of a cervical stump.

  d. 58120, 615.9, 622.4—**Correct Answer**
  The CPT code 58120 correctly describes the D&C as nonobestetric and therapeutic. Diagnosis code 615.9 lists the condition of pyometra under the code descriptor, and 622.4 correctly describes the stenosis of the cervix.

98. **Preoperative Diagnosis:** Endometrial hyperplasia with atypia and polyp, postmenopausal bleeding.
Postoperative Diagnosis: Same.
Nature of Operation: Gynecological oncology standby for 1 hour time.
Operative Indications: The patient is an 83-year-old female who was brought into the operating room by Dr. Niece and Dr. Michaels. I was asked to stand by in the event malignancy was diagnosed on frozen section.
Operative Procedure: The patient was brought to the operating room; she underwent a total abdominal hysterectomy (TAH) bilateral salpingo-oophorectomy (BSO) with frozen section that revealed no carcinoma.

  The total standby time was 1 hour. During this time, I [i.e., surgeon] was available solely for the purpose of this patient with no other patient care activities.

  Based on this report, the correct codes would be:

  a. 99360, 621.33—*Incorrect*
  The CPT code for the standby services should be reported in two units to capture the time of 1 hour.

  b. No codes should be reported, as the physician did not provide any service during the surgical procedure—*Incorrect*
  The physician did spend time solely for this patient in standby with no other patient activities. Standby codes are reported with CPT code 99360 and are reported in time increments of 30 minutes.

  c. 99360 × 2, 621.33—**Correct Answer**

The CPT code 99360 correctly identifies the standby services of the provider as being solely available to the patient in the case of a diagnosis of malignancy. The code would be reported in two units to capture the time of 1 hour. The diagnosis code identifies the endometrial hyperplasia with atypia.

  d. 99360, 621.33, 627.1—*Incorrect*
  The standby service code should be reported in two units to capture the time of 1 hour. ICD-9-CM code 627.1 for the postmenopausal bleeding would not be reported, as it is a sign/symptom of the endometrial hyperplasia.

99. A 58-year-old patient with a strangulated umbilical hernia underwent a hernia repair with mesh. The correct codes would be:

  a. 49582, 49568—*Incorrect*
  CPT code 49582 describes a strangulated umbilical hernia for a patient 5 years old or younger.

  b. 49582, 49568-51—*Incorrect*
  CPT code 49582 describes a strangulated umbilical hernia for a patient 5 years old or younger. CPT code 49568 for the implant of the mesh is an add-on code and does not require a modifier.

  c. 49587, 49568—**Correct Answer**
  CPT code 49587 correctly describes the repair for a strangulated umbilical hernia for a patient over the age of 5. No modifier was appended to the code for the mesh implant, as CPT code 49568 is an add-on code.

  d. 49587, 49568-51—*Incorrect*
  Although both CPT codes are correct, you would not append modifier 51 to an add-on code.

100. The following code represents a repeat transurethral resection of prostate tissue 3 years post–original procedure:

  a. 52500—*Incorrect*
  This code describes a transurethral resection of the bladder neck.

  b. 52630—**Correct Answer**
  This correctly identifies a "repeat" transurethral resection of the prostate.

  c. 52601—*Incorrect*
  This code does not describe the procedure as being performed for a regrowth.

  d. 52640—*Incorrect*
  This code describes a transurethral resection of postoperative bladder neck contracture.

101. A patient presented to the gastroenterologist complaining of weight loss and of blood in his stool. The physician performed a colonoscopy with removal of three colon polyps using hot biopsy forceps. The correct codes would be:

  a. 45384, 569.0—Correct Answer
The CPT code 45384 describes a colonoscopy, flexible, proximal to splenic flexure; with *removal of* tumor(s), *polyp(s)*, or other lesion(s) by *hot biopsy forceps* or bipolar cautery. The CPT code would be reported only once, as the code includes multiple polyps. You would report the diagnosis code for the anal or rectal polyp (569.0) and not the signs and symptoms of weight loss and blood in the stool.

  b. 45384 × 3, 569.0—*Incorrect*
This CPT code descriptor includes multiple polyps; therefore, you would report CPT code 45384 only once.

  c. 45384, 783.21, 578.1, 569.0—*Incorrect*
You would not report signs and symptoms (weight loss and blood in stool), as they are signs and symptoms of the polyps.

  d. 45384 × 3, 783.21, 578.1, 569.0—*Incorrect*
You would not report signs and symptoms (weight loss and blood in stool), as they are signs and symptoms of the polyps. The CPT code descriptor 45384 includes multiple polyps; therefore, you would report this code only once.

102. Select the correct code for a laparoscopic cholecystectomy with exploration of common duct:

  a. 47570—*Incorrect*
This code describes a laparoscopic cholecystoenterostomy.

  b. 47563—*Incorrect*
This code describes a laparoscopic cholecystectomy with cholangiography.

  c. 47564—Correct Answer
This code describes the correct procedure and describes the laparoscopic approach.

  d. 47610—*Incorrect*
This describes the correct procedure; however, it describes an open approach.

103 A diagnostic endoscopy is:

  a. Always reported as the primary procedure—*Incorrect*
When only a diagnostic endoscopy is performed with a surgical endoscopy, only the surgical endoscopy would be reported.

  b. Designated as an add-on code—*Incorrect*
The diagnostic endoscopy codes are designated as separate procedure codes.

  c. Always included in the surgical endoscopy—Correct Answer
This information can be found in the CPT manual under any of the endoscopy codes.

  d. Never reported alone—*Incorrect*
When only a diagnostic endoscopy is performed, it may be reported on its own.

104. A 55-year-old male new patient presented to the urologist for evaluation of dysuria. The physician documented an expanded problem-focused history and during the comprehensive examination performed a venipuncture for PSA and testosterone total. The postvoid residual by ultrasound revealed 22 mL, and the automated urine dipstick was positive for ketones and protein; specific gravity was 1.020, and pH was 7.0. A simple uroflow showed voided time 66 sec, straining to urinate present, prolonged urination time present, intermittency present, split stream absent and hesitancy absent. The assessment and plan included a diagnosis of benign prostatic hyperplasia (BPH) without significant obstruction, a transrectal ultrasound was ordered to measure the prostate size, and a prescription for Cialis was given for erectile dysfunction (moderate medical decision). The correct codes would be:

  a. 99202-25, 51736, 51798, 36415, 81003, 600.00, 788.1, 788.21—*Incorrect*
This code selection does not include the diagnosis code for erectile dysfunction. Incomplete bladder emptying would not be reported, as it is a sign and symptom of BPH.

  b. 99202-25, 51736, 51798, 36415, 81003, 600.00, 788.1, 607.84—Correct Answer
The level of service represented by CPT code 99202 is correct because documentation requirements for a new patient require that three of three key components be met or exceeded. In this case, the history was documented at the lowest level, expanded problem-focused (level 2), and was the determining factor in selecting the level of service. Modifier 25 was appended to the office visit to show it was a separate identifiable service from the other procedures performed (simple uroflow and postvoid residual). The simple uroflow is reported with CPT code 51736, the postvoid residual is reported with CPT code 51798, the venipuncture is reported with CPT code 36415, and the automated urinalysis without microscopy by dipstick is reported with CPT code 81003. The diagnosis codes are reported with 600.00 for the BPH, 788.1 for the dysuria, and 607.84 for the erectile dysfunction.

  c. 99202-25, 51736, 51798, 36415, 81002, 600.00, 788.1, 607.84—*Incorrect*

The CPT code 81002 represents a nonautomated urinalysis, whereas the physician performed an automated urinalysis.

d. 99204-25, 51736, 51798, 36415, 81003, 600.00, 788.1, 607.84—*Incorrect*
The level of service represented by the CPT code 99204 was not supported by the documentation. The level of history was expanded problem-focused level 2, the level of physical examination was comprehensive level 5, and the medical decision was moderate level 4. Documentation for a new patient requires that all three components be at the same level. You would need to select the level of service based on the lowest component, in this case, the history, level 2.

105. **Preoperative Diagnosis:** Hematuria.
Postoperative Diagnosis: Hematuria.
Patient presents for a cystourethroscopy. Flexible cystoscopy was performed with the 16-Fr flexible cystoscope after obtaining consent and explaining risks such as bleeding, dysuria, and infection. Patient was prepped with Betadine, and lidocaine jelly was instilled. The examination was done supine in the lithotomy position. The urethra was normal. Bladder examination reveals completely normal mucosa with normal ureteral orifices. Procedure was tolerated well. The patient was given an antibiotic after the procedure. Based on this report, the correct code(s) would be:

a. 52000, 96372, J1580—*Incorrect*
The note states the patient was given an antibiotic; however, it does not say it was injected. The antibiotic could have been in pill form and taken orally. Therefore, the documentation does not support the injection, and antibiotic should not be coded.

b. 52000-25, 96372, J1580—*Incorrect*
Modifier 25 is always appended to an E/M code and not to a procedure code. Documentation does not support the injection and drug code.

c. 52000, 96372—*Incorrect*
Documentation does not support an injection code.

d. 52000—Correct Answer
Only the cystourethroscopy is supported by documentation in the operative report.

106. The study of the motion and flow of urine is called:

a. Urodynamics—Correct Answer
Urodynamics is the study of the motion and flow of urine.

b. Urology—*Incorrect*
Urology is the branch of medicine that deals with the diagnosis and treatment of disorders of the urinary tract or urogenital system.

c. Uromotion—*Incorrect*
Uromotion is not a medical term.

d. Uroflowology—*Incorrect*
Uroflowology is not a medical term.

107. Under fluoroscopic guidance, Mr. Smith underwent a subcutaneous permanent pacemaker placement with transvenous placement of electrodes in the right atrium and right ventricle. The correct code(s) would be:

a. 33206, 71090—*Incorrect*
The CPT code 33206 code represents the insertion of a permanent pacemaker with a transvenous electrode; *atrial* only. CPT code 71090 correctly identifies the radiological guidance.

b. 33207, 71090—*Incorrect*
The CPT code 33207 represents the insertion of a permanent pacemaker with a transvenous electrode; *ventricular* only. The CPT code 71090 correctly identifies the radiological guidance.

c. 33208, 71090—Correct Answer
The CPT code 33208 represents the insertion of a permanent pacemaker with a transvenous electrode; *atrial and ventricular.* The CPT code 71090 correctly identifies the radiologic guidance.

d. 33210—*Incorrect*
The CPT code 33210 represents a temporary transvenous single-chamber cardiac, electrode, or pacemaker catheter.

108. Coronary artery bypass procedures using both venous grafts and arterial grafts during the same procedure are reported:

    a. Alone, as they represent both the arterial and venous grafting—*Incorrect*

    According to the CPT Guidelines for Combined Arterial-Venous Grafting for Coronary Artery Bypass, "These codes may NOT be used alone." Additionally, all the codes are designated as add-on codes.

    b. **In combination with the appropriate arterial graft code and the appropriate combined arterial-venous graft code— Correct Answer**

    According to the CPT Guidelines for Combined Arterial-Venous Grafting for Coronary Artery Bypass, "To report combined arterial-venous grafts it is necessary to report two codes: 1) the appropriate combined arterial-venous graft code (33517–33523) and 2) the appropriate arterial graft code (33533–33536)."

    c. A code from the coronary artery bypass–venous graft codes and a code from the arterial graft code—*Incorrect*

    According to the CPT Guidelines for Venous Grafting Only for Coronary Artery Bypass, **the venous grafting codes should not be used to report the performance of coronary artery bypass procedures using arterial grafts and venous grafts during the same procedure.**

    d. A code from the coronary artery bypass–venous graft codes and a code from the arterial graft code and the appropriate combined arterial-venous graft code—*Incorrect*

    According to the CPT Guidelines for Combined Arterial-Venous Grafting for Coronary Artery Bypass, **the two codes required to correctly report the service would be the appropriate combined arterial-venous graft code and the appropriate arterial graft code.**

109. Mrs. Escobar had continuous complaints of syncope and palpitations. Her cardiologist suspected arrhythmia and implanted a patient-activated cardiac event recorder with looping memory. The correct codes would be:

    a. **33282, 780.2, 785.1—Correct Answer**

    The CPT code 33282 represents the implantation of the event recorder, and the diagnosis codes correctly identify the syncope and palpitations.

    b. 33284, 780.2, 785.1—*Incorrect*

    The CPT code 33284 represents the *removal* of the event recorder.

    c. 33282, 785.1, 780.4—*Incorrect*

    Although the CPT code 33282 is correct and the ICD-9-CM code 785.1 correctly identifies the palpitations, the ICD-9-CM code 780.4 identifies dizziness and not syncope (fainting).

    d. 33828, 427.9—*Incorrect*

    Although the CPT code 33828 is correct, the ICD-9-CM 427.9 code identifies arrhythmia, which is only "suspected" and not listed as a definitive diagnosis and therefore should not be coded.

110. Travis, a 2-year-old boy, was born with an atrioventricular canal defect. Due to the child's inability to gain weight and dyspnea, Dr. Jones ordered a transesophageal echocardiogram to evaluate the defect. The correct codes would be:

    a. 93315, 783.41, 786.09—*Incorrect*

    The CPT code 93315 correctly identifies the transesophageal echocardiogram for the congenital cardiac anomaly; however, the diagnosis codes represent the signs and symptoms of the definitive diagnosis of atrioventricular canal defect.

    b. **93315, 745.69—Correct Answer**

    The CPT code 93315 correctly identifies the transesophageal echocardiogram for the congenital cardiac anomaly, and the diagnosis code represents the atrioventricular canal defect.

    c. 93312, 745.69—*Incorrect*

    This CPT code would not be used for conditions considered congenital (the patient had the condition since birth, so it is considered congenital).

    d. 99312, 783.41, 786.09—*Incorrect*

    This CPT code would not be used for conditions considered congenital (the patient had the condition since birth, so it is considered congenital), and the diagnosis codes represent the signs and symptoms of the definitive diagnosis of atrioventricular canal defect.

111. When a catheter is placed into an artery or vein and moved or manipulated from the original artery/vein punctured or from an artery that branches off the aorta, it is called:

    a. Nonselective catheter placement—*Incorrect*
    With nonselective catheter placement, the catheter is placed only into the aorta or placed into a vein or artery and not moved any further.

    b. Aorta catheter placement—*Incorrect*
    There is no such term.

    c. Branch catheter placement—*Incorrect*
    There is no such term.

    d. Selective catheter placement—Correct Answer
    With selective catheter placement, the catheter is moved or manipulated to a part of the arterial system other than the vessel punctured or the aorta.

112. A patient underwent a right arthroscopic anterior Bankart repair with a right posterior Bankart repair and a SLAP repair of the right shoulder with extensive débridement of degenerative joint disease and rotator cuff tear with a partial posterior superior synovectomy during one operative session. The correct codes would be:

    a. 29806-RT, 29806-59-RT, 29823-59-RT, 29820-59—*Incorrect*
    When a surgeon performs an arthroscopy of the shoulder and capsulorrhaphy (29806) anterior and posterior, it would be inappropriate to report this code twice, as just one capsule is being repaired. The partial synovectomy is bundled, and it would be inappropriate to code for the extensive débridement, as it was mainly performed in the same area referred to by CPT codes 29806 and 29807.

    b. 29806-RT, 29807-51-RT—Correct Answer
    Both the repair of the SLAP lesion and the capsulorrhaphy (29806) are separately reportable, and modifier 51 would be appended to the second surgical procedure to identify multiple surgical procedures. The HCPCS RT modifier would be reported to show the service was provided on the right side.

    c. 29806-RT, 29807-51-RT, 29823-59-51-RT—*Incorrect*
    It would be inappropriate to code for the extensive débridement (29823), as it was mainly performed in the same area as that referred to by the codes 29806 and 29807.

    d. 29806-RT, 29807-51-RT, 29820-51—*Incorrect*
    The CPT code 29820 representing the partial synovectomy is bundled into the code representing the shoulder capsulorrhaphy (29806).

113. A patient diagnosed with myalgia received bilateral trigger-point injections into the trapezius muscle. The correct code(s) would be:

    a. **20552—Correct Answer**
    Correctly identifies the injection(s) of single or multiple trigger point(s), into *1 or 2 muscle(s).*

    b. 20552 × 2—*Incorrect*
    This CPT code descriptor includes two muscles; therefore, the code should be reported only once.

    c. 20551 × 2—*Incorrect*
    This CPT code represents an injection into a *single tendon.*

    d. 20553—*Incorrect*
    This code represents single or multiple injections into *three or more muscles.*

114. A complete ultrasound examination of the retroperitoneum may be reported when documentation includes the following:

    a. Real-time scans of the kidneys, abdominal aorta, common iliac artery origins, and inferior vena cava, including any demonstrated retroperitoneal abnormality—*Incorrect*
    According to the CPT Guidelines, a complete ultrasound of the retroperitoneum may also be reported when a complete evaluation of the kidneys and urinary bladder along with clinical history suggest urinary tract pathology.

    b. Complete evaluation of the kidneys and urinary bladder, along with clinical history, suggests urinary tract pathology—*Incorrect*
    According to the CPT Guidelines, a complete ultrasound of the retroperitoneum may also be reported when real-time scans of the kidneys, abdominal aorta, common iliac artery origins, and inferior vena cava, including any demonstrated retroperitoneal abnormality.

    c. Complete single-organ evaluation with clinical history suggests urinary tract pathology—*Incorrect*
    A single-organ evaluation would be reported as a limited study. In addition, a complete study can be reported only when both the kidneys and urinary bladder, along with clinical history suggesting urinary tract pathology, are performed.

    d. Both a and b—Correct Answer
    This information is located in the CPT Guidelines in the Radiology subsection under Abdomen and Retroperitoneum.

115. **Radiology Report**

    Bone Age: Single AP view of the left wrist and hand was obtained. The patient is 9 years of age. This was compared with the hand of a patient 8 years and 10 months from the standard Greulich and Pyle atlas of skeletal development of the hand and wrist. Although the carpal bones, navicular lunate, triquetrum, greater multangular, lesser multangular, capitate, and hamate are all present in the patient's wrist, the standard shows moderately more maturation formation of these carpal bones, which would indicate some degree of retardation.

    Impression: There is some degree of retardation in the growth and development of the bones of the wrist in this patient when compared to the standard.

    Based on this report, the correct codes would be:

    a. **77072, 783.40—Correct Answer**
    The ICD-9-CM code 783.40 identifies the lack of normal physiological development, and CPT code 77072 bone age studies correctly describes the service performed.

    b. 77072, 783.42—*Incorrect*
    Although the CPT code is correct, the diagnosis code 783.42 describing delayed milestones does not correctly describe the diagnosis.

    c. 77073, 783.40—*Incorrect*
    Although the diagnosis code is correct, the CPT code 77073 describes a bone length study (measurement of the length of bones as opposed to the measurement of the wrist and hand in bone age studies).

    d. 77073, 783.42—*Incorrect*
    In this case, both the diagnosis code for delayed milestones and the CPT code for bone length studies are incorrect.

116. An asymptomatic postmenopausal patient was sent for a bone density DEXA of the axial skeleton. The study showed the patient to have osteopenia of the lumbar spine. The correct codes would be:

    a. 77081, 733.90, V49.81—*Incorrect*
    The CPT code 77081 is a DEXA of the appendicular skeleton, and the HCPCS code V49.81 does not have to be coded, because there is a definitive diagnosis of osteopenia.

    b. **77080, 733.90—Correct Answer**
    The CPT code 77080 correctly identifies the DEXA of the axial skeleton and the definitive diagnosis of osteopenia.

    c. 77082, 733.90, V49.81—*Incorrect*
    The CPT code 77082 identifies a DEXA for vertebral fracture assessment, and the HCPCS code V49.81 does not have to be coded, because there is a definitive diagnosis of osteopenia.

    d. 77082, 733.90—*Incorrect*
    Although the diagnosis code 733.90 is correct, the CPT code 77082 identifies a DEXA for vertebral fracture assessment.

117. Mrs. Kramer presented to the mental health clinic to see Dr. Felix for minimal psychotherapy and pharmacological management. The correct code(s) would be:

    a. 90862, 90804—*Incorrect*
    The CPT code 90804 is for 20 to 30 minutes of psychotherapy and would not be reported with CPT code 90862, which represents pharmacological management including minimal psychotherapy.

    b. 90805—*Incorrect*
    This CPT code would be reported when an E/M service is provided along with 20 to 30 minutes of psychotherapy.

    c. **90862—Correct Answer**
    This CPT code correctly describes the service provided as pharmacological management with no more than minimal psychotherapy.

    d. 90845—*Incorrect*
    This CPT code represents psychoanalysis.

118. The appropriate psychotherapy code is determined by:
- **a.** **The type of psychotherapy provided, the place of service, face-to-face time, and if E/M services were also provided— Correct Answer**
  This information is located in the CPT Guidelines in the Medicine subsection under Psychiatric Therapeutic Procedures.
- **b.** The type of psychotherapy provided, the status of the patient, face-to-face time, and if E/M services were also provided—*Incorrect*
  The status of the patient is not one of the key determining factors in the selection of the psychotherapy CPT code.
- **c.** The type of psychotherapy provided, the place of service, face-to-face time, and if pharmacological management was provided—*Incorrect*
  Pharmacological management is not one of the key determining factors in the selection of the psychotherapy CPT code; it is a separate service identified by a separate CPT code.
- **d.** The type of psychotherapy provided, who provided the service (e.g., MD or clinical social worker), face-to-face time, and if E/M services were also provided—*Incorrect*
  Who provided the service is not one of the key determining factors in the selection of the psychotherapy CPT code.

119. An intermediate ophthalmological service is described as:
- **a.** A general evaluation of the complete visual system—*Incorrect*
  According to the CPT Guidelines located in the Medicine subsection under Ophthalmology, **this describes a comprehensive ophthalmological service.**
- **b.** A low-level evaluation and management service—*Incorrect*
  Although ophthalmologists may use E/M codes, they also have specific ophthalmology codes located in the Medicine subsection of CPT.
- **c.** **An evaluation of a new or existing condition complicated with a new diagnostic or management problem, not necessarily relating to the primary diagnosis—Correct Answer**
  This information is found in the CPT Guidelines located in the Medicine subsection under Ophthalmology.
- **d.** A midlevel E/M service—*Incorrect*
  Although ophthalmologists may use E/M codes, they also have specific ophthalmology codes located in the Medicine subsection of CPT.

120. Dr. Franklin ordered an intermediate visual field examination for Mary Jones. During the examination, Mary was called away, and only one eye was tested. The correct code would be:
- **a.** 92083—*Incorrect*
  This code represents an extended visual field.
- **b.** 92083-52—*Incorrect*
  This code represents an extended visual field, and because the CPT code states "visual field examination *unilateral or bilateral*," there is no need to append modifier 52 for reduced services.
- **c.** **92082—Correct Answer**
  This code correctly identifies an intermediate visual field examination. Because the CPT code states "visual field examination *unilateral or bilateral*," there is no need to append modifier 52 for reduced services.
- **d.** 92082-52—*Incorrect*
  Although the CPT code is correct, there is no need to append modifier 52, as the CPT code states "visual field examination *unilateral or bilateral*."

121. **Radiology Report:** Right lower extremity venous duplex Doppler sonogram
Clinical History: Right leg swollen, ulcer in right ankle.
Protocol: Real-time images, spectral analysis and graded compressions.
Findings: The right lower extremity venous structures were evaluated from the level of the common femoral vein in the groin to the popliteal vein. The vessel walls appear normal. There is no evidence of wall thickening. Normal phasic venous flow was observed in each of the visualized venous vessels. The vessel walls are completely compressible and there is no evidence of intraluminal thrombus. Normal augmentation of flow was observed in each of the visualized areas. There is no evidence of retrograde flow or reflux noted.
Impression: No evidence of acute deep vein thrombosis.
   Based on this report, the correct codes would be:
- **a.** 93971-RT, 451.19—*Incorrect*
  Although the CPT code 93971 correctly identifies a duplex scan of extremity veins, unilateral or limited study, the diagnosis code of deep vein thrombosis is incorrect, as the impression indicates "no evidence of acute deep vein thrombosis." The RT modifier was correctly appended to indicate the right leg.

b. 93970-RT-52, 451.19—*Incorrect*
The CPT code 93970 represents a complete bilateral study, whereas the examination in this case was unilateral. Appending modifier 52 is not appropriate, as there is a specific CPT code to identify a unilateral study. The diagnosis code of deep vein thrombosis (451.19) is incorrect, as the impression indicates "no evidence of acute deep vein thrombosis."

c. 93970-RT, 729.81, 707.13—*Incorrect*
The CPT code 93970 represents a complete bilateral study, whereas the examination in this case was unilateral.

d. 93971-RT, 729.81, 707.13—Correct Answer
The CPT code correctly identifies the unilateral study, and the diagnosis codes represent both the swelling of the limb and the ulcer of the ankle. The RT modifier was correctly appended to indicate the right leg.

122. A patient with mastodynia presented for a bilateral mammogram with CAD (computer-aided detection). The correct codes would be:
a. 77056, 77051, 611.71—Correct Answer
The CPT code 77056 describes a bilateral diagnostic mammogram, and CPT code 77051 describes the CAD for a diagnostic mammogram.
b. 77057, 77052, 611.71—*Incorrect*
The CPT code 77057 describes a bilateral *screening* mammogram, and CPT code 77052 describes the CAD for a *screening* mammogram.
c. 77055, 77051, 611.71—*Incorrect*
The CPT code 77055 describes a *unilateral* mammogram.
d. 77056, 77052, 611.71—*Incorrect*
Although the CPT code 77056 is the correct code for the bilateral diagnostic mammogram, the CPT code for the CAD (77052) describes the CAD for a *screening* mammogram.

123. An 89-year-old male (new patient) presented to the physician's office for evaluation of scrotal discomfort, testicular tenderness, and urinary frequency. The patient never had this condition before and complains the symptoms are worse at night. He denies fever, chills, gross hematuria, nausea, or vomiting. The patient reports a bothersome testicular mass. He has no known drug allergies. A complete past, family, and social history was documented and reviewed with the patient along with a complete review of systems. A comprehensive physical examination was documented. A venipuncture and prostate-specific antigen (PSA) and testosterone total was performed. The patient was diagnosed with hypertrophy of prostate, hydrocele, and impotence of organic origin. The patient was sent to a radiology facility for a scrotal ultrasound. The medical decision was of moderate complexity. The correct codes would be:
a. 99204, 84403, 36415, 84153, 76870—*Incorrect*
All of the codes in this selection are correct with the exception of CPT code 76870 for the scrotal ultrasound. The patient was "sent to a radiology facility" for the scrotal ultrasound, and because this test was not performed at the physician's office, it should not be reported.
b. 99204, 84403, 36415, 84153—Correct Answer
The level of service was documented with all the components of a comprehensive history and physical examination. Because the medical decision was of moderate complexity, and because documentation for a new patient requires that all three key components be at the same level, this is considered a level 4 (99204) new patient office visit. The CPT code 84403 correctly identifies the testosterone, total; the CPT code 36415 identifies the venipuncture; and the CPT code 84153 identifies the PSA.
c. 99203, 84403, 36416, 84153—*Incorrect*
The documentation supports a level 4 (99204) new patient visit, and the CPT code 36416 identifies collection of a *capillary blood* specimen (e.g., finger, heel, ear stick).
d. 99204, 84403, 36416, 84153, 76870—*Incorrect*
The CPT code 36416 identifies collection of a *capillary blood* specimen (e.g., finger, heel, ear stick). Also, because the patient was "sent to a radiology facility" for the scrotal ultrasound, and this test was not performed at the physician's office, it should not be reported.

124. Context, duration, location, and associated signs and symptoms are all considered as elements of:
  a. The medical decision—*Incorrect*
  This consists of the number of diagnoses or management options, the amount and/or complexity of data to be reviewed, and the risk of complications and/or morbidity or mortality.
  b. The physical examination—*Incorrect*
  According to the 1995 Document Guidelines, the elements of the physical examination are the body areas and organ systems.
  c. **The history of presenting illness—Correct Answer**
  This information is located in the E/M Guidelines in the CPT manual under History of Presenting Illness.
  d. The review of systems—*Incorrect*
  This is an inventory of body systems obtained through a series of questions for the purpose of identifying signs and/or symptoms experienced by the patient.

125. A concise statement describing the symptom, problem, condition, diagnosis, or other factor that is the reason for the encounter is called:
  a. **Chief complaint—Correct Answer**
  This information is located in the E/M Guidelines under Chief Complaint.
  b. Referral—*Incorrect*
  A *referral* is made on the basis of the recommendation of a health-care professional. This term can refer to the act of a health-care professional sending a patient to another doctor or to the actual paper authorizing a visit to a specialist.
  c. Risk factor reduction—*Incorrect*
  A risk factor reduction is considered to be a contributing component of an E/M service.
  d. Prognosis—*Incorrect*
  ***Prognosis* refers to the prediction and probable course of the outcome of a disease.**

126. A patient underwent an excision of a subcutaneous right chest wall mass, 2.9 cm. The correct code would be:
  a. 21552—*Incorrect*
  This code represents a mass 3 cm or greater.
  b. **21555—Correct Answer**
  This code correctly identifies the service as excision, tumor, soft tissue of neck or anterior thorax, subcutaneous; less than 3 cm.
  c. 21556—*Incorrect*
  This code represents a *subfascial* excision.
  d. 21557—*Incorrect*
  This code represents a *radical resection.*

127. Jackie Franklin presented to the physician complaining of neck pain that radiated down her arms. To relieve her pain, the physician provided osteopathic manipulation to the following regions: cranial head, cervical spine, left hip, left and right shoulders, and left and right hands. According to the guidelines in CPT for osteopathic manipulative treatment (OMT), how many body regions were treated?
  a. Seven—*Incorrect*
  b. Three—*Incorrect*
  c. Five—*Incorrect*
  d. **Four—Correct Answer**
  Four regions were treated. The CPT manual defines the body regions as *head, cervical, thoracic, lumbar, sacral, pelvic, lower extremities, upper extremities, rib cage, abdomen,* and *viscera.* In this case, the patient received OMT in the following regions: *head, cervical, pelvis, and upper extremities* (the hands are part of the upper extremities), accounting for a total of four regions.

128. Ben Smith, 54 years old, underwent a flexible colonoscopy with polyp removal by snare technique under moderate conscious sedation; the procedure time was 25 minutes. The correct code(s) would be:
  a. **45385—Correct Answer**
  This code correctly identifies a colonoscopy, flexible, proximal to splenic flexure; with removal of tumor(s), polyp(s), or other lesion(s) by snare technique. You would not code additionally for the moderate conscious sedation, as it is included in the procedure. This is indicated in the CPT manual by the "bulls-eye" symbol that precedes the code.
  b. 45385, 99148—*Incorrect*
  You would not code additionally for the moderate conscious sedation, as it is included in the procedure. This is indicated in the CPT manual by the "bulls-eye" symbol that precedes the code.
  c. 45384, 99148—*Incorrect*
  This CPT code identifies a flexible colonoscopy with polyp removal by hot biopsy or bipolar cautery, and the moderate conscious sedation is included in the procedure and would not be separately reported.
  d. 45385, 99143—*Incorrect*
  Although the CPT code for the colonoscopy is correct, this moderate conscious sedation code is for a patient younger than 5 years of age, and moderate conscious sedation is included with the procedure.

129. The codes in Chapter 11 of the ICD-9-CM Manual are to be used:

  a. For both the mother's and the child's record—*Incorrect*
  Chapter 11 codes are used only on the maternal record, according to the ICD-9-CM Guidelines, Section 1, Conventions, General Coding Guidelines, and Chapter-Specific Guidelines, 11 (Chapter 11: Complications of Pregnancy, Childbirth, and the Puerperium [630–679], 2).

  b. Only for the child's record—*Incorrect*
  Chapter 11 codes are used only on the maternal record, according to the ICD-9-CM Guidelines, Section 1, Conventions, General Coding Guidelines and Chapter-Specific Guidelines, 11 (Chapter 11: Complications of Pregnancy, Childbirth, and the Puerperium [630–679], 2).

  c. Only for the mother's record—Correct Answer
  This information is located in the ICD-9-CM Guidelines, Section 1, Conventions, General Coding Guidelines and Chapter-Specific Guidelines, 11 (Chapter 11: Complications of Pregnancy, Childbirth, and the Puerperium [630–679], 2). **Here it is stated that Chapter 11 codes are used only on the maternal record.**

  d. In the mother's record; recording of the codes in Chapter 11 in the child's record is optional—*Incorrect*
  Chapter 11 codes are used only on the maternal record, according to the ICD-9-CM Guidelines, Section 1, Conventions, General Coding Guidelines and Chapter-Specific Guidelines, 11 (Chapter 11: Complications of Pregnancy, Childbirth, and the Puerperium [630–679], 2).

130. The fifth digit in ICD-9-CM category 948 Burns classified according to extent of body surface represents:

  a. The percentage of body surface burned—*Incorrect*
  The fourth digit in this category represents the percentage of body surface burned.

  b. The percentage of body surface with third-degree burn—Correct Answer
  This information is located by looking up category 948 and referencing the box containing the fifth digits, which states, "The following fifth-digit subclassification is for use with category 948 to indicate the percent of body surface with third-degree burn."

  c. The percentage of body surface with second-degree burn—*Incorrect*
  Second-degree burns are listed under each specific burn category and are not specifically identified by a percentage of body surface.

  d. The percentage of body surface with deep third-degree burn with loss of body part—*Incorrect*
  Deep third-degree burns with loss of body part are listed under each specific category and are not specifically identified by a percentage of body surface.

131. ICD-9-CM describes coding to the highest degree of specificity as:

  a. Coding signs and symptoms along with definitive diagnosis codes—*Incorrect*
  Signs and symptoms should be coded only when there is no definitive diagnosis.

  b. The inclusion of rule-out codes when a physician is formulating his or her diagnosis—*Incorrect*
  There are no specific rule-out diagnosis codes. When there is no definitive diagnosis, signs and symptoms should be coded.

  c. The coding of a diagnosis code to the highest number of digits available—Correct Answer
  This information is located in the ICD-9-CM Guidelines, Section 1 B.3, Level of Detail in Coding.

  d. Multiple coding for a single condition—*Incorrect*
  This refers to multiple coding scenarios such as "use additional code."

132. A patient received 30 minutes of acupuncture without electrical stimulation. The acupuncturist removed the needles and reinserted the needles to provide an additional 15 minutes of acupuncture with electrical stimulation. The correct codes would be:

   a. 97810 × 2, 97813—*Incorrect*

     Although the CPT code 97810 is the correct code for the initial acupuncture, it would not be reported twice, as there are add-on codes for the additional time if applicable (when the needles are reinserted). CPT code 97813 would not be reported, as the acupuncture guidelines state, "Only one initial code is reported per date."

   b. 97810, 97811, 97813—*Incorrect*

     Although the CPT code 97810 correctly identifies the first 15 minutes of acupuncture, the code 97811 would not be reported for the additional 15 minutes, as the needles would have had to have been reinserted to bill an additional 15 minutes of acupuncture. Acupuncture is reported based on 15 minute increments of personal (face-to-face) contact with the patient, *not the duration of acupuncture needle(s) placement.* CPT code 97813 would not be reported as the acupuncture guidelines state, "Only one initial code is reported per date."

   c. 97810, 97811, 97814—*Incorrect*

     Although CPT code 97814 is a correct selection, and although the CPT code 97810 correctly identifies the first 15 minutes of acupuncture, the code 97811 would not be reported for the additional 15 minutes, as the needles would have had to have been reinserted to bill an additional 15 minutes of acupuncture. Acupuncture is reported based on 15 minute increments of personal (face-to-face) contact with the patient, not the duration of acupuncture needle(s) placement.

   d. 97810, 97814—Correct Answer

     Only two codes are needed to correctly report the services. CPT code 97810 identifies the first 15 minutes of acupuncture without electrical stimulation, and the additional 15 minutes of acupuncture without electrical stimulation would not be reported, as the needles were not reinserted. CPT code 97814 correctly identifies the additional 15 minutes of acupuncture with electrical stimulation with the reinsertion of needles. This add-on code is used instead of CPT code 97813, as the acupuncture guidelines state, "Only one initial code is reported per date."

133. Select the CPT code for Graves' disease with thyrotoxic crisis or storm:

   a. 242.01—Correct Answer

     This code describes Graves' disease (toxic diffuse goiter) with thyrotoxic crisis or storm.

   b. 242.00—*Incorrect*

     This code describes Graves' disease (toxic diffuse goiter) *without* thyrotoxic crisis or storm.

   c. 242.90—*Incorrect*

     This code describes *thyrotoxicosis* without mention of goiter or other cause and without mention of thyrotoxic crisis or storm.

   d. 242.91—*Incorrect*

     This code, although describing thyrotoxic crisis or storm, describes these in the context of *thyrotoxicosis,* not Graves' disease.

134. To treat 7-year-old Johnny's continuous ear infections, Dr. Kildare inserted bilateral ventilating tubes. The service was provided under general anesthesia. The correct code would be:

   a. 69436—*Incorrect*

     Although this is the correct CPT code, the service was performed bilaterally; therefore, you would need to append modifier 50 (bilateral procedure).

   b. 69436-50—Correct Answer

     The CPT code correctly identifies the service performed, and appending modifier 50 indicates that the procedure was performed bilaterally.

   c. 69433—*Incorrect*

     This CPT codes describes the service (tympanostomy) performed under *topical or local anesthesia.*

   d. 69433-50—*Incorrect*

     Although the correct modifier was appended, this CPT code indicates that the service (tympanostomy) was performed under *topical or local anesthesia.*

135. A patient diagnosed with hypertensive retinopathy underwent an intracapsular cataract extraction with insertion of intraocular lens prosthesis. The correct codes would be:

a. **66983, 362.11—Correct Answer**
This CPT code identifies the intracapsular cataract extraction with insertion of intraocular lens prosthesis and the hypertensive retinopathy.

b. 66983, 362.12—*Incorrect*
Although the CPT code 66983 is correct, the diagnosis code 362.12 describes *exudative* retinopathy and is therefore incorrect.

c. 66982, 362.11—*Incorrect*
Although the diagnosis code 362.11 is correct, the CPT code 66982 describes an *extracapsular* cataract removal with insertion of intraocular lens prosthesis and is therefore incorrect.

d. 66982, 362.12—*Incorrect*
In this case, both the CPT code and diagnosis code are incorrect. The CPT code describes an *extracapsular* cataract removal, and the diagnosis code describes exudative retinopathy.

136. The patient (post–Mohs' surgery) presented to the plastic surgeon for a reconstruction of a defect in the left lateral lower lid and canthus repaired with an orbicularis myocutaneous flap. The correct code(s) would be:

a. 17311, 15732—*Incorrect*
The CPT code 17311 describes a Mohs' surgery, which this physician did not perform. The plastic surgeon performed the myocutaneous flap.

b. 17311, 14060—*Incorrect*
The CPT code 17311 describes a Mohs' surgery, which this physician did not perform. The plastic surgeon performed the myocutaneous flap. CPT code 14060 describes an adjacent tissue transfer.

c. 15732—**Correct Answer**
The plastic surgeon performed only the myocutaneous flap of the eyelid.

d. I13150—*Incorrect*
This describes a complex repair; the plastic surgeon performed a myocutaneous flap of the eyelid.

137. According to the CPT Guidelines for Critical Care Services, the following is not true:

a. Services for a patient who is not critically ill but is located in a critical care unit are reported using other appropriate E/M codes—*Incorrect*
This is true, and the question asks for what is not stated as true in the critical care guidelines.

b. Critical care time provided by the physician does not have to be continuous—*Incorrect*
This is true, and the question asks for what is not stated as true in the critical care guidelines.

c. **Time spent in activities that occur outside of the unit or off the floor may be reported as critical care time as long as the time spent directly contributes to the treatment of the patient—Correct Answer**
This is not true regarding the critical care. As per the guidelines, time spent in activities that occur outside of the floor/unit may not be counted as critical care time, as the physician is not immediately available to the patient.

d. Time spent on the floor/unit documenting critical care services in the medical record may be counted as critical care time—*Incorrect*
This is true, and the question asks for what is not stated as true in the critical care guidelines.

138. CPT codes for anticoagulant management (99363–99364) may be reported:

a. **Only in the outpatient setting—Correct Answer**
The guidelines state, "These services are outpatient services only."

b. Only in the hospital setting—*Incorrect*
The guidelines state, "These services are outpatient services only."

c. In any setting the service takes place—*Incorrect*
The guidelines state, "These services are outpatient services only."

d. In the hospital setting for the first time, followed by outpatient setting thereafter—*Incorrect*
The guidelines state, "These services are outpatient services only."

139. Mrs. Jones was seen by her primary care physician for strep throat. She was given amoxicillin. Three days later, she called the doctor's office and asked to speak to her physician, as she was not feeling any relief from the antibiotic. The physician spent 15 minutes on the phone with Mrs. Jones, reassuring her that she needed to give the antibiotic time to work and to set a return appointment to the office upon completion of her prescription if she did not feel better at that time. The correct code would be:

a. 99441—*Incorrect*
Although this CPT code represents a telephone service that was provided, this code describes 5 to 10 minutes of telephone service. Additionally, no CPT code would be reported, as the guidelines for all telephone services state they are to be reported when the telephone call did not originate from a related E/M service provided within the previous 7 days.

b. 99442—*Incorrect*
This CPT code represents a telephone service from 11 to 15 minutes; however, no CPT code would be reported, as the guidelines for all telephone services state they are to be reported when the telephone call did not originate from a related E/M service provided within the previous 7 days.

c. 99443—*Incorrect*
This CPT code represents a telephone service for 21 to 30 minutes. Additionally, no CPT code would be reported, as the guidelines for all telephone services state they are to be reported when the telephone call did not originate from a related E/M service provided within the previous 7 days.

d. **No CPT code should be reported—Correct Answer**
No CPT code would be reported, as the guidelines for all telephone services state they are to be reported when the telephone call did not originate from a related E/M service provided within the previous 7 days. This information is located in the E/M section in the CPT manual under Telephone Services.

140. Mrs. Peters was followed in the clinic for her antepartum and postpartum care by Dr. Michaels. Her 6 lb 3 oz baby boy was delivered by cesarean by Dr. Franklin, a hospital physician who was not affiliated with Dr. Michaels' practice. Code for the services of Dr. Franklin would be:

a. 59400—*Incorrect*
This code represents the entire obstetric package (antepartum care, vaginal delivery, and postpartum care). Dr. Franklin performed only the delivery by cesarean.

b. 59409—*Incorrect*
This code represents a vaginal delivery. Dr. Franklin performed a cesarean delivery.

c. 59510—*Incorrect*
This code represents the entire obstetric package (antepartum care, cesarean delivery, and postpartum care). Dr. Franklin performed only the delivery by cesarean.

d. **59514—Correct Answer**
This code represents the cesarean delivery only.

141. A condition in which gastric juices containing acid travel back from the stomach up into the esophagus is called:

a. **Gastroesophageal reflux disease (GERD)—Correct Answer**

b. Diverticulosis—*Incorrect*
Diverticulosis is a condition marked by small sacs or pouches (diverticula) in the walls of an organ such as the stomach or colon.

c. Diverticulitis—*Incorrect*
Diverticulitis is an inflammation of the small sacs or pouches (diverticula) in the walls of an organ such as the stomach or colon.

d. Ulcerative Colitis—*Incorrect*
Ulcerative colitis is a disease that causes ulcers and inflammation in the inner lining of the colon and rectum.

142. A patient presenting for a radiological procedure was positioned to lie on his right side. This position is called:

a. Right recumbent—*Incorrect*
This identifies the patient as lying down (recumbent) but does not indicate that he is lying on his side (lateral).

b. **Right lateral recumbent—Correct Answer**
This identifies the patient as lying down (recumbent) on his right side (lateral).

c. Right prone—*Incorrect*
Prone **indicates the patient is lying with his face downward.**

d. Right supine—*Incorrect*
Supine indicates the patient is lying on his back with his face upward.

143. In radiology, the term "projection" refers to:
  a. How the patient is placed for the examination—*Incorrect*
  This would be described by the term *position*.
  b. The path the x-ray beam travels—Correct Answer
  This is called the *projection*.
  c. The various planes of the body—*Incorrect*
  Planes refer to points of reference by which positions are indicated.
  d. The radiological technique—*Incorrect*
  This refers to the type of service provided (e.g. MRI, x-ray).

144. CPT defines code 88300 as level 1–Surgical pathology, gross examination only. The term "gross" for this purpose is defined as:
  a. Examination of the specimen by sight—Correct Answer
  b. A disgusting specimen—*Incorrect*
  In this context, the term gross refers to an examination of the specimen by sight.
  c. Examination of the specimen before removal—*Incorrect*
  Surgical pathology refers to specimens that have been removed and are submitted for examination.
  d. A unit amount—*Incorrect*
  In this context, the term gross refers to an examination of the specimen by sight.

145. Mrs. Brown, a 68-year-old established Medicare patient, presented to the gynecologist for her routine preventive Pap test and breast examination. The physician sent the specimen out to the laboratory for testing. The correct codes would be:
  a. G0101, Q0091—Correct Answer
  The service was provided to a Medicare patient; therefore, HCPCS codes would be selected. G0101 identifies the Pap test and breast examination, and Q0091 describes the collection and preparation of the specimen to be sent to the laboratory.
  b. 99397, 99000—*Incorrect*
  The CPT code 99397 describes a preventive visit for a non-Medicare patient, and the CPT code 99000 describes a specimen-handling code.
  c. 99397, 88164—*Incorrect*
  The CPT code 99397 describes a preventive visit for a non-Medicare patient, and the CPT code 88164 describes the processing of the specimen. In this scenario, the specimen was sent to the laboratory for processing and was not processed by the physician.
  d. G0101, P3000—*Incorrect*
  Although the HCPCS code G0101 correctly identifies the Pap test and breast examination, the HCPCS code P3000 describes the processing of the specimen for a Medicare patient. In this scenario, the specimen was sent to the laboratory for processing and was not processed by the physician.

146. Diagnosis codes for sunburns are located in which chapter of the ICD-9-CM?
  a. Injury and Poisoning—*Incorrect*
  Sunburns are not classified as an injury.
  b. Skin and Subcutaneous Tissue—Correct Answer
  c. External Causes—*Incorrect*
  In the ICD-9-CM, this is an index to the external causes of injury and poisoning (E codes).
  d. Symptoms, Signs, and Ill-Defined Conditions—*Incorrect*
  Sunburns are classified as definitive diagnosis codes and are located in the Skin and Subcutaneous Tissue section.

147. According to the ICD-9-CM Coding Guidelines, how many codes are required to completely describe a pressure ulcer?

a. One—*Incorrect*
In the ICD-9-CM Coding Guidelines, Section 1, Chapter 12, a. 1), "Two codes are needed to completely describe a pressure ulcer. A code from subcategory 707.0 Pressure ulcer, to identify the site of the pressure ulcer, and a code from subcategory 707.2 Pressure ulcer stages."

b. Two—**Correct Answer**
In the ICD-9-CM Coding Guidelines, Section 1, Chapter 12, a. 1), "Two codes are needed to completely describe a pressure ulcer. A code from subcategory 707.0 Pressure ulcer, to identify the site of the pressure ulcer, and a code from subcategory 707.2 Pressure ulcer stages."

c. Three—*Incorrect*
In the ICD-9-CM Coding Guidelines, Section 1, Chapter 12, a. 1), "Two codes are needed to completely describe a pressure ulcer. A code from subcategory 707.0 Pressure ulcer, to identify the site of the pressure ulcer and a code from subcategory 707.2 Pressure ulcer stages."

d. One, with an additional code if applicable—*Incorrect*
In the ICD-9-CM Coding Guidelines, Section 1, Chapter 12, a. 1), "Two codes are needed to completely describe a pressure ulcer. A code from subcategory 707.0 Pressure ulcer, to identify the site of the pressure ulcer, and a code from subcategory 707.2 Pressure ulcer stages."

148. Wound closure utilizing adhesive strips as the sole method of repair is coded by using:

a. **The appropriate E/M code—Correct Answer**
The Integumentary Guidelines, under Repair (Closure), state, "Wound closure utilizing adhesive strips as the sole repair material should be coded using the appropriate E/M code."

b. The appropriate classification of repair code—*Incorrect*
The Integumentary Guidelines, under Repair (Closure), state, "Wound closure utilizing adhesive strips as the sole repair material should be coded using the appropriate E/M code."

c. A simple repair code—*Incorrect*
A simple repair requires a simple, one-layer closure and involves primarily the epidermis or dermis or subcutaneous tissues.

d. An E/M code with a modifier 22—*Incorrect*
As per the CPT Guidelines in Appendix A, under modifier 22, "This modifier should not be appended to an E/M service."

149. A patient encounter for the complaint of headache, diagnosis given as probable migraine headache, possible gastroenteritis, would be coded as:

a. **784.0—Correct Answer**
Only the headache would be coded, as both the migraine and gastroenteritis were listed as probable and not as definitive diagnoses.

b. 346.90—*Incorrect*
The migraine was not a definitive diagnosis and therefore should not be coded.

c. 346.90, 558.9—*Incorrect*
Both the migraine and gastroenteritis were listed as probable and not as definitive diagnoses and therefore should not be coded.

d. 558.9—*Incorrect*
The gastroenteritis was not a definitive diagnosis and therefore should not be coded.

150. The term "metastatic" is used to indicate:

a. **The site mentioned is the secondary site—Correct Answer**
Metastasis is the spreading of a disease (especially cancer) to another part of the body.

b. The site is not specific to primary or secondary—*Incorrect*
Metastatic refers to the secondary site.

c. The site mentioned is the primary site—*Incorrect*
Metastatic refers to the secondary site.

d. The site mentioned is for carcinoma in situ—*Incorrect*
Carcinoma in situ refers to an early stage of cancer in which the tumor is confined to the organ where it first developed.

Index